Human Embryo Adoption

Human Embryo Adoption

Volume 2

Catholic Arguments For and Against

Edited by Trent Horn and Kent Lasnoski

∞

The National Catholic Bioethics Center
Broomall, PA

Published by
The National Catholic Bioethics Center
600 Reed Road, Suite 102, Broomall, PA 19008

© The National Catholic Bioethics Center 2025

All rights reserved

No part of this publication may be reproduced, stored in a retrieval system, or transmitted, in any form or by any means, without the prior permission in writing of The National Catholic Bioethics Center, or as expressly permitted by law, by license, or under terms agreed upon with the appropriate reproduction rights organization. Inquiries concerning reproduction outside the scope of the above should be sent to The National Catholic Bioethics Center at the address above.

Nihil Obstat
Msgr. Joseph G. Prior, Censor Librorum
February 9, 2025

Imprimatur
✠ Most Rev. Nelson J. Perez, DD, Archbishop of Philadelphia
February 24, 2025

The nihil obstat and imprimatur are official declarations that a book or pamphlet is free of doctrinal or moral error. There is no implication that those who have granted the nihil obstat and imprimatur agree with the content, opinions, or statements expressed therein. The nihil obstat and imprimatur apply to the text of the book as submitted. They were granted prior to the addition of the bibliography and index and prior to proofreading and corrections of the text by the editors for mechanics and editorial style and for basic fact-checking unrelated to matters of faith and morals.

Unless otherwise noted, scripture quotations are from the Revised Standard Version of the Bible (RSV) © 1946, 1952, 1971, National Council of the Churches of Christ in the United States of America, and quotations from official Church documents are from the Vatican English translation, published online at www.vatican.va © Dicastero per la Comunicazione—Libreria Editrice Vaticana.

Block quotes from *Donum veritatis*, *Donum vitae*, *Dignitas personae*, the *Catechism of the Catholic Church*, the Wednesday catechesis of Pope St. John Paul II, an address of John Paul II, and an address of Pope Francis in chapters 3 and 15 © Dicastero per la Comunicazione—Libreria Editrice Vaticana. Used with permission. Chapter 10 based on "Frozen Embryos, Unwanted Pregnancies, and Artificial Wombs: Which Options Are Morally Licit?," *Nova et Vetera* 19.4 (Fall 2021) © *Nova et Vetera* 2021. Used with permission. Revisions © The National Catholic Bioethics Center 2025.

Library of Congress Control Number: 2025932463

ISBN 978-0-935372-82-3 (paperback)

Cover design by Nicholas Furton

Contents

Introduction		ix
	Trent Horn and Kent Lasnoski	

Part 1: The Context of Embryo Adoption

1.	Medical Aspects of Embryo Adoption Cara Buskmiller, MD	3
2.	The Social Context and Experience of Embryo Donation and Adoption Jeffrey Keenan, MD	17
3.	Prenatal Adoption and the Magisterium Jimmy Akin	25

Part 2: Objections to Embryo Adoption

4.	Embryo Transfer after Adoption and the Extended Inseparability Argument: Objections that Appeal to the Generative Faculty Rev. Fr. Nicanor Pier Giorgio Austriaco, OP	53
5.	Children's Rights to Love and Life Christopher Bobier	63
6.	Embryo Adoption and Becoming a Parent Charles Robertson	81
7.	The Feminine Act of Admission Mary Gormally	105
8.	Argument against Embryo Adoption from the Perspective of Theology of the Body Kent Lasnoski	115
9.	Some Moral Contraindications to Human Embryo Adoption Rev. Tadeusz Pacholczyk	125

10.	The Next Steps If Embryo Adoption Is Illicit Irene Alexander	151

Part 3: Defenses of Embryo Adoption

11.	The Procreative Dimension of Marital Union and Embryo Transfer Christopher Tollefsen	173
12.	Protecting the Dignity of the Child: Understanding the Rationale for the Inseparability Norm in the Context of the Embryo Adoption Debate Melissa Moschella	195
13.	Adoption as a Spiritual Status and a Social Practice: Contextualizing the Catholic Practice of Prenatal and Postnatal Adoption John Berkman	219
14.	The Annunciation and Embryo Adoption Francis Etheredge	241
15.	The Theology of the Body and the Morality of Embryo Adoption: What Does the Magisterium of the Catholic Church Teach? Elizabeth Bothamley Rex	265
16.	The Rescue of Embryonic Persons and Organ Transplants: Corporal Works of Mercy Janet Smith	293
17.	Throw Open the Doors: Next Steps in Embryo Adoption Christopher M. Reilly	313

Bibliography	331
Index	379

Editors

Trent Horn, MS, MA, is a staff apologist for Catholic Answers.

Kent Lasnoski, PhD, is the president of San Damiano College for the Trades in Springfield, Illinois. Previously he was an associate professor of theology at Wyoming Catholic College in Lander, Wyoming.

Contributors

Jimmy Akin is the senior apologist at Catholic Answers.

Irene Alexander, PhD, is an associate professor of theology at the University of Dallas in Irving, Texas.

Rev. Fr. Nicanor Pier Giorgio Austriaco, OP, PhD, SThD, is a professor of biological sciences and sacred theology at the University of Santo Tomas in Manila and a professorial lecturer in philosophy at the University of the Philippines, Diliman, both in the Philippines.

John Berkman, PhD, is a professor ordinarius of moral theology at the Regis-St. Michael's Faculty of Theology, University of Toronto, in Toronto, Canada.

Christopher Bobier, PhD, is an associate professor of foundational sciences at Central Michigan University College of Medicine in Mount Pleasant, Michigan.

Cara Buskmiller, MD, MS, is an assistant professor of fetal intervention at Baylor College of Medicine in Houston, Texas.

Francis Etheredge, MA, is an author and freelance writer living in Gloucestershire, the United Kingdom.

Mary Gormally (née Geach), PhD, is a philosopher and writer residing in the United Kingdom.

Jeffrey Keenan, MD, is the president and medical director at the National Embryo Adoption Center in Knoxville, Tennessee.

Melissa Moschella, PhD, is a professor of the practice, philosophy, at the McGrath Institute for Church Life, University of Notre Dame, in Notre Dame, Indiana.

Rev. Tadeusz Pacholczyk, PhD, is the senior ethicist at the National Catholic Bioethics Center in Broomall, Pennsylvania.

Christopher M. Reilly, ThD, is an independent scholar and author in the Washington, DC, area.

Elizabeth Bothamley Rex, PhD, MBA, is a bioethicist and an associate scholar at the Charlotte Lozier Institute in Arlington, Virginia, and a former adjunct professor of Catholic bioethics at Holy Apostles College and Seminary in Cromwell, Connecticut.

Charles Robertson, PhD, is an instructor at the St. Theresa Institute of Faith and Mission in Bruno, Saskatchewan, Canada.

Janet Smith, PhD, is a former professor of moral theology at Sacred Heart Major Seminary in Detroit, Michigan.

Christopher Tollefsen, PhD, is a professor of philosophy at the University of South Carolina in Columbia, South Carolina.

Introduction

Trent Horn and Kent Lasnoski

It is often said the Catholic Church thinks in centuries, not years. For better or worse, this assessment rings true in the case of pondering the ethics of embryo adoption. The first birth of a person conceived through in vitro fertilization (IVF) occurred in 1978,[1] yet faithful Catholic laity and ordained clergy alike have no clearly articulated, definitive conclusion from Catholic magisterial teaching ultimately defining embryo adoption as intrinsically evil or as morally permissible. The faithful sit in a kind of limbo on the question, morally frozen and unable to act for the life of these young prisoners who sit in freezers and bring in payments to the fertility clinics that keep them in their undead-but-not-quite-living state. Many feel the call to set the captives free, to give shelter to the homeless, to feed the hungry, to give the gift of their body for the sake of these forgotten, marginalized persons, yet they can do little beyond praying and lobbying for the injustice of IVF to cease. At the same time, theologians continue to plumb the depths of the theological and spiritual tradition of the Church for clear answers to aid the magisterium in its duty to teach the faithful what the truth requires of us.

The pressure to find a definitive answer for this moral crisis has only grown in the last fifty years. In America alone, in 2021 more than eighty-six thousand infants were born using artificial reproductive technologies, and

---

1. See Katharine Dow, "Looking into the Test Tube: The Birth of IVF on British Television," *Medical History* 63.2 (April 2019): 189–208, doi: 10.1017/mdh.2019.6.

99 percent of these births were achieved through IVF. That number represents 2 percent of all births in the United States.[2] As people marry later, as they delay having children, as insurance companies firm up their commitment to IVF as standard of care, and with the rise of same-sex couples desiring parenthood through gestation, the numbers will only continue to rise. As the births rise, so, too, will the number of imprisoned and frozen children. At this time in 2024, more than one million frozen embryos languish in the United States alone.[3] The way forward for faithful Catholics must be clarified.

Two books considering the ethics of embryo adoption from a Catholic perspective already exist: *Human Embryo Adoption* published by the National Catholic Bioethics Center itself in 2009 and *The Ethics of Embryo Adoption and the Catholic Tradition*, edited by Sarah-Vaughan Brakman and Darlene Fozard Weaver, in 2007. Why is this new book even necessary? First of all, these two previous volumes were published before moral theologians could adequately think through the release of the CDF's instruction *Dignitas personae* in 2008. *Dignitas personae* is the closest the Church has come to a definitive statement on the moral liceity of embryo adoption, yet even faithful Catholic moral theologians have not reached a consensus on whether the CDF intended to close the question by its statements in that instruction. Some strongly argue that, in combination with a previous instruction, *Donum vitae*, the conversation has been closed, while others believe the CDF has intentionally left the question open, especially since the CDF has not reinserted itself into the scholarly dialogue to clarify its own dogmatic intention in the text. Thus, by 2010 a new round of scholarly thinking addressing the issues raised in *Dignitas personae* and its use of a speech by Pope St. John Paul II exploded into the world of peer-reviewed

---

2. US Department of Health and Human Services, "Fact Sheet: In Vitro Fertilization (IVF) Use across the United States," news release, March 13, 2024, https://www.hhs.gov/about/news/2024/03/13/fact-sheet-in-vitro-fertilization-ivf-use-across-united-states.html.
3. See Zoe Sottile, "Alabama Ruled Frozen Embryos Are Children. Here's What It Could Mean for Embryos Frozen across the State," CNN, updated February 26, 2024, https://www.cnn.com/2024/02/26/us/ruling-impact-alabama-ivf-embryos/index.html.

theological journals.[4] Since then, a round of articles contending with one another has shown up every couple of years. New argumentative strategies warrant a sustained and balanced hearing. Perhaps the most compelling reason for a new edition is the astounding 2024 supreme court ruling in Alabama, which recognized the personhood of frozen embryos, giving them protection under the law in accord with a 2018 amendment to the Alabama Constitution. In this volume, we have gathered together a variety of approaches in one place for dialogue and discernment.

The strategy of this volume has been to organize the analyses topically or thematically and pair arguments from one side of the debate with corresponding arguments from the other side. The themes have been drawn from the current state of the question. Authors from each side were given a chance to review the manuscripts for chapters written by authors on their own side as well as by the authors in part 1, to make sure they did not cover the same ground. But they were not able to review the manuscripts for chapters written by authors on the other side. Thus, the essays in this volume are not direct responses to other essays in this volume. They are positive presentations of positions, arguments, and replies as they currently stand and as they are poised to move forward.

When discussing the ethical status of embryo adoption (EA), some people may be tempted to rush into an examination of the arguments for and against this procedure. But part 1 of this anthology is meant to curb that tendency and provide a crucial medical, sociological, and theological backdrop for this important debate. In "Medical Aspects of Embryo Adoption," Cara Buskmiller, MD, walks us through the medical procedures EA entails as well as their physical and psychological consequences for the woman undergoing this procedure. Then Jeffrey Keenan explores "The Social Context and Experience of Embryo Donation and Adoption" by surveying the experiences of both donor couples and adopting couples.

Jimmy Akin, a Catholic apologist who has published on how to interpret the teachings of the Catholic Church, then walks us through how the Church views this subject. In his essay, "Prenatal Adoption and the

---

4. See John Paul II, Address to the Participants in the Symposium on *"Evangelium vitae* and Law" and the Eleventh International Colloquium on Roman and Canon Law (May 24, 1996), *AAS* 88 (1996): 943–944.

Magisterium," Akin surveys the different authoritative levels of Church teaching and how they are applied to the subject of adoption, especially prenatal adoption. He concludes, "The CDF thus does not offer a bottom-line assessment of the adoption of frozen embryos. It notes positive and negative factors but does not rule the practice to be ultimately morally licit or illicit" (46). This would be expected given that the editors and contributors to this volume strive to be faithful to the magisterium, and so debate on this issue is possible only because the magisterium has, for now, left it an open question.

With this background knowledge in place, the discussion shifts in part 2 to authors who present various objections to EA.

Rev. Nicanor Pier Giorgio Austriaco, OP, says in his essay, "Embryo Transfer after Adoption and the Extended Inseparability Argument," that EA is precluded even if the act of becoming pregnant is exclusively reserved to the marital covenant and that such reasoning would also preclude ectogenesis, that is, artificial wombs. Charles Robertson makes a similar argument in his essay, "Embryo Adoption and Becoming a Parent," because EA makes a woman become a mother apart from the actions of her spouse, even if the act of EA does not itself make her a mother.

Other contributors ground their objections to EA in appeals to the nature and theology of the body.

Mary Gormally's essay, "The Feminine Act of Admission," focuses on what she calls the female marriage act and says, "For a woman to allow an intromission of impregnating kind is for her to imitate the marriage act" in a way that is contrary to the virtue of chastity (105). Gormally also addresses the objection that the Blessed Virgin Mary, in allowing herself to become pregnant through the miraculous intervention of the Holy Spirit, violates this principle or provides a warrant for EA. In his chapter, Kent Lasnoski offers "Arguments against Embryo Adoption from the Perspective of Theology of the Body" grounded in the problem of EA's cohering with the necessity that procreation be an authentic gift of self between the couple that leads to pregnancy.

Rev. Tadeusz Pacholczyk of the National Catholic Bioethics Center presents "Some Moral Contraindications to Human Embryo Adoption." Pacholczyk argues that when EA is used to initiate pregnancy, it involves a "misuse of the goods of marriage" and involves an "alternative to the procreative act" that is intrinsically evil (129, 131). He also offers a proposal for what should practically be done with the million or more frozen embryos that currently exist in the United States alone and cannot be morally gestated. Irene Alexander continues that theme in her essay, "The Next Steps If Embryo Adoption Is Illicit."

Christopher Bobier's essay, "Children's Rights to Love and Life," provides an important voice in this discussion to make the case that adoptive parents ought to give preference to adopting postnatal children who are in state custody over adopting frozen human embryos, based on weighing the harms of not adopting in each case.

Our anthology then shifts to part 3, where various defenses of EA are offered and answers mapping onto the previous objections are given.

In "The Procreative Dimension of Marital Union and Embryo Transfer," Christopher Tollefsen answers arguments that claim EA separates the unitive and procreative dimensions of marriage and the marriage act. Melissa Moschella likewise engages the inseparability argument against EA, contending that procedures which create children apart from the marital act (such as IVF) do not respect the child's rights or dignity. EA does not inflict injustice on the child but remedies past harms. Hence her essay's title—"Protecting the Dignity of the Child." John Berkman's essay, "Adoption as a Spiritual Status and a Social Practice," places EA approvingly in the historical context of Catholic support for adoption, saying that "a full defense of prenatal adoption will include a vision of the good of prenatal adoption in relationship to Catholic social teaching" (239).

In contrast to Lasnoski's chapter, Elizabeth Bothamley Rex's essay, "The Theology of the Body and the Morality of Embryo Adoption," argues for a coherence between the anthropology of the human person found in the magisterial teaching of John Paul II (as well as Benedict XVI and Francis) and EA. In addition, Francis Etheredge offers an alternative perspective to Gormally's earlier piece by focusing on the Incarnation as being positive evidence for the morality of EA in "The Annunciation and Embryo Adoption." Finally, Janet Smith defends EA as a corporal work of mercy in "The Rescue of Embryonic Persons and Organ Transplants," and Christopher Reilly calls us to "Throw Open the Doors" and offers several practical next steps when it comes to EA.

It cannot be our intention to finally settle the question with this volume, for that is not the task of the moral theologian. We have, instead, gathered the best arguments from a variety of approaches on both sides of the debate and considered what Catholics might do next once the truth of the matter is known. We humbly submit this work for the edification of the reader, for the advancement of knowledge on the topic, and ultimately at the service of the magisterial teaching authority of the Church, whose mission it is to explain and defend the truth of God's revelation, especially as it relates to matters of faith and morals. Though the Church thinks in centuries, the problem of IVF and embryo freezing demands action today. Its amassing injustice weighs heavily on the consciences of Catholics around the world. We pray that this volume will aid in the Church's discernment of a definitive teaching on this matter. May God grant us this grace.

Part 1:
The Context of Embryo Adoption

1

Medical Aspects of Embryo Adoption
Cara Buskmiller, MD

Medicine is a moral enterprise.
—Edmund Pellegrino

As of 2024, there are an uncounted number of embryos in some type of cryostorage across the world. In 2013, there were an estimated 1.4 million frozen embryos in the United States alone, with some experts claiming that this number could be as high as four million.[1] Physicians at the National Embryo Donation Center have estimated that this number grows at approximately 20 percent per year, meaning that, in 2024, there may be more than ten million cryopreserved embryos. For comparison, the worldwide death toll of COVID-19, one of the more visible and ethically important health disasters of the twenty-first century, was seven million.[2]

A minority of parents with frozen embryos, estimated in one study at about 13 percent, desire to donate them so that another party can build

---

1. Geoffrey P. Lomax and Alan O. Trounson, "Correcting Misperceptions about Cryopreserved Embryos and Stem Cell Research," *Nature Biotechnology* 31.4 (April 5, 2013): 288–290, doi: 10.1038/nbt.2541; and Dave Snow et al., "Contesting Estimates of Cryopreserved Embryos in the United States," *Nature Biotechnology* 33.9 (September 2015): 909, doi: 10.1038/nbt.3342.
2. World Health Organization, "WHO COVID-19 Dashboard," accessed January 22, 2023, https://covid19.who.int/.

Part 1: The Context of Embryo Adoption

a family.³ In contrast, 79 percent express vague plans for ongoing storage, 29 percent desire to donate embryos for research, and 14 percent plan to directly discard their embryos. A relatively new embryo disposition is referred to as compassionate transfer, in which the remainder of a couples' embryos, sometimes ten or more, are moved into the uterus at an unfavorable time of the menstrual cycle to accord with the parents' desires.⁴ The prevalence of this technique is not well studied at the present time.

This chapter aims to fully equip the reader with a physician's understanding of embryo adoption, from the gynecologic, obstetric, and psychiatric aspects.

Terminology

The term *embryo adoption* is discouraged in medicine, because regarding embryos as true persons is considered a fallacy within the profession at large.⁵ Instead, *embryo donation* is the preferred term, which fits with the treatment of embryos as tissue, like blood products or gametes, and only potential lives.⁶

The justification for this choice in terminology is ostensibly based in positive law, such as state statutes regarding the status of embryos, and social norms that require screening standards, unlike in postnatal adoption. But even when policy exceptions or some subcultures (e.g., Catholicism) treat embryos as persons, the term *embryo adoption* is dismissed as being obsolete.⁷

---

3. Alison E. Zimon et al., "Embryo Donation: Survey of In-vitro Fertilization (IVF) Patients and Randomized Trial of Complimentary Counseling," *PLoS One* 14.8 (August 15, 2019), e0221149, doi: 10.1371/journal.pone.0221149.
4. Ethics Committee of the American Society for Reproductive Medicine, "Compassionate Transfer: Patient Requests for Embryo Transfer for Nonreproductive Purposes," *Fertility and Sterility* 113.1 (January 2020): 62–65. doi: 10.1016/j.fertnstert.2019.10.013.
5. Bonnie G. Patel and Brooke V. Rossi, "Embryo Donation: Medical Aspects," in *Third Party Reproduction: A Comprehensive Guide*, ed. James M. Goldfarb (New York: Springer, 2014), 96.
6. Susan Crockin and Lauren M. Nussbaum, "Embryo Donation: Legal Aspects," in Goldfarb, *Third Party Reproduction*, 101–111.
7. Patel and Rossi, "Embryo Donation: Medical Aspects," 96.

This chapter, written within the context of Catholic bioethics, continues to use the term *embryo adoption*, given the identical status of embryos, fetuses, neonates, and children within that moral framework.

The Circumstances

Embryo freezing has undergone several changes in the decades since the use of in vitro fertilization (IVF) became widespread. The most notable changes have occurred within the culture of reproductive infertility and endocrinology, the subspecialty of obstetrics and gynecology that practices assisted reproductive technology (ART), including IVF. It has been a humbling thirty years to be a provider in this field.

Single-embryo transfer became more common, because of the morbidity of higher-order multiple gestation caused by out-of-control practices of multiple embryo transfer.[8] Preimplantation genetic diagnosis, a technique that was applied to 30–40 percent of pregnancies in the United States, was shown to be suboptimal at detecting conditions besides single-gene disorders and aneuploidy, as mosaic embryos (previously discarded as abnormal) often result in normal children if implanted and are often genetically normal even if simply re-biopsied.[9] A host of other techniques came into fashion and then faded, including almost every endometrial preparation method[10] and intracytoplasmic sperm injection

---

8. Jocelyn Stairs et al., "In Vitro Fertilization and Adverse Pregnancy Outcomes in the Elective Single Embryo Transfer Era," *American Journal of Perinatology*, e-pub December 26, 2022, doi: 10.1055/a-1979-8250.
9. Nathan R. Treff and Diego Marin, "The 'Mosaic' Embryo: Misconceptions and Misinterpretations in Preimplantation Genetic Testing for Aneuploidy," *Fertility and Sterility* 116.5 (November 2021): 1205–1211, doi: 10.1016/j.fertnstert.2021.06.027; and Rachel Theobald et al., "The Status of Preimplantation Genetic Testing in the UK and USA," *Human Reproduction* 35.4 (April 28, 2020): 986–998, doi: 10.1093/humrep/deaa034.
10. Sarah Lensen et al., "A Randomized Trial of Endometrial Scratching before In Vitro Fertilization," *New England Journal of Medicine* 380.4 (January 24, 2019): 325–334, doi: 10.1056/NEJMoa1808737; and Demiá Glujovsky et al., "Endometrial Preparation for Women Undergoing Embryo Transfer with Frozen Embryos or Embryos Derived from Donor Oocytes," *Cochrane Database of Systematic Reviews* 10.10 (October 28, 2020), CD006359, doi: 10.1002/14651858.CD006359.pub3.

PART 1: THE CONTEXT OF EMBRYO ADOPTION

for unexplained infertility.[11] Perhaps most unfortunately, many clinics began to protocolize embryo discard, rather than ongoing storage, as the default disposition choice, a somewhat expected move in the face of the liability attached to a growing quantity of stored and abandoned embryos.

In a happier but still humbling vein, live births continue to result from poor quality embryos and embryos frozen for up to thirty years,[12] with several studies showing that embryos can survive even older freezing methods for more than a decade.[13] Technological advances occurred as well, notably, with faster freezing methods being associated with better embryo survival rates, compared with traditional slow embryo freezing.[14]

---

11. Panagiotis Drakopoulos et al., "ICSI Does Not Offer Any Benefit over Conventional IVF across Different Ovarian Response Categories in Non-Male Factor Infertility: A European Multicenter Analysis," *Journal of Assisted Reproduction and Genetics* 36.10 (August 2019): 2067–2076, doi: 10.1007/s10815-019-01563-1; and Jianjuan Song et al., "ICSI Does Not Improve Live Birth Rates but Yields Higher Cancellation Rates Than Conventional IVF in Unexplained Infertility," *Frontiers in Medicine* 7 (February 10, 2021), 614118, doi: 10.3389/fmed.2020.614118.
12. Yaling Xiao et al., "Transfer of A Poor-Quality along with A Good-Quality Embryo on In Vitro Fertilization / Intracytoplasmic Sperm Injection-Embryo Transfer Clinical Outcomes: A Systematic Review and Meta-Analysis," *Fertility and Sterility* 118.6 (December 2022): 1066–1079, doi: 10.1016/j.fertnstert.2022.08.848; and Jen Christensen and Nadia Kounang, "Parents Welcome Twins from Embryos Frozen 30 Years Ago," CNN, November 21, 2022, https://www.cnn.com/2022/11/21/health/30-year-old-embryos-twins/index.html.
13. Stefano Canosa et al., "The Effect of Extended Cryo-Storage Following Vitrification on Embryo Competence: A Systematic Review and Meta-Analysis," *Journal of Assisted Reproduction and Genetics* 39.4 (April 2022): 873–882, doi: 10.1007/s10815-022-02405-3; and Yuling Mao et al., "Effects of Vitrified Cryopreservation Duration on IVF and Neonatal Outcomes," *Journal of Ovarian Research* 15.1 (September 8, 2022): 101, doi: 10.1186/s13048-022-01035-8.
14. Martin Graham Wilding et al., "Human Cleavage-Stage Embryo Vitrification Is Comparable to Slow-Rate Cryopreservation in Cycles of Assisted Reproduction," *Journal of Assisted Reproduction and Genetics* 27.9–10 (September 2010): 549–554, doi: 10.1007/s10815-010-9452-1; and Ana S. Lopes et al., "Re-Expansion and Cell Survival of Human Blastocysts following Vitrification

In addition to this, embryologists have continued to optimize embryo storage and incubation conditions.[15]

The tumult of humbling discoveries indicating that dreamed-up techniques do not help, the cold reality of massive excess embryo buildup, and the surprising resilience of the human embryo are interesting circumstances for the medical professional commenting on embryo adoption in the 2020s. Outside this historical moment, the couples considering embryo adoption are usually doing so for treatment of infertility, usually as a lower-cost option than using donor gametes or going through another stimulated cycle. Often, couples have had many previous failed ART attempts and have been trying for longer than the average ART patient.[16] Less commonly, there are couples in the United States who adopt embryos with a mission-like attitude of rescuing them, through collaboration with like-minded organizations. Within this treatment option, the recipients of embryo donation, like those

---

and Warming Using Two Vitrification Systems," *Journal of Assisted Reproduction and Genetics* 32.1 (January 2015): 83–90, doi: 10.1007/s10815-014-0373-2.

15. Maria Rendón Abad et al., "The Influence of Oxygen Concentration during Embryo Culture on Obstetric and Neonatal Outcomes: A Secondary Analysis of a Randomized Controlled Trial," *Human Reproduction* 35.9 (September 1, 2020): 2017–2025, doi: 10.1093/humrep/deaa152; Devorah Heymann et al., "The Effect of Hyaluronic Acid in Embryo Transfer Media in Donor Oocyte Cycles and Autologous Oocyte Cycles: A Systematic Review and Meta-Analysis," *Human Reproduction* 37.7 (June 30, 2022): 1451–1469, doi: 10.1093/humrep/deac097; Mária Ángeles Valera et al., "A Propensity Score-Based, Comparative Study Assessing Humid and Dry Time-Lapse Incubation, with Single-Step Medium, on Embryo Development and Clinical Outcomes," *Human Reproduction* 37.9 (August 25, 2022): 1980–1993, doi: 10.1093/humrep/deac165; and Giuseppe Gullo et al., "Closed vs. Open Oocyte Vitrification Methods Are Equally Effective for Blastocyst Embryo Transfers: Prospective Study from a Sibling Oocyte Donation Program," *Gynecologic and Obstetric Investigation* 85.2 (April 2020): 206–212, doi: 10.1159/000506803.

16. Viveca Söderström-Anttila et al., "Embryo Donation: Outcome and Attitudes among Embryo Donors and Recipients," *Human Reproduction* 16.6 (June 2001): 1120–1128, doi: 10.1093/humrep/16.6.1120; and Fiona MacCallum et al., "Parenting and Child Development in Families with a Child Conceived through Embryo Donation," *Journal of Family Psychology* 21.2 (June 2007): 278–287, doi: 10.1037/0893-3200.21.2.278.

of oocyte or sperm donation, typically undergo screening and make choices about the genetic content of the tissue they accept. Of course, given that the consequence of embryo donation effectively is the adoption of a genetically unrelated child, there are typically additional psychological screenings and waiting periods required.[17]

The Act Itself: Gynecology

Embryo adoption involves embryo transfer. ET is a procedure that involves intervention outside of nature for the sake of a patient. If there are grounds for objecting to embryo adoption by ET into the uterus of an adoptive mother, the objection cannot be founded on the degree of artifice or risk involved, since the art of medicine commonly employs artificial means, so long as these are not intrinsically evil.

ET occurs after the process of IVF has concluded. This is an important factual point: fertilization, the process of steps that being with gametes and conclude with an independent human organism, is over. It is extremely inaccurate, for example, to speak of a child "conceived through embryo donation." Thus, embryo adoption does not involve fertilization, the beginning of new life, or cocreation in any medical sense of the word, although perhaps *procreation* can colloquially embrace cocreation and pregnancy.

Instead, embryo adoption begins steps of gestation which were never extended to the frozen embryo. The first step in gestation is the movement of the zygote from the location of fertilization (usually the fallopian tube) to the location of implantation (usually the endometrial cavity). This change of location in vivo is due in large part to maternal cilia wafting the embryo along the reproductive tract, since the embryo has no moving extremities and is still enclosed in the semirigid zona pellucida. Since a maternal reproductive tract has been withheld from the frozen embryo, this step is replaced with the procedure aptly called embryo transfer. This procedure moves the embryo from its location at the close of fertilization (plus some incubation), which is the embryology lab, and into the location of implantation (the endometrial cavity).

---

17. Crockin and Nussbaum, "Embryo Donation: Legal Aspects," 101–111.

This is an important artificial difference between frozen embryos and embryos in vivo: "to become pregnant" for most women occurs at the same time as fertilization, even though these are biologically and logically separate events. However, for women receiving frozen embryos, fertilization and "becoming pregnant" are separated and uncoupled in other additional ways, notably in time. It is vital to maintain the rather sharp logical and medical distinctions between fertilization, local movement of the embryo, and becoming pregnant, even though they are usually part of a confluence of events.

Given the unusual separation between these events, it is important to clearly restate: ET for frozen embryos occurs after the embryonic person begins to exist and cannot strictly be called part of the creation of a new person, except in a casual sense where this refers to all of reproduction. Instead, ET replaces a part of gestation, which is local motion of the embryo into the endometrial cavity prior to implantation. If ET is under discussion as intrinsically evil, then discussion should be on the grounds of gestation or pregnancy not on the grounds of conception, fertilization, or procreation, which is a "coming to be" that finished at the end of the process of fertilization. ET or local motion of the embryo is a "becoming [in the uterus]," which is a different type of change.

Embryos are transferred either as cleavage-stage or as blastocysts. Cleavage-stage refers to embryos on day 2 or 3 after fertilization between the two-cell stage and the more compacted morula of as many as sixteen cells. Blastocysts are day 5–6 embryos and are characterized by a separated trophectoderm and inner cell mass, a level of organization not seen in younger embryos.

Depending on the prospective mother's ovulatory status, she may undergo a natural cycle or a stimulated cycle following any number of protocols. In the latter and more traditional path, exogenous hormones are used to prepare the endometrium to receive the embryo. In a natural cycle or in other mini, or minimal, stimulation protocols, zero or very little such stimulation is added to a predictable endogenous hormonal milieu (e.g., in a healthy woman of proven fertility with regular cycles). Exogenous hormones may be oral, transdermal, or vaginal. Often, a woman's response to these hormones or her natural cycle is monitored with serum estrogen measurements and ultrasound examination of the endometrial stripe—a measurement of the thickness of the uterine lining that will receive the embryo.

Embryos are kept in storage until the time of transfer, when they are actively thawed with several prepared solutions and a warming device. Just over half of embryos preserved with older slow-freeze methods survive thawing, while over 90 percent of embryos survive thawing after fast-freezing, or vitrification. Embryos are then placed in a particular region near the tip of a transfer catheter. The prospective mother is placed in a dorsal lithotomy position, as with other gynecologic exams, and a speculum is introduced to allow visualization of the cervix. Under ultrasound guidance, the embryo is introduced into the center of the uterine cavity, with care taken to place the embryo within the cavity and not beneath the surface of the endometrium. The woman is then asked to remain supine for about one hour, then given follow-up precautions to avoid rapid acceleration-deceleration activities.

The embryo hatches from the zona pellucida on days 5 to 7, so a cleavage embryo will hatch and implant two to five days after ET, and a blastocyst will hatch one to three days after placement. Following this, a pregnancy test done between nine and fourteen days after ET can assess whether the embryo has successfully established himself or herself in a detectable clinical pregnancy.

The Consequences: Obstetrical

Pregnancy after embryo adoption is much like pregnancy after ET of any other frozen embryo, most of which occur outside the setting of embryo adoption. There is a 30–50 percent rate of clinical pregnancy after ET of a frozen embryo, where *clinical pregnancy*, means a positive pregnancy test with ongoing pregnancy symptoms into the first trimester, as opposed to a *chemical pregnancy* which is a positive pregnancy test followed by normal female gynecologic cycling. After ET with a frozen embryo, there is a 10–30 percent rate of miscarriage and a 25–60 percent live-birth rate, depending on the embryo, maternal age, and the cycle protocol. In contrast, spontaneous fertilization is followed by an 82 percent rate of clinical pregnancy (18 percent rate of chemical pregnancy),[18] a 10 percent rate of

---

18. N. J. Ellish et al., "A Prospective Study of Early Pregnancy Loss," *Human Reproduction* 11.2 (February 1996): 406–412, doi: 10.1093/humrep/11.2.406.

miscarriage after clinical pregnancy is recognized,[19] and an approximately 71 percent chance of live birth (less than 1 percent stillbirth),[20] usually at term after thirty-seven weeks. With ET of one embryo, the rate of multiple gestation is about 2 percent; with ET of two embryos, the rate of multiples is 15–20 percent. Even if ET results in a singleton pregnancy, there is still a higher rate of pathologies related to placental function in these pregnancies, compared with pregnancies from spontaneous fertilization.

When the embryo has no genetic material related to the mother or any previous men with whom she has conceived children, the mother's body has no prior exposure to the embryo's antigens (the molecules that all human cells express). This is a theoretical explanation for pregnancy loss but also for the higher rates of placenta previa, placental abruption, placenta accreta, pregnancy-induced hypertensive disorders (including gestational hypertension and preeclampsia), preterm birth, fetal growth restriction, and low birth weight.[21] These complications are also related to maternal age.[22]

When there are twins, there are additional risks. Twins are the most common multiple gestation that results from frozen ET. Twin gestations have a higher risk of preterm birth, with the average gestational age at delivery dropping from thirty-eight weeks to between thirty-five and thirty-six

---

19. American College of Obstetricians and Gynecologists (ACOG) Committee on Practice Bulletins—Gynecology, "ACOG Practice Bulletin No. 200: Early Pregnancy Loss," *Obstetrics and Gynecology* 132.5 (November 2018): e197–e207, doi: 10.1097/AOG.0000000000002899.
20. ACOG et al., "Obstetric Care Consensus #10: Management of Stillbirth," *Journal of Obstetrics and Gynecology* 135.3 (March 2020): e110–e132, doi: 10.1097/AOG.0000000000003719.
21. Fei Kong et al., "Placental Abnormalities and Placenta-Related Complications following *In-Vitro* Fertilization: Based on National Hospitalized Data in China," *Frontiers in Endocrinology* 13 (June 30, 2022), 924070, doi: 10.3389/fendo.2022.924070; and Suleena Kansal Kalra and Thomas A. Molinaro, "The Association of In Vitro Fertilization and Perinatal Morbidity," *Seminars in Reproductive Medicine* 26.5 (September 2008): 423–435, doi: 10.1055/s-0028-1087108.
22. Baha M. Sibai et al., "Hypertensive Disorders in Twin versus Singleton Gestations, *American Journal of Obstetrics and Gynecology* 182.4 (April 2000): 938–942, doi: 10.1016/s0002-9378(00)70350-4.

weeks.[23] Twins who result from IVF are eight times more likely to deliver preterm.[24] The risk of pregnancy-induced hypertension is also higher in twins generally,[25] and the risk is even higher in twins from IVF—as many as 10–15 percent of mothers carrying IVF twins will get hypertensive disorders.[26] Twins may result in the need for cesarean delivery, a major abdominal surgery for the woman, depending on the presentation of the first twin.[27]

Dichorionic twins (each twin having his or her own placenta) are lower risk than are monochorionic twins (twins sharing a placenta), because of the unique complications that arise when two fetuses share the major organ they use for nutrition and respiration. The rate of monochorionic twins after ET of a single frozen blastocyst is about 2 percent; the rate of monochorionic twins after ET of two frozen blastocysts is lower, but the rate of dichorionic twins is about 15 percent.[28] Monochorionic twins experience complications of their shared placenta in about 15 percent of cases, some of which lead to the death of one or both twins, permanent neurological

---

23. Saed M. Ziadeh, "The Outcome of Triplet versus Twin Pregnancies," *Gynecologic and Obstetric Investigation* 50.2 (August 2000): 96–99, doi: 10.1159/000010290.
24. Yali Zhang, "A Comparison of Preterm Birth Rate and Growth from Birth to 18 Years Old between In Vitro Fertilization and Spontaneous Conception of Twins," *Twin Research and Human Genetics* 24.4 (August 2021): 228–233, doi: 10.1017/thg.2021.33.
25. J. Villar et al., "Eclampsia and Preeclampsia: A Worldwide Health Problem for 2000 Years," in *Preeclampsia*, ed. H. Critchley et al. (London: Royal College of Obstetricians and Gynaecologists Press, 2003), 57–72; and Sibai, "Hypertensive Disorders," 938–942.
26. Rania Okby et al., "Preeclampsia Acts Differently in In Vitro Fertilization versus Spontaneous Twins," *Archives of Gynecology and Obstetrics* 297.3 (March 2018): 653–658, doi: 10.1007/s00404-017-4635-y.
27. Henry C. Lee et al., "Trends in Cesarean Delivery for Twin Births in the United States: 1995–2008," *Obstetrics and Gynecology* 228.5 (November 2011): 1095–1101, doi: 10.1097/AOG.0b013e3182318651.
28. Atsushi Yanaihara et al., "Clinical Outcome of Frozen Blastocyst Transfer; Single vs. Double Transfer," *Journal of Assisted Reproduction and Genetics* 25.11–12 (November–December 2008): 531–534, doi: 10.1007/s10815-008-9275-5.

injury in one or both twins, or milder problems that require neonatal and pediatric care or therapy.[29]

Hypertensive disorders have small but measurable long-lasting effects on the mother, increasing her risk of cardiovascular disease, stroke, end-stage renal disease, and metabolic disease such as diabetes.[30] Preterm delivery also has long-lasting consequences into childhood, especially when there are effects on neurological function, such as those from intraventricular hemorrhage, a common complication of extreme prematurity.[31]

Needless to say, obstetric risks after ET of frozen embryos, regardless of whether they are adopted, are higher than risks of spontaneous pregnancy.

The Consequences: Psychiatry

Despite being called embryo donation by the secular medical profession, embryo adoption is obviously unlike other tissue donations, because an independent person who results from it (the child) may reflect on it as more like an adoption and less like a kidney transplant. In fact, children from various forms of autologous ART typically think of donors as parent-like and want to identify them.[32] Fittingly, an early survey of ART-clinic workers

---

29. Thomas Trevett and Anthony Johnson, "Monochorionic Twin Pregnancies," *Clinics in Perinatology* 32.2 (June 2005): 475–494, doi: 10.1016/j.clp.2005.02.007.
30. Mark W. Cunningham Jr. and Babbette LaMarca, "Risk of Cardiovascular Disease, End-Stage Renal Disease, and Stroke in Postpartum Women and Their Fetuses after a Hypertensive Pregnancy," *American Journal of Physiology—Regulatory, Integrative, and Comparative Physiology* 315.3 (September 2018): R521–R528, doi: 10.1152/ajpregu.00218.2017.
31. Jill Glennis Zwicker and Susan Richardson Harris, "Quality of Life of Formerly Preterm and Very Low Birth Weight Infants from Preschool Age to Adulthood: A Systematic Review," *Pediatrics* 121.2 (February 2008): e366–e376, doi: 10.1542/peds.2007-0169; and Betty R. Vohr, "Neurodevelopmental Outcomes of Premature Infants with Intraventricular Hemorrhage across A Lifespan," *Seminars in Perinatology* 46.5 (August 2022), 151594, doi: 10.1016/j.semperi.2022.151594.
32. Margaret K. Nelson et al., "Gamete Donor Anonymity and Limits on Numbers of Offspring: The Views of Three Stakeholders," *Journal of Law and Bioscience* 3.1 (April 2016): 39–67, doi: 10.1093/jlb/lsv045.

also thought that couples planning to accept donated embryos needed more counselling than couples planning to accept donated sperm or eggs.[33]

Several aspects of the psychology of couples who aim to receive donated embryos for treatment of infertility have been explored. Some of these aspects include couples' belief that these children will be *superior* to children available for adoption because of the typically higher socioeconomic status of IVF patients who have leftover embryos,[34] fear that adopted embryos will be *inferior* because they were not chosen by their parents for family building,[35] attraction to the egalitarian fact that neither partner has a greater genetic relation to the child,[36] and belief that the ability to experience pregnancy is additive to the mother's self-image.[37] Of families who received donor embryos for infertility, many develop parental overinvolvement, although this is similar to other IVF families.[38]

The psychological effects of being an adopted embryo are inappropriately underemphasized. In a sample of British families used in several studies on psychological health of these families, only one-third of parents had told

---

33. Laura Machin, "A Hierarchy of Needs? Embryo Donation, In Vitro Fertilisation and the Provision of Infertility Counselling," *Patient Education and Counseling* 85.2 (November 2011): 264–268, doi: 10.1016/j.pec.2010.09.014.
34. Sonja Goedeke and Deborah Payne, "Embryo Donation in New Zealand: A Pilot Study," *Human Reproduction* 24.9 (August 2009): 1939–1945, doi: 10.1093/humrep/dep116.
35. Vohr, "Neurodevelopmental Outcomes of Premature Infants."
36. Linda Applegarth, "Embryo Donation: Counseling Donors and Recipients," in *Infertility Counseling: A Comprehensive Handbook for Clinicians*, ed. Sharon N. Covington and Linda Hammer Burns (Cambridge: Cambridge University Press, 2006), 356–369.
37. Heather Widdows and Fiona MacCallum, "Disparities in Parenting Criteria: An Exploration of the Issues, Focusing on Adoption and Embryo Donation," *Journal of Medical Ethics* 28.3 (June 2002): 139–142, doi: 10.1136/jme.28.3.139.
38. MacCallum et al., "Parenting and Child Development in Families," 285 table 2; and Fiona MacCallum and Sarah Keeley, "Embryo Donation Families: A Follow-Up in Middle Childhood," *Journal of Family Psychology* 22.6 (December 2008): 799–808, doi: 10.1037/a0013197.

or were planning to tell their child about his or her origins, compared with 100 percent of adoption families and 93 percent of IVF families. When interviewed during the child's early life, forty-three percent of families planned *not* to tell the child, a number that *rose* to 47 percent during interviews that took place when children were school aged. (In the meantime, all of the adoption families had already disclosed the adoption to their children.)[39] This is despite the fact that, in the same sample, a shocking 72 percent of these parents had disclosed the child's origins to *other family members*. A Finnish sample was slightly more encouraging with 69 percent planning to disclose, but in the subset of persons who had information about the embryo's biological parents, only 29 percent of couples planned to disclose.[40] Information about adolescents and young adults who were adopted as embryos is extremely limited, but this is expected by experts to be a tumultuous time, especially if an accidental disclosure occurs.

Framework of Fertilization and Gestation

Embryo adoption, a term mostly used by ethicists who view the embryo as a human person, is a procedure that largely consists of optional endometrial preparation for the prospective mother, thawing for the embryo, and transfer of the embryo into the endometrial cavity. There are risks to mother and embryo during this early part of the process, and there are ongoing risks throughout the remainder of gestation. Consequences of adverse outcomes such as preeclampsia and preterm birth may echo into later life for both persons, and psychological aspects probably continue to have effects throughout life.

Medical science draws a sharp distinction between the process of creating a new person (which is certainly located either throughout or within the steps of fertilization) and gestation (which has defined borders between

---

39. MacCallum et al., "Parenting and Child Development in Families," 286 table 3; and Fiona MacCallum and Susan Golombok, "Embryo Donation Families: Mothers' Decisions regarding Disclosure of Donor Conception," *Human Reproduction* 22.11 (November 2007): 2888–2895, doi: 10.1093/humrep/dem272.
40. Viveca Söderström-Anttila et al., "Embryo Donation: Outcome and Attitudes among Embryo Donors and Recipients," *Human Reproduction* 16.6 (June 2001): 1112–1128, doi: 10.1093/humrep/16.6.1120.

the end of fertilization and delivery). Frozen embryos are temporarily or forever barred from beginning gestation, which embryo adoption purposes to restore. Embryo transfer is a procedure similar in risks and benefits to mother and child as other fetal interventions, and so objections to it based on risk, artificialness, or invasiveness are unpersuasive to physicians. The very legitimate debate about the ethics of embryo adoption must find other grounds about the moral status of this act.

2

The Social Context and Experience of Embryo Donation and Adoption

Jeffrey Keenan, MD

Although embryo donation and adoption (EA) has only recently gained widespread popularity and recognition, it is not a new concept or phenomenon. For example, in 1989 Paul Devroey and colleagues reported already having transferred ninety-five donated oocytes and embryos.[1] In considering this topic, both the donor and the recipient must be borne in mind. Of course, there would be no embryo donation without embryo donors, couples with embryos remaining from their in vitro fertilization (IVF) cycles. Those embryos who are not implanted are either discarded or placed into cryostorage. Although there is no census of the quantity of frozen embryos in the United States, the number is estimated to be over 1.5 million.[2]

Embryos' ambiguous status in society and under the law dominates the social context and personal experience of embryo donation and adoption. This shapes the perception of EA as an alternative to IVF or traditional adoption on the part of both prospective donors and prospective adoptive parents. Unsurprisingly, this tension is felt most acutely by donor couples, who must navigate competing emotions and motivations regarding

---

1. P. Devroey et al., "Establishment of 22 Pregnancies after Oocyte and Embryo Donation," *British Journal of Obstetrics and Gynaecology* 96.8 (August 1989): 900–906, doi: 10.1111/j.1471-0528.1989.tb03343.x.
2. Gerard Letterie, "In Re: The Disposition of Frozen Embryos: 2022," *Fertility and Sterility* 117.3 (March 2022): 479, doi: 10.1016/j.fertnstert.2022.01.001.

the future of their embryos. Additionally, technological developments and evolving cultural views related to anonymous donation of genetic material further complicate this choice. Couples who adopt embryos also can face difficult emotional and moral decisions. Outcomes for EA compare favorably with IVF, the processes being largely similar, except for variations caused by implanting previously frozen embryos instead of fresh embryos. Beyond technology and personal motivations, unclear or nonexistent law in most jurisdictions place the status of the frozen embryo in limbo, although few, if any, concerns arise about family building once a decision to adopt has been made.

Experience of Donor Couples

A large proportion of frozen embryos will never be used by their genetic parents, so the potential for births from the donation of such embryos is quite high. However, most parents who have these embryos in cryostorage do not intend to donate them. There are many reasons for this, and despite the growing popularity of EA, it appears that the inventory of frozen embryos will continue to increase faster than the number who are adopted by other couples, unless significant governmental or professional regulation is enacted.

Paradoxically, the reasons for placing embryos for adoption or not are often the same. A sense of altruism is positively associated with the preference for donating embryos for both research as well as adoption: "The powerful impulse to give back to society and to help others may make research morally preferable to individuals whose sense of responsibility precludes their allowing their embryos to become children in any family except their own. For those less strongly moved by the particular and intimate sense of responsibility, altruism leads them to donate embryos to another couple."[3] However, despite more than two decades of research, no treatments utilizing embryonic stem cells are approved by the US Food and Drug Administration (FDA), and only a handful of clinical trials are active in this area.

Similarly ironic, "expressions of 'parental' responsibility," that is, "concern about or responsibility for the health or welfare of the embryo or child it

---

3. Anne Drapkin Lyerly et al., "Fertility Patients' Views about Frozen Embryo Disposition: Results of a Multi-Institutional U.S. Survey," *Fertility and Sterility* 93.2 (February 2010): 507, doi: 10.1016/j.fertnstert.2008.10.015.

could become," were negatively associated with the preference for donating embryos to another couple but positively associated with thawing and disposing of them, freezing them forever, and so-called compassionate transfer, wherein the embryos are placed back into the uterus at a time when it is not possible for them to implant, thus ensuring their death.[4] Strangely, many couples do not have a plan for what to do with their embryos. Because the United States does not limit how long embryos can be cryopreserved, this could equate to parents' keeping their embryos in cryostorage indefinitely, apparently with no thought or concern about the fact that they will not live indefinitely and that these embryos will become an inheritance to some unwilling relation, clinic, or friend.[5]

A possible reason for these apparently incoherent preferences is that couples who create embryos through IVF are often underinformed. Although standard consent processes contain all pertinent information regarding medical and legal risks, many couples do not delve into important issues, such as how many children they desire, their feeling on the fate of unused embryos, long-term storage costs, and the option of freezing eggs rather than embryos. Furthermore, some clinics require preimplantation genetic testing, which informs the couple about the genetic normalcy and sex of their embryos. This information can make donating their embryos more difficult. Couples who do choose to donate embryos must decide whether to do so anonymously (closed adoption) or openly. The National Embryo Donation Center allows either method.[6] This is akin to how traditional adoption was

---

4. Lyerly et al., "Fertility Patients' Views about Frozen Embryo Disposition," 507.
5. See Alison E. Zimon et al, "Embryo Donation: Survey of *In-Vitro* Fertilization (IVF) Patients and Randomized Trial of Complimentary Counseling," *PLoS One* 14.8 (August 15, 2019), e0221149, doi: 10.1371/journal.pone.0221149.
6. Currently, the National Embryo Donation Center is the nation's largest provider of EA services, with approximately fourteen hundred births. The first national program for embryo donation and adoption was started in 1996 by the Snowflakes program of Christian Nightlight Adoptions, then located in California. EA received wide national attention in 2005, when President George W. Bush hosted children born through this program at an event on the controversies surrounding embryonic stem cell research. See National Embryo Adoption Center, "About," National Embryo Adoption Center, accessed February 29, 2024, https://www.embryodonation.org/about;

practiced for decades, if not centuries, and is guided by the knowledge that many couples will donate their embryos only anonymously or on an open basis. Lacking access to the option of their choice, parents often choose to destroy their embryos, donate them for destructive research, or, at the very least, opt for indefinite storage. However, this practice is the exception to the norm. Most private clinics practice only closed EA. Other organizations, such as the Snowflakes program, allow only open adoption.

Anonymous donation has been complicated by technology and is subject to changing state and national laws. In 1985, Sweden became the first country to outlaw anonymous sperm donation. Germany, Switzerland, the United Kingdom, and many other countries have followed suit, generally applying the same rule to eggs and embryos as well.[7] Shifting societal norms in the United States could also result in laws which allow donor-conceived children to find their genetic parents. Even without that, direct-to-consumer DNA testing has resulted in many donor-conceived children finding their genetic parents who wished to remain anonymous.[8] As more and more people make their DNA part of the public record through the use of such companies, it is probable that many, possibly a significant majority of, anonymous donors will not remain so.

Nightlight Christian Adoptions, "Embryo Adoption-Donation," Snowflakes Embryo Adoption Program, accessed February 29, 2024, https://nightlight.org/snowflakes-embryo-adoption-donation/; and George W. Bush White House, "President Discusses Embryo Adoption and Ethical Stem Cell Research," news release, May 24, 2005, https://georgewbush-whitehouse.archives.gov/news/releases/2005/05/text/20050524-12.html.

7. Claes Gottlieb et al., "Disclosure of Donor Insemination to the Child: The Impact of Swedish Legislation on Couples' Attitudes," *Human Reproduction* 15.9 (September 2000): 2052–2056, doi: 10.1093/humrep/15.9.2052; and Editorial, "Sperm Donation Laws by Country 2024, World Population Review, accessed February 28, 2024, https://worldpopulationreview.com/country-rankings/sperm-donation-laws-by-country. See also International Federation of Fertility Societies, "Chapter 8: Donation," in "IFF Surveillance 07," ed. H. Jones Jr. and J. Cohen, special issue, *Fertility and Sterility* 87.4 suppl 1 (April 2007): S28–S32, doi: 10.1016/j.fertnstert.2007.01.092.
8. See Emily Bazelon, "Why Anonymous Sperm Donation Is Over, and Why That Matters," *New York Times*, December 3, 2023, https://www.nytimes.com/2023/12/03/magazine/anonymous-sperm-donation-genetic-testing.html/.

Experience of Adopting Couples

The motivation of recipients to adopt these embryos are many. Based on our experience at the National Embryo Donation Center, the most common reason for EA is infertility and the desire to start or build a family. Some of these couples choose EA because all other methods have failed. Many couples who lack either sperm or eggs choose EA rather than donor eggs or sperm because of the moral implications of allowing a third party into the marital relationship. Others are uncomfortable with the so-called genetic disequilibrium which occurs in the family when a child is related to one parent and not the other. Other reasons couples cite for choosing to adopt embryos include severe genetic problems which would probably be transmitted to children, having a heart for adoption, being adopted themselves, and simply having a calling to adopt these orphaned embryos. Regardless of the specific motivation to adopt, the burden of childlessness is simultaneously a spiritual, emotional, and psychological struggle. These couples should be offered counseling with both an experienced infertility counselor and a member of the clergy.

Another challenge for many of these couples is the financial barrier to treatment. Most insurance companies do not cover EA or other infertility treatments, and by the time couples consider the option of EA, they are often financially depleted. EA compares very favorably with any of these other options with regard to pregnancy rates. Moreover, it is much less expensive than either IVF or donor-egg treatments, which require not only IVF but also a paid donor and preparatory treatment for the recipient. On average, EA is 60–80 percent the cost of IVF.[9] Therefore, EA allows couples with lesser means to rescue these embryos or pursue this family building option.

The treatment itself is straightforward, and since most couples undergoing EA have been through other infertility therapies, they typically have little difficulty navigating the evaluation process and treatment protocols. Nevertheless, an EA program requires several administrative procedures and significant staff time and effort. Furthermore, the FDA has imposed significant regulations on EA and maintains the right to inspect all facilities which

---

9. Caroline Lester, "Embryo 'Adoption' Is Growing but It's Getting Tangled in the Abortion Debate," *New York Times*, February 17, 2019, https://www.nytimes.com/2019/02/17/health/embryo-adoption-donated-snowflake.html.

perform this process. This combination of factors serves to discourage clinics from participating in the process. Perhaps as a consequence of a long track record of safety, in 2016 the FDA eased some of the restrictions and infectious-transmission testing requirements for centers involved in embryo donation and adoption.[10]

Prospective recipients are screened to make certain that they have no medical contraindications to becoming pregnant, such as uncontrolled hypertension or diabetes. An exam and imaging are performed to be certain that there are no uterine or pelvic abnormalities, which could complicate a pregnancy or result in miscarriage. Transfer of the embryos must be performed at a time when the uterus is receptive to implantation. This can be accomplished either by timing the recipient's natural cycle to the transfer or by briefly stopping her cycle and replacing her estrogen and progesterone until a pregnancy test is performed. If the test is positive, the estrogen and progesterone must be continued until the tenth or twelfth week of pregnancy, at which time the placenta takes over hormonal production. Pregnancies conceived from frozen embryo transfer are at slightly higher risk for complications such as higher birth weight, maternal hypertension, and placental implantation anomalies, compared with pregnancies conceived through fresh embryo transfer. However, the great majority of these pregnancies are easily managed and result in healthy full-term births.[11]

---

10. Revisions to Exceptions Applicable to Certain Human Cells, Tissues, and Cellular and Tissue-Based Products, 81 Fed. Reg. 40512 (August 22, 2016). It should be noted that there has never been a reported case of infectious transmission resulting from frozen embryo transfer in either humans or animals.
11. A. M. Terho et al., "High Birth Weight and Large-for-Gestational Age in Singletons Born after Frozen Compared to Fresh Embryo Transfer, by Gestational Week: A Nordic Register Study from the CoNARTaS Group," *Human Reproduction* 36.4 (March 18, 2021): 1083–1092, doi: 10.1093/humrep/deaa304; Caroline J. Violette et al., "Assessment of Abnormal Placentation in Pregnancies Conceived with Assisted Reproductive Technology," *International Journal of Gynecology and Obstetrics* 163.2 (November 2023): 555–562, doi: 10.1002/ijgo.14850; and Abha Maheshwari et al., "Is Frozen Embryo Transfer Better for Mothers and Babies? Can Cumulative Meta-Analysis Provide a Definitive Answer?," *Human Reproduction Update* 24.1 (January–February 2018): 35–58, doi: 10.1093/humupd/dmx031.

Finally, a mention should be made of issues related to cryopreservation of embryos and the likelihood for an ensuing pregnancy. Cryopreservation methods have changed dramatically over the last two decades. The preferred method used now is called vitrification. This process results in even higher survival rates for frozen embryos, and so pregnancy rates are higher as well. Pregnancy rates vary from over 50 percent per transfer to under 20 percent per transfer, depending on the number of embryos transferred, the age of the mother at the time of the creation of the embryos, the skill of the embryologists and physicians, and how well the embryos survived the warming procedure. What does not have an effect is the length of time which the embryos have been frozen. In fact, a new record was set in October 2022, when twins were born after having been frozen for thirty years.[12]

Legal Status of Embryo Donation and Adoption

At least four states have laws recognizing and codifying embryo adoption and donation and structuring a legal framework under which it may operate. Tennessee, for example, has passed legislation which makes EA a legal entity, prevents children born from this process from claiming inheritance rights from their genetic parents, and disallows genetic parents from claiming such children as their own or requesting rights of parenthood.[13] Absent a specific law codifying this process, most states recognize the birth mother as the child's legal mother and her partner or husband as the child's father.[14] Yet despite the absence of laws in every state, there are no cases in which a child has been taken from a birth mother and given to genetic parents, nor has an embryo-adopted child obtained inheritance rights from his or her genetic parents.

Unfortunately, embryos are considered property under most state laws and judicial assessments. This is problematic when a couple separates

---

12. Kristen Gallant, "Twins Born from Embryos Frozen Nearly 30 Years Ago Break Record," WATE 6, November 21, 2022, https://www.wate.com/news/top-stories/twins-born-from-embryos-frozen-nearly-30-years-ago-break-record/.
13. Tennessee Code §36-2-401.
14. See Douglas NeJaime, "Who Is a Parent?," American Bar Association, May 10, 2021, https://www.americanbar.org/groups/family_law/publications/family-advocate/2021/spring/who-a-parent/.

or divorces and disagrees about the fate of their remaining embryos. For the most part, the disposition decision on remaining embryos has been granted to the spouse or partner who does not want to use them for pregnancy.[15] Death of a spouse does not preclude the surviving spouse from donating embryos for adoption.[16]

Uncertain Future

Embryos are innocent nascent children who had no say in their conception or current status. There is no way to save them from destruction or indefinite freezing without thawing them and placing them in the womb of a willing mother. Whether couples participate in EA as a rescue mission or a family building mission, they face several challenges ranging from cultural and psychological factors to economic barriers due to high cost and the absence of insurance coverage. Religious people have and will continue to address these needs and spearhead embryo donation and adoption. Considering Catholicism's continued opposition to IVF, even as other Christians have welcomed it, the Roman Catholic Church could play a substantial role if internal debate resolves in favor of EA.

---

15. See Naomi Cahn, "Who Gets the Frozen Embyos?," *Forbes*, February 4, 2020, https://www.forbes.com/sites/naomicahn/2020/02/04/who-gets-the-frozen-embryos/?sh=684b54156cfd.
16. See Ethics Committee of the American Society for Reproductive Medicine, "Posthumous Retrieval and Use of Gametes or Embryos: An Ethics Committee Opinion," *Fertility and Sterility* 110.1 (July 2018): 45–59, doi: 10.1016/j.fertnstert.2018.04.002.

3

Prenatal Adoption and the Magisterium

Jimmy Akin

In 2008, when discussing what could be done with the thousands of frozen embryos housed in fertility clinics around the world, the Congregation for the Doctrine of the Faith (CDF) noted in *Dignitas personae*, "It has also been proposed, solely in order to allow human beings to be born who are otherwise condemned to destruction, that there could be a form of '*prenatal adoption*.'"[1] In context, this was envisioned as the transfer of a previously frozen embryo into a willing woman who would then become the adoptive mother of the child. This procedure and the magisterium's teaching on it will be at the center of our discussion, but it exists within a broader context. For that reason, we will look first at the magisterium and then at adoption in general and prenatal adoption, including the form envisioned in *Dignitas personae*.

The Magisterium

Christ willed that certain individuals have the ability to teach authoritatively in his name. Thus, when he sent out the seventy-two disciples, he told them, "Whoever listens to you listens to me, and whoever rejects you rejects me, and whoever rejects me rejects the one who sent me" (Luke 10:16). The seventy-two disciples were a temporary institution in the Church, but Christ expressed the same will for the more enduring group of twelve apostles, telling them to go among the nations "teaching them to obey everything that

---

1. Congregation for the Doctrine of the Faith (CDF), *Dignitas personae* (September 8, 2008), n. 19.

Part 1: The Context of Embryo Adoption

I have commanded you" (Matt. 28:20). He thus intended that his Church have a teaching authority or magisterium. (*Magister* is Latin for teacher.)

When the apostles died, this function was inherited by their successors, the bishops: "Bishops, as successors of the apostles, receive from the Lord, to whom was given all power in heaven and on earth, the mission to teach all nations and to preach the Gospel to every creature."[2] Thus, today the Church's magisterium consists of the bishops of the world teaching in union with the Pope, the head of the episcopal college.

The substance of Christian faith and practice was delivered by Christ and the apostles at the beginning of the Church's history as "the faith which was once for all delivered to the saints" (Jude 3). Consequently, it is referred to as the *deposit of faith*, which is found in both Scripture and Tradition: "Sacred tradition and Sacred Scripture form one sacred deposit of the word of God, committed to the Church."[3] The deposit of faith, which is the primary object of the magisterium's teaching, contains both doctrines handed on explicitly by Christ and the apostles and the implications that can be drawn from these.

The primary subject matter on which the magisterium teaches is classically described as *res fidei et morum*. This phrase is commonly translated "matters of faith and morals." However, scholars have noted that the Latin word *mores* (singular, *mos*) means more than just what English speakers think of as matters of morality. This creates a broader scope for magisterial teachings than might otherwise be suspected. Francis Sullivan explains, "*Mores* includes far more than what we would call 'morals'; actually it includes everything that the gospel reveals about the Christian way of life: How to live, how to pray, how to worship God. ... Perhaps the English word that comes closest to the Tridentine sense of *mores* is 'practices,' so that *res fidei et morum* would be better translated 'matters pertaining to (Christian) faith and practice.'"[4]

The concept of prenatal adoption as the transfer of previously frozen embryos was not imaginable in the age of the apostles, so it would not seem

---

2. Vatican Council II, *Lumen gentium* (November 21, 1964), n. 24.
3. Vatican Council II, *Dei verbum* (November 18, 1965), n. 10.
4. Francis A. Sullivan, *Magisterium: Teaching Authority in the Catholic Church* (Eugene, OR: Wipf and Stock, 2002), 128.

to be part of the deposit of faith. However, the broader recognition of *res fidei et morum* as matters of Christian faith and practice may be seen as allowing the magisterium to teach on whether it is a practice that is acceptable as part of Christian life.

The magisterium can teach on matters of faith and morals with different levels of authority. In extraordinary cases, it can teach under the Church's charism of infallibility.[5] When this happens, the resulting teaching is spoken of as *infallible, definitive,* or *irreformable.* These three terms apply to the same set of teachings. However, in some cases, the magisterium goes further than infallibly defining that a teaching is *true.* It may also define that it has been divinely *revealed.* When this happens, we refer to the resulting teaching as a *dogma.* Dogmas are thus a subset of infallible teachings.[6]

When a dogma is declared, the Church indicates that it is taught explicitly or implicitly in the deposit of faith by virtue of the fact it is divinely revealed. Since it was the deposit of faith that Christ principally commissioned his Church to teach, divine revelation itself is referred to as the *primary* object of infallibility. However, experience has shown that the Church also needs the ability to define certain truths closely connected to revelation (e.g., whether a Pope was validly elected, whether a council was genuinely ecumenical, or whether a teaching has been infallibly declared): "According to Catholic doctrine, the infallibility of the Church's Magisterium extends not only to the deposit of faith but also to those matters without which that deposit cannot be rightly preserved and expounded."[7] Because these latter truths are not revealed, they are not part of the Church's primary teaching mission, and for this reason, they are referred to as the secondary object of infallibility.

The limits of the secondary object have not yet been fully clarified. An open question concerns the natural moral law, which is distinct from moral principles revealed in Scripture and Tradition. Because it is not part of divine revelation, the natural law—which includes both positive precepts ("do this") and negative ones ("do not do this")—is not part of the primary

---

5. Vatican Council II, *Lumen gentium,* n. 25.
6. Jimmy Akin, *Teaching with Authority: How to Cut through Doctrinal Confusion & Understand What the Church Really Says* (El Cajon, CA: Catholic Answers Press, 2018), n. 86.
7. CDF, *Mysterium ecclesiae* (June 24, 1973), n. 3.

object of infallibility, and it might or might not be considered part of the secondary object. Some light was shed on this question in 1999, when representatives of the CDF—including Joseph Cardinal Ratzinger—were asked about the negative moral norms. They replied, "Given that the observance of all negative moral norms that concern intrinsically evil acts (*intrinsece mala*) is necessary for salvation, it follows that the Magisterium has the competence to teach infallibly and make obligatory the definitive assent of the members of the faithful with regard to the knowledge and application in life of these norms. This judgment belongs to the Catholic doctrine on the infallibility of the Magisterium."[8]

The opinion at the CDF thus has been that the Church is capable of teaching infallibly at least on the negative moral norms of natural law that concern intrinsically evil acts. This entails the ability also to teach with lesser degrees of authority than infallibility. Therefore, if it turns out that the form of prenatal adoption that we are principally concerned with (transfer of a previously frozen embryo) involves an intrinsically evil act, this would allow the magisterium to teach on the subject with levels of authority up to and including infallibility. Cases where the magisterium teaches infallibly are historically rare—at least compared with the total volume of magisterial teachings—and the infallibility of a teaching is not to be presumed. The *Code of Canon Law* provides that "no doctrine is understood as defined infallibly unless this is manifestly evident."[9]

When—as is ordinarily the case—the magisterium teaches noninfallibly, the teaching may have varying levels of authority: "Here the theologian will need, first of all, to assess accurately the authoritativeness of the interventions which becomes clear from the nature of the documents, the insistence with which a teaching is repeated, and the very way in which it is expressed"[10] These criteria—(1) the nature of the documents that contain a teaching, (2) the frequency with which it is proposed, and (3) the language with which it is proposed—are the keys to assessing the authority of a non-infallible teaching.

---

8. CDF, *Proclaiming the Truth of Jesus Christ: Papers from the Vallombrosa Meeting* (Washington, DC: US Catholic Conference, 2000), 66.
9. *Code of Canon Law*, can. 749 §3.
10. CDF, *Donum veritatis* (May 24, 1990), n. 24.

A special note pertaining to the nature of documents concerns those issued by the Congregation for the Doctrine of the Faith or CDF (today the Dicastery for the Doctrine of the Faith or DDF). Because the magisterium consists *only* of the bishops of the world teaching in union with the Pope, a document must be written or authorized by a bishop in order to have doctrinal authority. No other individuals are capable of binding the faithful to believe particular doctrines, for "the task of interpreting the Word of God authentically has been entrusted solely to the Magisterium of the Church, that is, to the Pope and to the bishops in communion with him."[11]

However, an individual bishop is capable only of authoritatively teaching his own flock: "In fact, only the faithful entrusted to the pastoral care of a particular bishop are required to accept his judgment given in the name of Christ in matters of faith and morals, and to adhere to it with a religious assent of soul."[12] Consequently, for documents issued by Vatican dicasteries to have doctrinal authority for the whole Church, they must be approved by the Pope—the only individual bishop who has authority over the whole Church.

Thus, the CDF acknowledges, "The Roman Pontiff fulfills his universal mission with the help of the various bodies of the Roman Curia and in particular with that of the Congregation for the Doctrine of the Faith in matters of doctrine and morals. Consequently, the documents issued by this Congregation *expressly approved by the Pope* participate in the ordinary magisterium of the successor of Peter."[13] This approval is typically indicated by a note at the end of a CDF document. Documents that do not carry papal authorization represent the opinions of their authors but do not themselves carry doctrinal authority (e.g., the *Doctrinal Commentary* issued by Ratzinger and Archbishop Tarcisio Bertone in 1998).[14] The instructions of the CDF with which we are principally concerned—*Donum vitae* (1987) and *Dignitas personae* (2008)—received papal approval and thus constitute acts of the magisterium.

---

11. Catechism of the Catholic Church, 2nd ed. (Washington, DC: US Conference of Catholic Bishops/Libreria Editrice Vaticana, 2018 update), n. 100.
12. John Paul II, *Apostolos suos* (May 21, 1998), n. 11.
13. CDF, *Donum veritatis*, n. 18, emphasis added.
14. CDF, *Doctrinal Commentary on the Concluding Formula of "Professio Fidei"* (June 29, 1998).

When the magisterium teaches authoritatively, different responses from the faithful can be called for. When a dogma is defined, the proper response is described as "divine and catholic faith"[15] or as "theological faith."[16] When an infallible teaching is not a dogma, the response called for is "firm and definitive assent." When the magisterium teaches noninfallibly, the response called for is "religious assent," which is also described as "religious submission of mind and will."[17] The degree of assent varies depending on the level of authority invested in a teaching, which is determined by applying the three criteria named above.

However, this does not mean that all magisterial teachings will be received without difficulty:

> The willingness to submit loyally to the teaching of the Magisterium on matters *per se not irreformable must be the rule. It can happen, however, that a theologian may, according to the case, raise questions regarding the timeliness, the form, or even the contents of magisterial interventions.* ... When it comes to the question of interventions in the prudential order, it could happen that some Magisterial documents might not be free from all deficiencies. Bishops and their advisors have not always taken into immediate consideration every aspect or the entire complexity of a question. But it would be contrary to the truth, if, proceeding from some particular cases, one were to conclude that the Church's Magisterium can be habitually mistaken in its prudential judgments.[18]

The CDF then discusses what a theologian should do if he finds himself unable to accept a noninfallible teaching: "If, despite a loyal effort on the theologian's part, the difficulties persist, the theologian has the duty to make known to the Magisterial authorities the problems raised by the teaching in itself, in the arguments proposed to justify it, or even in the manner in which it is presented. He should do this in an evangelical spirit and with a profound desire to resolve the difficulties. His objections could then contribute to real progress and provide a stimulus to the Magisterium

---

15. *Code of Canon Law*, can. 750 §1.
16. CDF, *Doctrinal Commentary*, nn. 5–6.
17. Vatican Council II, *Lumen gentium*, n. 25.
18. CDF, *Donum veritatis*, n. 24, emphasis added.

to propose the teaching of the Church in greater depth and with a clearer presentation of the arguments."[19]

It is important to note that a theologian who feels unable to accept a particular magisterial teaching should not automatically be accused of dissent. The CDF defines the term *dissent* as "public opposition to the Magisterium of the Church."[20] Consequently, dissent is not the same thing as merely having a disagreement. The US bishops' Committee on Doctrine notes,

> [*Donum veritatis*] restricts the meaning of the word *dissent* to "public opposition to the Magisterium of the Church, which must be distinguished from the situation of personal difficulties." This should be noted because in American usage the term *dissent* is used more broadly to include even the private expression of rejection of reformable magisterial teaching. ... Obviously, "public opposition" does not encompass the private denial of teaching on the part of an individual.
>
> More important, however, it does not seem appropriate to apply the term *public* to the professional discussions that occur among theologians within the confines of scholarly meetings and dialogues or to the scholarly publication of views.[21]

This recognition creates intellectual space for scholars to discuss difficulties with noninfallible magisterial teachings without being accused of dissent. As we will see, the magisterium has not issued a firm teaching on the adoption of frozen embryos, so no one should be accused of dissent. However, even if the magisterium, at some point, issues a firm teaching on this subject (pro or con), those who disagree and discuss the matter in scholarly venues should not be charged with dissent.

The Nature of Adoption

Adoption refers to the procedure by which one person legally becomes the child of someone who is not his biological parent. Adoption has taken many

---

19. CDF, *Donum veritatis*, n. 30.
20. CDF, *Donum veritatis*, n. 32.
21. National Conference of Catholic Bishops, Committee on Doctrine, *The Teaching Ministry of the Diocesan Bishop: A Pastoral Reflection* (Washington, DC: NCCB, 1992), 18.

forms in history, and the motives for it have varied. One motive is the care of children who have been orphaned or abandoned or whose parents are unable or unwilling to properly care for them. However, there have been other ways of providing for the care of children (e.g., guardianship and fosterage) that do not involve transferring the title of legal parentage. Consequently, in many cultures, the mere need to care for children has not been seen as sufficient for adoption.

Another motive for adoption is the continuation of a family line, such as for couples who are infertile or who have not been able to produce a suitable male heir. The continuation of family lines was a principal reason for adoption in Rome, where it was used to create a legal basis for inheritance and the continuation of the family. A notable form of Roman adoption was *adrogation*, in which a person who was already a legal adult (*sui iuris* or "under his own authority") voluntarily agreed to become the son of an older man in order to become his heir. This form of adoption was practiced in the imperial family, such as when Augustus adopted the three sons of his daughter Julia. When death and exile prevented them from serving as future emperors, Augustus adopted Tiberius, who was a grown man. Later Claudius adopted Nero, though Claudius already had a biological son, Britannicus.

Ancient Israelite society did not commonly practice adoption. This is partly because of the Hebrew practices of polygamy and the levirate marriage (Deut. 25:5–10), which often made it possible to continue family lines without adoption.[22] However, there are instances in the Hebrew Scriptures that reflect the practice, most notably Genesis 48:5, where the patriarch Jacob declares of his biological grandsons, "Ephraim and Manasseh shall be mine, as Reuben and Simeon are."

The tribal organization of Israel also resulted in a form of posthumous adoption whereby a person or group could be adopted into the tribe of a long-dead patriarch:

> The newcomer is attached "in name and in blood" to the tribe; this means that he acknowledges the tribe's ancestor as his own, that he will marry within the tribe and raise up his family

---

22. Lewis N. Dembitz and Kaufmann Kohler, "Adoption," in *The Jewish Encyclopedia*, ed. Isodore Singer (Funk and Wagnalls, 1901–1906; JewishEncyclopedia.com, 2002), https://www.jewishencyclopedia.com/articles/852-adoption In a levirate marriage, a man marries his brother's widow.

inside it. The Arabs say that he is "genealogized" (root: *nasaba*). With a whole clan the fusion takes longer, but the result is the same, and the newcomers are finally considered as being of the same blood. ... The tribes of Israel were not exempt from such changes, and they absorbed groups of different origin. Thus the tribe of Judah eventually welcomes to its own ranks the remnants of the tribe of Simeon, and incorporated foreign groups like the Calebites and Yerahmeelites.[23]

With the New Testament—which was written after Israelites had substantial contact with the Greco-Roman world—the concept of adoption becomes named. For example, "Pharaoh's daughter adopted (Greek, *aneilato*) [Moses] and brought him up as her own son" (Acts 7:21). The concept of adoption (Greek, *huiothesia*) also becomes a theme in St. Paul's letters, which refer repeatedly to our adoption as sons of God (Rom. 8:15, 9:4; Gal. 4:5; Eph. 1:5).

Adult adoption, as in the case of Roman *adrogation*, and posthumous adoption, as in the case of Israelite absorption into tribes, are very different from the understanding of adoption used in contemporary developed societies. This illustrates the need to think carefully about adoption and the different ways it can manifest. The form of adoption we are here concerned with is prenatal adoption.

Precisely how adoption is handled legally varies from one jurisdiction to another. Currently, in the United States, there are strong protections for the right of biological mothers to change their minds, and adoptions do not become final and irrevocable until sometime after birth. However, while this is praiseworthy, it is not an essential feature of adoption. Also, what are commonly called embryo adoptions are often handled not as adoptions per se but as property transfers—whereby a frozen embryo is legally treated as a piece of property that is transferred to a new couple. This legal maneuver also is not essential to the process.

Here we will prescind from the details of particular legal systems and refer to any procedure that finishes with the result of an individual's being considered the legal child of someone who is not the biological parent as an adoption. This will apply regardless of whether the adoption becomes legally binding only after birth and whether it is handled as a property transfer

---

23. Roland de Vaux, *Ancient Israel: Its Life and Institutions* (London: Darton, Longman and Todd, 1961), 6.

or something else. It is the end result we are concerned with, not the state of discussions or arrangements prior to birth.

With that in mind, prenatal adoption could happen in at least four ways:

1. *Without Embryo Transfer* (WET): This would occur when, prior to birth, the child's biological mother determines that she is unable or unwilling to raise the child, and arrangements are initiated for another person to become the child's legal parent after birth. The embryo is not transferred into another woman's womb but gestates in the biological mother's womb.

2. *Crisis Embryo Transfer* (CET): This would occur when a medical emergency occurs before the child can survive outside the womb. The embryo would then be transferred from the womb of the biological mother to the womb of another woman who could carry it to term and become its legal mother. The condition of becoming the child's legal mother is required for this to be a form of prenatal adoption. One could also envision a situation where, as the result of a crisis where the biological mother cannot carry the child, another woman brings it to term but then returns it to the biological mother. This embryo transfer without adoption would not be a form of prenatal adoption, and so we will not further consider it here.

3. *Voluntary Embryo Transfer* (VET): This would occur when there is no medical emergency and the parties voluntarily transfer the embryo into the womb of a woman who is not its biological mother but who then becomes its legal mother. This state of affairs would apply whether the embryo had previously been in the womb of the biological mother or had been stored outside her womb (e.g., in cryopreservation).

4. *With Extrauterine Gestation* (WEG): This would occur when, prior to birth, arrangements are initiated for someone other than the biological parents of the embryo to become its legal parent and when the embryo is never placed into the womb of a woman but is gestated in an artificial womb. This form of prenatal adoption has not occurred as of the time of writing, but it is on the horizon, and moralists should be thinking about it.

The most detailed magisterial statement on prenatal adoption is found in *Dignitas personae*. However, to set this document's teaching in a broader framework, we will also look at what the magisterium has said about adoption in general and what it has said that bears on these forms of prenatal adoption.

Adoption in General

The writings of Scripture represent divine revelation rather than teachings of the magisterium per se. However, the appearance and acceptance of adoption in the Old Testament—such as Jacob's adoption of Ephraim and Manasseh—would create at least a presumption in favor of adoption's moral liceity. This presumption is strongly reinforced in the New Testament, where adoption becomes a way in which Christians' relationship to God the Father is described.

In its long history, the magisterium has addressed adoption numerous times. We will not review these in detail, but we will note a passage from the *Catechism of the Catholic Church* that reflects the general tone of magisterial interventions on the topic: "The Gospel shows that physical sterility is not an absolute evil. Spouses who still suffer from infertility after exhausting legitimate medical procedures should unite themselves with the Lord's Cross, the source of all spiritual fecundity. They can give expression to their generosity by adopting abandoned children or performing demanding services for others" (n. 2379).

This appreciative statement indicates the fundamental moral liceity of adoption. The absence of exceptions in statements like this creates a general presumption in favor of the liceity and positive value of adoption. However, this does not mean that all forms of adoption are acceptable, and it would be possible to overcome the presumption of liceity by citing one or more specific factors that render a particular form morally illicit.

Prenatal Adoption without Embryo Transfer

Although one may exist, I am unaware of an occasion when the magisterium has addressed the specific form of prenatal adoption where arrangements are initiated before birth but the biological mother carries the baby to term. However, this is a common procedure. Mothers may determine before birth that they cannot or do not wish to raise the child with which they are pregnant, and they may initiate adoption arrangements prior to birth. This can include contacting an adoption agency, finding appropriate adoptive parents, and, in some jurisdictions, making preliminary legal arrangements, though the adoption does not become final and irrevocable until after birth. The fact that the magisterium has not condemned this common practice would thus suggest the fundamental moral liceity of at least one form of what may be considered prenatal adoption.

Prenatal Adoption with Crisis Embryo Transfer

It could appear that the magisterium has addressed and rejected this form of prenatal adoption as a type of surrogate motherhood. The relevant passage is found in *Donum vitae*. While this document does reject surrogate motherhood, it provides a very specific definition of this practice, stating,

> By "surrogate mother" the Instruction means:
>
> a) the woman who carries in pregnancy an embryo implanted in her uterus and who is genetically a stranger to the embryo because it has been obtained through the union of the gametes of "donors." She carries the pregnancy with a pledge to surrender the baby once it is born to the party who commissioned or made the agreement for the pregnancy.
>
> b) the woman who carries in pregnancy an embryo to whose procreation she has contributed the donation of her own ovum, fertilized through insemination with the sperm of a man other than her husband. She carries the pregnancy with a pledge to surrender the child once it is born to the party who commissioned or made the agreement for the pregnancy.[24]

This definition makes it clear that the practice being condemned does not correspond to prenatal adoption with CET. The gestational mother, in this case, does not contribute her own ovum to the embryo she receives, so the second situation does not apply, and neither situation applies to CET, since the gestational mother does not pledge to surrender the baby but

---

24. CDF, *Donum vitae* (February 22, 1987), II.A.3.

instead becomes its legal mother. CET thus is not the same practice as the surrogate motherhood that the document rejects.

This means that the magisterium appears not to have addressed CET, and so there is room for moralists to debate its status. The general presumption in favor of adoption already documented would create an initial presumption in favor of CET, but moralists might be able to identify factors that would overcome this presumption. Because it has common elements with surrogate motherhood, those factors might be found in *Donum vitae*'s critique of the latter practice. In response to the question "Is 'surrogate' motherhood licit?," the CDF states,

> No, for the same reasons which lead one to reject heterologous artificial fertilization: for it is contrary to the unity of marriage and to the dignity of the procreation of the human person. Surrogate motherhood represents an objective failure to meet the obligations of maternal love, of conjugal fidelity and of responsible motherhood; it offends the dignity and the right of the child to be conceived, carried in the womb, brought into the world and brought up by his own parents; it sets up, to the detriment of families, a division between the physical, psychological and moral elements which constitute those families.[25]

For opponents of CET, this paragraph would be a promising source of factors that might render it illicit. Their burden would then be to argue that the reasons for rejecting surrogate motherhood also apply to CET in the relevant respects. For proponents of CET, the burden would then be to argue that the criticisms of surrogate motherhood do not apply to CET in the relevant respects.

For both parties, this will involve a careful reading of the text. For example, a too-absolute understanding of the right of the child "to be conceived, carried in the womb, brought into the world and brought up by his own parents" would prohibit not only CET and all forms of prenatal adoption but also postnatal adoption. Therefore, this must be read in a qualified way that at least allows for postnatal adoption. An opponent of CET might argue that postnatal adoption is *all* that should be allowed, but a proponent might argue that, if postnatal adoption is justified in a particular

---

25. CDF, *Donum vitae*, II.A.3.

Part 1: The Context of Embryo Adoption

case, a medical emergency might justify a crisis embryo transfer to ensure the survival of the child, possibly including the adoption of the child by a nonbiological mother who is able and willing to care for it.

Prenatal Adoption with Voluntary Embryo Transfer

The form of prenatal adoption on which the magisterium has primarily focused involves VET. It also involves in vitro fertilization. An important development leading to IVF was embryo transfer (ET). In 1890, British embryologist Walter Heape performed the first mammalian embryo transfer in rabbits.[26] In 1932, Aldous Huxley published his science fiction novel *Brave New World*, which involved the concept of IVF and helped popularize the idea. In 1934, Gregory Pinchus and Ernst Enzmann attempted IVF in rabbits, which resulted in successful births.[27] However, later analysis suggested that the conceptions actually occurred in vivo rather than in vitro. In the late 1950s, Min Chueh Chang successfully impregnated a rabbit through IVF, but the technique would not be used succesfully in humans until the 1970s.[28]

The first human born as a result of IVF was the Englishwoman Louise Brown, and one of the physicians who performed the procedure—Robert Edwards—was awarded the Nobel Prize in Physiology or Medicine in 2010. (His colleagues, Patrick Steptoe and Jean Purdy, did not receive the award, because they had died.) Afterward, IVF became increasingly common. By 2018 it was estimated that more than eight million children had been born through IVF.[29]

As the process of IVF developed, doctors began harvesting numerous oocytes from prospective mothers and producing multiple embryos, only

---

26. Walter Heape, "Preliminary Note on the Transplantation and Growth of Mammalian Ova within a Uterine Foster-Mother," *Proceedings of the Royal Society of London* 48 (January 1891): 457–458, doi: 10.1098/rspl.1890.0093.
27. G. Pincus and E.V. Enzmann, "Can Mammalian Eggs Undergo Normal Development In Vitro?," *Biological Sciences* 20.2 (February 1934): 121–122, doi: 10.1073/pnas.20.2.121.
28. Tian Zhu, "In Vitro Fertilization," Embryo Project Encyclopedia, Arizona State University, July 22, 2009, https://embryo.asu.edu/pages/vitro-fertilization.
29. European Society of Human Reproduction and Embryology, "More Than 8 Million Babies Born from IVF since the World's First in 1978," *Science Daily*, July 3, 2018, https://www.sciencedaily.com/releases/2018/07/180703084127.htm.

some of which were reimplanted for gestation. The remainder were stored indefinitely in cryopreservation, and soon there were hundreds of thousands of frozen embryos in fertility clinics across the world.

It should be noted that VET need not involve frozen embryos or even IVF. It would be possible in principle—without a medical emergency—to transfer a naturally conceived embryo from one woman to another as part of an adoption process. Further, even when IVF is used, the embryos are not always frozen, and VET could take place. However, because IVF with the cryopreservation of embryos has become common, this scenario has dominated the discussion.

John Paul II on Embryo Production

An early magisterial intervention regarding these embryos occurred in 1996 when—after recalling the rights inherent in the unborn from the moment of conception—Pope St. John Paul II stated,

> I consider it my duty once again to assert these inviolable rights of the human being from his conception on behalf of all the embryos which are often subjected to freezing (cryo-preservation), in many cases becoming an object of sheer experimentation or, worse, destined to programmed destruction backed by law.
>
> Likewise, I confirm that it is gravely illicit, because of the dignity of the human person and of his having been called to life, to use methods of procreation which the Instruction *Donum vitae* has defined as unacceptable to moral doctrine. The illicitness of these interventions on the origin of life and on human embryos has already been stated (cf. Instruction *Donum vitae*, I, 5; II), but it is necessary that the principles on which the same moral reflection is based be taken up at the legal level.
>
> I therefore appeal to the conscience of the world's scientific authorities and in particular to doctors, that the production of human embryos be halted, taking into account that there seems to be no morally licit solution regarding the human destiny of the thousands and thousands of "frozen" embryos which are and remain the subjects of essential rights and should therefore be protected by law as human persons. I also call on all jurists to work so that States and international institutions will legally recognize the natural rights of the very origin of human life and will likewise defend the inalienable rights which these thousands of

Part 1: The Context of Embryo Adoption

"frozen" embryos have intrinsically acquired from the moment of fertilization.[30]

Here John Paul II does a number of things. First, he recalls the situation of frozen embryos and names two of the fates that may befall them: (1) becoming objects of "sheer experimentation" and (2) the "worse" fate of being destroyed. Second, he recalls the illicitness of the means of procreation condemned in *Donum vitae* and says the moral principles must be "taken up at the legal level." Third, he appeals to scientific authorities to cease producing human embryos, "taking into account that there seems to be no morally licit solution regarding the human destiny of the thousands and thousands of 'frozen' embryos, which are and remain the subjects of essential rights and should therefore be protected by law as human persons." It is noteworthy that what the Pontiff calls for is a ban on the production of human embryos in general and that he backs up the need for this ban by appealing specifically to the state of frozen embryos. The fact that *Donum vitae* had already condemned methods by which embryos are produced means that the situation of frozen embryos did not have to be appealed to. However, the situation of so many frozen embryos creates special urgency.

When it comes to the frozen embryos themselves, the Pontiff notes that there seems to be no morally licit solution for them. Unfortunately, John Paul II does not explicitly state which options he sees as illicit. However, it may be possible to infer them from the context. He has already mentioned two unacceptable fates—experimentation and destruction—and he has appealed to the illicit means of producing them described in *Donum vitae*, so these are probably what he is thinking of. However, the fact that he says there does not *seem* to be a solution is cautionary language that does not rule one out. It merely indicates that one is not obvious. (In Italian, *non si intravede* means "it is not visible/glimpsed.")

Fourth, John Paul II recalls that frozen embryos remain "the subjects of essential rights" and "should therefore be protected by law as human persons."

---

30. John Paul II, Address to the Participants in the Symposium on "*Evangelium Vitae* and Law" and the Eleventh International Colloquium on Roman and Canon Law, EWTN, May 24, 1996, https://www.ewtn.com/catholicism/library/i-appeal-to-worlds-scientific-authorities-halt-the-production-of-human-embryos-8784.

He thus calls on states and institutions to recognize these rights and "defend the inalienable rights which these thousands of 'frozen' embryos have intrinsically acquired from the moment of fertilization." However, he does not explore what form this protection would take. Hypothetically, the context might suggest that he is calling for a *prospective* defense of their rights (i.e., by not creating them). However, the language he uses suggests a *retrospective* defense (i.e., now that they are created, they must be defended).

When assessing the level of authority of this teaching, we must apply the three criteria named by the CDF: "The nature of the documents, the insistence with which a teaching is repeated, and the very way in which it is expressed." John Paul II's teaching is not found in a high-level teaching document, like an apostolic constitution or an encyclical, but in an address to a gathering of professionals. This is a sign of lower authority. This teaching has been repeated on other occasions, such as in *Dignitas personae* (see below), but not with great frequency. And we have seen that part of the teaching is formulated using tentative language ("seems," *non si intravede*). All of this points to it's having a lower level of authority in the broader sweep of magisterial teachings.

As a point of reference, it may be helpful to recall that the entire subject of IVF is new in the experience of the Church, and the magisterium has not yet made infallible pronouncements regarding it. The US bishops' Committee on Doctrine notes, "An example of teaching that is non-definitive and calls for *obsequium religiosum* [religious submission] is the teaching of the instruction *Donum vitae* against such practices as artificial insemination, surrogate motherhood, and *in vitro* fertilization."[31] John Paul II's intervention thus expresses a binding but noninfallible teaching that has not yet been invested with a high level of authority.

Following John Paul II's call for a cessation to the in vitro production of human embryos, pro-lifers continued to seek ways that the situation of existing frozen embryos might be morally resolved, including prenatal adoption with VET. The first person born as a result of this procedure was the American woman Hannah Strege. This took place in 1998, and such children were popularly dubbed "snowflake babies" because of their having been cryogenically preserved. Nightline Christian Adoptions and other agencies then

---

31. Committee on Doctrine, *Teaching Ministry of the Diocesan Bishop*, 24n25.

facilitated more than fifteen hundred such VET adoptions between 1998 and 2018.[32]

Dignitas personae

In 2008, the CDF published a document titled "Instruction *Dignitas personae* on Certain Bioethical Questions." This document contains a section that reviews the causes for the creation of so many thousands of frozen embryos and states,

> Cryopreservation is *incompatible with the respect owed to human embryos*; it presupposes their production *in vitro*; it exposes them to the serious risk of death or physical harm, since a high percentage does not survive the process of freezing and thawing; it deprives them at least temporarily of maternal reception and gestation; it places them in a situation in which they are susceptible to further offense and manipulation.
>
> The majority of embryos that are not used remain "orphans." Their parents do not ask for them and at times all trace of the parents is lost. This is why there are thousands upon thousands of frozen embryos in almost all countries where *in vitro* fertilization takes place.[33]

The first paragraph presents cryopreservation as itself an offense against the human embryo, and the second introduces the problem of orphaned frozen embryos. The document then turns to how the latter situations might be resolved: "With regard to the large number of *frozen embryos already in existence* the question becomes: what to do with them? Some of those who pose this question do not grasp its ethical nature, motivated as they are by laws in some countries that require cryopreservation centers to empty their storage tanks periodically. Others, however, are aware that a grave injustice has been perpetrated and wonder how best to respond to the duty of resolving it." The document then considers three options:

> Proposals to *use these embryos for research* or *for the treatment of disease* are obviously unacceptable because they treat the embryos

---

32. Nightlight Christian Adoptions, "The Beginning of Embryo Adoption," accessed March 22, 2024, https://nightlight.org/testimonial/the-beginning-of-embryo-adoption/.
33. CDF, *Dignitas personae*, n. 18, emphasis original.

as mere "biological material" and result in their destruction. The proposal to thaw such embryos without reactivating them and use them for research, as if they were normal cadavers, is also unacceptable.

The proposal that these embryos could be put at the disposal of infertile couples as a *treatment for infertility* is not ethically acceptable for the same reasons which make artificial heterologous procreation illicit as well as any form of surrogate motherhood; this practice would also lead to other problems of a medical, psychological and legal nature.

It has also been proposed, solely in order to allow human beings to be born who are otherwise condemned to destruction, that there could be a form of *"prenatal adoption."* This proposal, praiseworthy with regard to the intention of respecting and defending human life, presents however various problems not dissimilar to those mentioned above.[34]

The three proposals considered are thus (1) research or the treatment of disease, (2) infertility treatment, and (3) prenatal adoption. The congregation states that the first proposal is "obviously unacceptable," and if the embryos are treated as normal cadavers, it "is also unacceptable." The congregation states that the second proposition "is not ethically acceptable," and it alludes to a passage in *Donum vitae* for a discussion of principles. When it comes to the third proposal, the congregation notes that this proposal has been made "solely in order to allow human beings to be born who are otherwise condemned to destruction," and it takes a notably different tone. The first two options were summarily dismissed in entirely negative terms. However, here the document introduces a positive note, saying that the proposal is "praiseworthy with regard to the intention of respecting and defending human life." However, it embeds this within the statement that the proposal "presents however problems not dissimilar to those mentioned above."

The phrase *not dissimilar* is ambiguous. It indicates that the problems are at least somewhat similar to the previously named ones. However, it is not specific about which individual problems the prenatal adoption of frozen embryos would raise or the extent to which they are the same or different from parallel problems in the first two proposals. All of this is

---

34. CDF, *Dignitas personae*, n. 19, emphasis original.

left to the conjecture of the individual reader, and the document provides no more than a general statement. However, this does not amount to a condemnation of the practice. Stating that problems exist does not mean that they cannot be overcome, mitigated, or tolerated. There is a difference in kind between saying that a practice is "obviously unacceptable," "also unacceptable," or "not ethically acceptable" and that a practice "presents ... problems not dissimilar." The former are unequivocal rejections, while the latter is not.

Instead of exploring the principles further, the congregation pivots and makes a top-level summary statement: "All things considered, it needs to be recognized that the thousands of abandoned embryos represent a *situation of injustice which in fact cannot be resolved*. Therefore John Paul II made an 'appeal to the conscience of the world's scientific authorities, and in particular to doctors, that the production of human embryos be halted, taking into account that there seems to be no morally licit solution regarding the human destiny of the thousands and thousands of "frozen" embryos which are and remain the subjects of essential rights and should therefore be protected by law as human persons.'"[35]

This statement is composed of two sentences, the first of which expresses the congregation's view and the second of which contains a quotation from John Paul II's 1996 address, which is introduced to back up the congregation's view. The top-level statement can be taken in at least two ways. The first is to read it as rejecting the practice of the prenatal adoption of frozen embryos. On this reading, the statement that the abandoned embryos "represent a *situation of injustice which in fact cannot be resolved*" would be taken to mean that prenatal adoption will not resolve their situation in a moral manner, and therefore, it should not be pursued.

However, there are problems with this reading. The first is a conceptual difficulty, because this interpretation seemingly envisions a morally irresolvable situation in which no moral action can be taken with respect to frozen embryos. The idea that God would place the faithful in morally irresolvable situations in which all of the alternatives are sinful is in tension with classic Christian morality, which has held that there is always a moral solution to a situation, even if it is a difficult and costly one. This view seems to be endorsed in sacred Scripture, as Paul tells his readers, "God is faithful,

---

35. CDF, *Dignitas personae*, n. 19, emphasis original, citing John Paul II, Address to the Participants in the Symposium on "*Evangelium Vitae* and Law," n. 6.

and he will not let you be tempted beyond your ability, but with the temptation he will also provide the way of escape, that you may be able to endure it" (1 Cor. 10:13). It thus would seem that—at least in the case of individual frozen embryos—there *must be* a moral course of action with respect to them, whether that would be (1) leaving them frozen indefinitely (perhaps until they cease to be viable), (2) allowing them to thaw and experience natural death (perhaps baptizing them first), (3) having them prenatally adopted, or (4) something else.

A second problem with this interpretation is textual. The first sentence is introduced by the clause "all things considered." This indicates that we are shifting to a summary of a situation. Since there has been no discussion of the problems raised by prenatal adoption, this appears to indicate that the first sentence is thinking not specifically of prenatal adoption but of how the situation is left after considering all three of the proposed solutions to the problem of frozen embryos.

A third problem is that this interpretation would create a discontinuity between the first sentence and the quotation from John Paul II that is offered to support it. The Pope only said that there seems to be no morally licit solution—that is, that one is not obvious (*non si intravede*). The congregation would thus be making a more absolute statement than the Pontiff did and doing so without providing a justification for the stronger position. The statement from John Paul II would thus provide only partial support for the congregation's conclusion.

A fourth problem would be that the adoption of previously frozen embryos was not one of the options that John Paul II considered and rejected. He did not name it—the only fates he mentioned for such children were experimentation and destruction—and the first cryopreserved embryo was not gestated until two years after his 1996 statement. It would thus be odd or inappropriate to cite this statement as an argument against an option that John Paul II was not discussing.

A fifth problem would be that John Paul II was addressing a collective problem not an individual one. The situation that he said seemed to lack a morally licit solution was that of "the human destiny of the thousands and thousands of 'frozen' embryos." Similarly, the congregation spoke of the situation of "the thousands of abandoned embryos" not being resolvable. It would be odd or inappropriate to take an irresolvable collective situation to mean that no individual cases can be morally solved.

A sixth problem would be that John Paul II seemed to envision the possibility of solutions at least in individual cases. He stated that the frozen embryos "are and remain the subjects of essential rights and should therefore be protected by law as human persons." In addition, he said, "I also call on all jurists to work so that States and international institutions ... will likewise defend the inalienable rights which these thousands of 'frozen' embryos have intrinsically acquired from the moment of fertilization." This strongly suggests that there *are* moral actions that can be taken with respect to frozen embryos, even if the Pontiff did not explore what they might be.

In view of these difficulties, it is highly problematic to interpret the congregation's final statement as saying that the prenatal adoption of frozen embryos will not morally resolve individual cases, because they are *all* morally insoluble.

We thus must consider the second way of taking the statement. On this view, the congregation has already offered its thoughts on the individual practice of the prenatal adoption of frozen embryos: it is praiseworthy with respect to intent, and it presents problems that are "not dissimilar" to the other two options. Rather than seeking to go further in assessing the practice, the congregation then pivots to considering the overall situation and the overall solution: stop making frozen embryos! The congregation thus makes a general assessment that the overall, collective situation of thousands of abandoned embryos cannot be practically solved—there certainly will not be enough prenatal adoptions to do so, and the other options are clearly illicit—and then quotes John Paul II making the same point that frozen embryo production needs to be stopped.

This reading avoids the problems associated with the first interpretation, and it makes sense in context. A careful reading of the document thus supports the understanding of its offering a partial assessment of the prenatal adoption of frozen embryos—it has a praiseworthy intent but involves problems somewhat similar to other solutions—and then focusing on the overall solution of stopping the production of frozen embryos. The CDF thus does not offer a bottom-line assessment of the adoption of frozen embryos. It notes positive and negative factors but does not rule the practice to be ultimately morally licit or illicit. We thus are in a situation where the magisterium has offered thoughts on the practice but has not established a firm teaching regarding it.

This assessment is consistent with remarks made by Archbishop Rino Fisichella, then president of the Pontifical Academy of Life, at the press conference introducing *Dignitas personae*, when he "told reporters that 'the discussion is still open' and the Vatican has not ruled out the possibility of embryo adoption completely, although it is leaning toward a completely negative judgment because embryo adoption involves the future parents in an immoral process."[36] The US bishops also offered a similar assessment in 2009:

> "Embryo adoption" refers to having an abandoned embryo transferred to the uterus of a woman willing to gestate this child to save his or her life. Many have asked whether this might be a legitimate way for conscientious couples to respond, in a potentially life-affirming way, to the terrible problem of thousands of abandoned embryos at IVF clinics in the United States. However, serious moral concerns have been raised about embryo adoption, particularly as it requires the wife in the adopting couple to receive into her womb an embryonic child who was not conceived through her bodily union with her husband. The Church's teaching authority has acknowledged the moral concerns associated with this practice. The terrible plight of abandoned frozen embryos underscores the need for our society to end practices such as IVF that regularly produce so many "spare" or unwanted human beings.[37]

Here the US bishops note that the magisterium "has acknowledged moral concerns associated with this practice" but without saying a firm judgment has been made. They also refer to the "terrible plight of abandoned frozen embryos" and the need to "end practices such as IVF" that lead to them.

Prenatal Adoption with Extrauterine Gestation

Finally, we will look briefly at prenatal adoption with extrauterine gestation. In this scenario, one or more artificial wombs would be used to gestate the child, who would be adopted before birth by a new parent

---

36. Cindy Wooden, "Adopting Embryos Raises Moral Questions, Vatican Officials Say," Catholic News Service, December 12, 2008, https://web.archive.org/web/20110112204018/http:/www.catholicnews.com/data/stories/cns/0806229.htm.
37. US Conference of Catholic Bishops, "Life-Giving Love in an Age of Technology," USCCB, 2009, https://www.usccb.org/beliefs-and-teachings/what-we-believe/love-and-sexuality/life-giving-love-in-an-age-of-technology.

or couple. This scenario has not yet taken place, because of the primitive state of artificial womb technology. However, in 2019, Dutch scientists estimated that artificial wombs for humans would be available within ten years.[38] Since our purpose is looking at prenatal adoption, we may set aside the general issues of safety and success that would inevitably attend the first artificial wombs. How might the development of safe and reliable artificial wombs affect the issue?

They might avoid the concerns of some with implanting a heterologous (biologically unrelated) embryo in a woman. Further, the development of such wombs would create a new avenue for bringing previously frozen embryos who would otherwise die to term. In 2023, Rev. Tadeusz Pacholczyk of the National Catholic Bioethics Center told the *National Catholic Register* that "'it will probably always be the case that there will be no morally licit solution regarding the fate of frozen embryos' unless the Church were to one day sanction artificial wombs, which he called 'improbable.'"[39]

A brief mention of artificial wombs is found in *Donum vitae*: "Techniques of fertilization *in vitro* can open the way to other forms of biological and genetic manipulation of human embryos, such as attempts or plans for fertilization between human and animal gametes and the gestation of human embryos in the uterus of animals, or the hypothesis or project of constructing artificial uteruses for the human embryo. *These procedures are contrary to the human dignity proper to the embryo, and at the same time they are contrary to the right of every person to be conceived and to be born within marriage and from marriage.*"[40]

While this reference is clearly negative, it is not clear that it would apply to all use of artificial wombs. It is introduced in the context of highly problematic practices such as IVF, which may even be heterologous, and this passage envisions the fusion of human and animal gametes and the apparent nonemergency use of gestating human embryos in animal uteruses.

---

38. Kayleen Devlin, "The World's First Artifical Womb for Humans," video, BBC, October 15, 2019, https://www.bbc.com/news/av/health-50056405.
39. Lauretta Brown, "Frozen in Time: Catholic Ethicists Discuss the Fate of the Estimated 1 Million Human Embryos on Ice," *National Catholic Register*, January 17, 2023, https://www.ncregister.com/news/frozen-in-time-catholic-ethicists-discuss-the-fate-of-the-estimated-1-million-human-embryos-on-ice.
40. CDF, *Donum vitae*, I.6, emphasis original.

It may thus be envisioning the use of artificial wombs in such morally problematic circumstances—as opposed to their use as a lifesaving measure when the child will otherwise die.

Further clarification from the magisterium would be needed to establish that *all* use of artificial wombs is to be prohibited. In particular, it is worth noting that the neonatal incubators used to keep premature children alive are essentially first generation artificial wombs. They serve as a replacement for uterine gestation when this becomes impossible and thus function as artificial wombs. In fact, infant incubators have been used at least as early as 1835.[41]

The fact that the magisterium has not reacted negatively to the widespread use of neonatal incubators suggests that there is not an intrinsic moral problem with them, and there is not a difference in kind between these devices and ones that would extend their usefulness further back toward conception. There would be concerns with the safety and reliability of artificial wombs from early stages of embryonic development, and there would be personalistic concerns involving "the right of the child to be conceived, carried in the womb, brought into the world and brought up by his own parents."[42] However, the magisterium appears to have tacitly accepted the use of artificial means of allowing a child to develop outside the biological mother's womb, at least in situations like the crisis of a premature birth or the incapacity of the mother to carry a child to term. This thus appears to be another area in which—in the absence of a firm magisterial teaching—the subject may be debated.

---

41. Kelsey Rebovich, "The Infant Incubator in Europe (1860–1890)," Embryo Project Encyclopedia, Arizona State University, November 2, 2017, https://keep.lib.asu.edu/items/173300.
42. CDF, *Donum vitae*, II.A.3.

Part 2: Objections to Embryo Adoption

4

Embryo Transfer after Adoption and the Extended Inseparability Argument

Objections That Appeal to the Generative Faculty

Rev. Fr. Nicanor Pier Giorgio Austriaco, OP

Since time immemorial, a woman could become pregnant only via an act of sexual intercourse.[1] If she became pregnant through an act of sexual intercourse with her husband, her becoming pregnant was judged to be virtuous and morally licit. On the other hand, if she became pregnant through an act of sexual intercourse with a man other than her husband, her becoming pregnant was then judged to be vicious and morally illicit.

Today, a woman can become pregnant via an act of embryo transfer. Therefore, we can now ask whether her becoming pregnant via this nonsexual act is to be judged as virtuous or vicious, as morally licit or illicit. There have been many objections raised against embryo adoption, but I believe that the objection that appeals to the generative faculty is the central question at the heart of the decades-old debate among Catholic ethicists over embryo transfer after adoption.[2]

---

1. An earlier version of this chapter was published as "Embryo Adoption and the Extended Inseparability Argument," *National Catholic Bioethics Quarterly* 21.1 (Spring 2021): 29–35, doi: 10.5840/ncbq20212114.
2. For the pro-embryo-adoption position in the Catholic moral tradition, see Sarah-Vaughan Brakman and Darlene Fozard Weaver, "Embryo Adoption before and after *Dignitas Personae*: Defending an Argument of Limited Permissibility," in *Contemporary Controversies in Catholic Bioethics*, ed. Jason T.

PART 2: OBJECTIONS TO EMBRYO ADOPTION

In this chapter, I propose that this Catholic debate over embryo adoption is at a genuine impasse awaiting resolution from the magisterium of the Catholic Church, because both sides have reached a point where there is a fundamental disagreement over whether the act of becoming pregnant—which I argue is a telos of the generative faculties of the couple—is reserved to the marital covenant. This can be resolved not by further argumentation but by authoritative definition in response to the question, Should the principle of inseparability be extended to the act of becoming pregnant?

The Extended Inseparability Argument

As I noted at the outset, since time immemorial, becoming pregnant was judged to be morally virtuous or vicious by ascertaining the identity of the man who impregnated the woman. How a woman became pregnant was a morally salient question for people, both ancient and modern, whether they were ethicists or not.

Why was this so? Why is it still so? One possibility is that, for ordinary folk who believe in the exclusivity of the marriage bond, making a woman pregnant, like having sex with her, and making a baby with her, was one of the acts that should be reserved to her husband, because these acts can be realized only through the exercise of his causality during the conjugal act.

Some could object to this folk logic by proposing that having sex is the only act truly reserved to spouses. Becoming pregnant by another man was forbidden from time immemorial because becoming pregnant was used as a proxy for having sex. If a woman became pregnant by another, she had had sex with another. The former was forbidden not because it is intrinsically vicious but because the latter is illicit.

How should we respond to this objection? One way is by examining an analogous situation that has already been clarified in Catholic sexual ethics. Let us, therefore, consider the relationship between making a baby and having sex. Again, since time immemorial, making a baby with a woman was thought to be the prerogative of her husband. Would the objection

---

Eberl (Cham, CH: Springer, 2017), 147–167. For the anti-embryo adoption position, see Catherine Althaus, "Establishing the Moral Object of Heterologous and Homologous Embryo Transfer," in Eberl, *Contemporary Controversies in Catholic Bioethics*, 169–187.

apply that making a baby with another man was forbidden only because the act of making a baby with another was used as a proxy for the act of having sex with him?

For many in the developed world today, the causal link between making a baby and having sex is only an accidental one and a morally innocuous one at that. In their view, a woman can make a baby with a man other than her husband as long as she does not have sex with him—hence, the widespread public support for heterologous artificial fertilization, where a woman's egg is fertilized by the sperm of a donor who is not her husband. These individuals from the developed world would affirm that the immemorial objection against a woman's making a baby with someone other than her husband is unsound. This act was forbidden only because the act of making a baby with another man was used as a proxy for the act of having sex with him. The former is morally licit, while the latter is morally illicit.

In contrast, the Catholic Church has determined that the teleological ordering of the act of having sex, an act that unites the couple as they exercise their generative faculties, demands that one not separate it from the act of making a baby, an act that transmits life.[3] In Catholic sexual ethics, this is called the inseparability principle.[4] Thus, a woman can make a baby only with her husband. She cannot make one with another man without violating

---

3. See Paul VI, *Humanae vitae* (July 25, 1968), n. 16. Pope St. Paul VI distinguishes couples who postpone pregnancy by abstaining from sex during fertile periods and couples who do the same using contraception by explicitly appealing to the teleological ordering of the sexual faculty: "In reality, these two cases are completely different. In the former the married couple rightly use a faculty provided them by nature. In the later they obstruct the natural development of the generative process. It cannot be denied that in each case the married couple, for acceptable reasons, are both perfectly clear in their intention to avoid children and wish to make sure that none will result."
4. See *Catechism of the Catholic Church*, 2nd ed. (Washington, DC: United States Conference of Catholic Bishops/Libreria Editrice Vaticana, 2018 update), n. 2363: "The spouses' union achieves the twofold end of marriage: the good of the spouses themselves and the transmission of life. These two meanings or values of marriage cannot be separated without altering the couple's spiritual life and compromising the goods of marriage and the future of the family. The conjugal love of man and woman thus stands under the twofold obligation of fidelity and fecundity."

her marital covenant, *even if she does not have sex with him*.⁵ Thus, for the Catholic moral tradition, the act of making a baby with a man other than one's husband, like having sex with him, is morally illicit, because making a baby is an act that is reserved to the marital covenant by the very teleological ordering and meaning of the conjugal act. Making a baby by another man and having sex with him were forbidden from time immemorial, in the Catholic view, not because the former was a proxy for the latter but because both acts are reserved to the marital covenant.

Several Catholic ethicists, and I am one of them, have argued that the ethical reasoning linking the acts of having sex and of making a baby and, therefore, reserving both to the causality of a husband should be extended to the act of becoming pregnant, therefore ruling out embryo transfer in all its manifestations.⁶ Indeed, I would propose that this trinity of acts are

---

5. Congregation for the Doctrine of the Faith, *Donum vitae* (February 22, 1987), II.A.2. "Recourse to the gametes of a third person, in order to have sperm or ovum available, constitutes a violation of the reciprocal commitment of the spouses and a grave lack in regard to that essential property of marriage which is its unity. ... Furthermore, it offends the common vocation of the spouses who are called to fatherhood and motherhood: it objectively deprives conjugal fruitfulness of its unity and integrity."
6. See Nicanor Pier Giorgio Austriaco, "On the Catholic Vision of Conjugal Love and the Morality of Embryo Transfer," in *Human Embryo Adoption*, ed. Thomas V. Berg and Edward J. Furton (Philadelphia: National Catholic Bioethics Center, 2006), 115–134; Nicholas Tonti-Filippini, "The Embryo Rescue Debate: Impregnating Women, Ectogenesis, and Restoration from Suspended Animation," *National Catholic Bioethics Quarterly* 3.1 (Spring 2003): 111–137, doi: 10.5840/ncbq20033181; Steven A. Long, "An Argument for the Embryonic Intactness of Marriage," *Thomist* 70.2 (April 2006): 267–288, doi: 10.1353/tho.2006.0019; E. Christian Brugger, ed., "Symposium on *Dignitas Personae*," *National Catholic Bioethics Quarterly* 9.3 (Autumn 2009): 470–474, doi: 10.5840/20099333; Catherine Althaus, "Human Embryo Transfer and the Theology of the Body," in *Embryo Adoption and the Catholic Tradition*, ed. Sarah-Vaughan Brakman and Darlene Fozard Weaver (Dordrecht, NL: Springer, 2007), 43–67; Tracy Jamison, "Embryo Adoption and the Design of Human Nature: The Analogy between Artificial Insemination and Artificial Impregnation," *National Catholic Bioethics Quarterly* 10.1 (Spring 2010): 111–122, doi: 10.5840/ncbq201010175;

actually distinct moments of a single movement that realizes the potency of the conjugal act and the exercise of a couple's generative faculties. By having sex, making a baby, and becoming pregnant, a couple attains the perfection of the marital act they have shared. They have realized the fruitfulness of the conjugal covenant in its fullness. I will call this proposal the extended inseparability argument, because it proposes to extend the principle of inseparability from two acts (having sex and making a baby) to three acts (having sex, making a baby, and becoming pregnant).

Responding to the Extended Inseparability Argument

Over the past nearly twenty years, opponents have used three logical and rhetorical strategies to respond to the extended inseparability argument and affirm the liceity of embryo transfer after adoption. I do not think that any of them have defeated the argument.

First, critics have pointed to the great good of embryo transfer after adoption.[7] Embryo adoption saves the life of an abandoned child, it gives him a family, it is an act of mercy, it is an act of charity, it is an act that is truly pro-life, and so on. Therefore, critics argue, the extended inseparability argument is flawed, because it does not acknowledge or even minimizes this great good that should be embraced by society and the Church.

Paschal Corby, "Estranged Fathers: The Alienation of Men in Heterologous Embryo Transfer," *National Catholic Bioethics Quarterly* 13.2 (Summer 2013): 287–297, doi: 10.5840/ncbq201313250; Charles Robertson, "A Thomistic Analysis of Embryo Adoption," *National Catholic Bioethics Quarterly* 14.4 (Winter 2014): 673–695, doi: 10.5840/ncbq201414470; Charles Robertson, "Navigating an Impasse in the Embryo Adoption Debate: A Response to Elizabeth Rex," *National Catholic Bioethics Quarterly* 16.3 (Autumn 2016): 409–417, doi: 10.5840/ncbq201616339; Irene Alexander, "Is Artificial Impregnation Opposed to the Unity of Marriage? A New Look at the Question of Embryo Adoption," *Nova et Vetera* 16.1 (Winter 2018): 47–80; and Michael Arthur Vacca, "Equivalence of the Moral Objects in Embryo Adoption and Heterologous IVF," *National Catholic Bioethics Quarterly* 22.3 (Autumn 2022): 437–446, doi: 10.5840/ncbq202222340.

7. For a recent example of this view, see Christopher M. Reilly, "Rescuing the Good Samaritan in Embryo Adoption and Beyond," *National Catholic Bioethics Quarterly* 20.3 (Autumn 2020): 487–498, doi: 10.5840/ncbq202020345.

Part 2: Objections to Embryo Adoption

This objection is irrelevant to the extended inseparability argument. For the Catholic moral tradition, affirming the inseparable link between having sex and making a baby is the outcome of recognizing the teleological structure of the conjugal act and the generative faculties of the couple and, therefore, what it means for one spouse to give himself or herself to the other in the sexual embrace. The principle of inseparability is not the conclusion of a utilitarian or consequentialist argument that is determined by the goodness or badness of personal or social outcomes, though we can now acknowledge and recognize the individual and social ills that have occurred after societies ignored the inseparability principle. Similarly, the extended inseparability argument cannot be defeated by utilitarian or consequentialist claims.

Second, critics have argued that the extended inseparability argument devalues adoption or restricts the meaning of parenthood in a way that is an injustice to an authentic theology of adoption. Sarah-Vaughan Brakman and Darlene Fozard Weaver raise this objection against opponents of embryo adoption (EA) who would want to evaluate the morality of embryo transfer apart from the context of adoption: "Inherent Wrongness Arguments therefore consider EA on morally limited terms that abstract EA from the intention of the adopters, from the larger context of EA, and from relevant normative commitments of Catholic moral tradition."[8] The act of becoming pregnant, in their view, must be evaluated within the constellation of acts that constitutes the social practice of adoption and the kind of familial relationships and goods that it entails.

However, the extended inseparability argument has nothing to do with adoption or parenthood. If acknowledging the inseparable link between having sex and making a baby does not devalue adoption or parenthood—and no one to my knowledge has made that argument against the principle of inseparability—then acknowledging the inseparable link between having sex, making a baby, and becoming pregnant would not either. Even if the extended inseparability argument were valid and true, any individual or any couple could still adopt an abandoned embryonic child and become his parents. One could just cannot become pregnant with him.

---

8. Brakman and Weaver, "Embryo Adoption before and after *Dignitas Personae*," 157.

Third, opponents have argued that the Catholic Church has linked the conjugal act only with procreation—that is, she has linked only having sex and making a baby. Since becoming pregnant is not a constituent act of having sex or making a baby, then the Church's prohibitions against separating sex and procreation are not applicable to the ethical debate surrounding embryo adoption.[9]

This objection is valid and true. However, it fails to appreciate the reasoning of the extended inseparability argument, which proposes that having sex, making a baby, and becoming pregnant are teleologically linked and, therefore, should be understood as one movement that actualizes the full potency of the conjugal act and the generative faculties of the couple. This is not an argument moving from first principles in the morality of human sexuality and procreation to some further moral conclusion. Rather, it is a proposal for establishing a moral first principle that extends the inseparability principle that already links having sex and making a baby to include becoming pregnant, once again, because of the ontological structure and potency of the conjugal act.

In my view, therefore, the only legitimate way to object to the extended inseparability argument is to propose that the reasoning used in its defense is irredeemably flawed. One would have to argue either that the teleological foundation undergirding the extended inseparability argument is invalid or that the teleological foundation is not applicable if it is extended past the acts of having sex and making a baby to the act of becoming pregnant.

For the first strategy, one could simply affirm that the teleological ordering in nature is morally irrelevant. Many contemporary secular ethicists, heirs of David Hume, would heartily embrace this critique, which has been called the naturalistic fallacy. However, no Catholic ethicist who is aware of the teleological framework that is central to the Catholic Church's sexual ethics could go down this path.[10] For the Catholic moral tradition,

---

9. See, for example, Reilly, "Rescuing the Good Samaritan," 494.
10. I am aware that Catholic ethicists who embrace the new natural law theory would similarly eschew the teleological argumentation that has been used by the Catholic moral tradition for millennia. For example, Melissa Moschella has opined that the classical account of natural law in the Catholic moral tradition is unsound, because "it fails to recognize that the notion of 'according to nature' does *not* contain the notion of 'good.'" See her "Sexual Ethics, Human

teleology in nature is a legitimate source for moral reflection regarding normative human behavior.[11]

As for the second strategy, it is not clear to me how one could justify fragmenting the teleological movement of the conjugal act to affirm that the link between having sex and making a baby is essential while the link between having sex, making a baby, and becoming pregnant is not. If the act of making a baby is a legitimate telos for the conjugal act that reveals the fecundity of the spouses, then the act of becoming pregnant should be one as well. In the natural order, having sex leads to making a baby, which then leads to becoming pregnant. All of these reveal the fruitfulness of the act of self-giving that occurs in marriage in all its perfection.

In the end, therefore, I propose that the debate over embryo adoption is at a genuine impasse awaiting resolution from the magisterium of the Catholic Church, because both sides have reached a point where there is a fundamental disagreement over whether the act of becoming pregnant, as a telos of the generative faculties of a couple, should be reserved to the marital covenant. This can be resolved not by further moral argumentation but by

---

Nature, and the 'New' and 'Old' Natural Law Theories," *National Catholic Bioethics Quarterly* 19.2 (Summer 2019): 251–278, 277, emphasis added, doi: 10.5840/ncbq201919218. For a robust discussion and defense of the Catholic Church's use of a teleological framework to ground her sexual ethics, an account that exposes the errors of Moschella's new natural law view, see Edward Feser, "In Defense of the Perverted Faculty Argument," in *Neo-Scholastic Essays* (South Bend, IN: St. Augustine Press, 2015), 378–415. Also see Carlos A. Casanova, "The Underlying Assumptions of Germain Grisez's Critique of the Perverted Faculty Argument," *Espiritu* 69.159 (2020): 95–126.

11. In *Persona humana* (December 29, 1975), n. 5, the Congregation for the Doctrine of the Faith explicitly links the foundational moral principle for sexual ethics to the finality of the sexual act: "Speaking of 'the sexual nature of man and the human faculty of procreation,' the Council noted that they 'wonderfully exceed the dispositions of lower forms of life.' It then took particular care to expound the principles and criteria which concern human sexuality in marriage, and which are based upon the finality of the specific function of sexuality. ... These final words briefly sum up the Council's teaching—more fully expounded in an earlier part of the same Constitution—on the finality of the sexual act and on the principal criterion of its morality: it is respect for its finality that ensures the moral goodness of this act."

authoritative definition in response to the question, Should the principle of inseparability be extended to the act of becoming pregnant?

Implications of the Extended Inseparability Argument

If the extended inseparability argument is valid and true, as I think it is, then the act of becoming pregnant has to be reserved to the agency of a husband. This would rule out embryo transfer, both heterologous and homologous, in any of its manifestations, because here it is the physician who makes the woman pregnant.[12] Once again, however, I note that this does not rule out embryo adoption. Any individual or any couple could still adopt an abandoned embryonic child and become his parents. One could just cannot become pregnant by transferring him into his mother's womb.

Finally, the extended inseparability argument would explain why the ectogenesis or gestation outside the uterus of a human being from the moment of conception onward is vicious and morally illicit. This action attacks not only the dignity of the child, who should be gestated in the womb of his mother, but also the integrity of the conjugal covenant, because it deprives the husband of the privilege of making his wife pregnant, that is, with child.

---

12. I remain open to the moral permissibility of a physician-husband who performs embryo transfer on his wife with their own embryo or an embryo that they have adopted, but I am still considering the implications of this nonsexual act on the teleological structure and meaning of the conjugal act.

5

Children's Rights to Love and Life
Christopher Bobier

Abortion opponents argue in broad strokes that abortion is immoral because it involves the intentional killing of another human being. Although human embryos are nascent, they *are* human beings, and since intentionally killing another human being is generally wrong, it is generally wrong to intentionally kill a human embryo. Kate Finley argues that abortion opponents have a compelling reason to also be proponents of adoption. To defend an anti-abortion position with integrity requires that abortion opponents bear the cost of their convictions by taking action, and adoption, she argues, "Is a particularly powerful way for them [abortion opponents] to 'live out' their commitments with integrity."[1] While she does not mention it explicitly, Finley's argument extends to the practice of embryonic adoption (i.e., heterologous embryo transfer, a procedure that involves the implantation into a woman's womb of an embryo that is not her own but has been abandoned by another). If embryos are human beings, and opponents of abortion should be proponents of adoption, then opponents of abortion should be proponents of embryonic adoption. After all, abortion opponents claim to defend helpless and vulnerable embryonic children, and there are many helpless and vulnerable embryonic children who are left over from in vitro fertilization procedures and who will probably die if they are not adopted.

---

1. Kate Finley, "Abortion, Adoption and Integrity," in *Agency, Pregnancy and Persons*, ed. Nicholas Colgrove et al. (New York: Routledge, 2023), 153.

PART 2: OBJECTIONS TO EMBRYO ADOPTION

This chapter offers arguments in favor of adoption from the perspectives of both parents and children, and shows that many of these assertions also extend to embryonic adoption. However, I suggest that would-be adoptive parents have compelling reasons to pursue traditional adoption, that is, adoption of a postnatal child in state custody, rather than an embryonic child. The chapter proceeds as follows: In section 1, I offer arguments for positing a pro tanto moral duty to adopt.[2] In section 2, I offer an argument for why children have a right to be adopted. Then, in section 3, I offer arguments showing that would-be adoptive parents should pursue traditional adoption, not embryonic adoption.

Parental Rights

A number of scholars have argued in defense of what many agree to be common sense: parenting contributes to one's well-being in a variety of ways. Christine Overall observes that "the creation of the mutually enriching, mutually enhancing love that is the parent-child relationship" offers a strong reason to have a child.[3] The claim is that adults, not just children, benefit from entering into the parent-child relationship. It is a unique relationship, after all, one of asymmetrical power, care, sacrifice, and love. It is a relationship that offers a distinctive sort of intimacy and dependence, for parents relate to their children differently than they relate to each other, their friends, and other children. To have a child opens up a whole new world of experiences, thereby creating opportunity for parents to grow in virtue and knowledge as well as to experience a new outlook on life. To love, care for, and engage with a vulnerable child fosters a unique relationship that contributes to a meaningful, good life. Rosalind Hursthouse, accordingly, observes that parenthood can be "partially constructive of a flourishing life,"[4] while Harry Brighouse and Adam Swift claim that it "produces

---

2. A pro tanto moral duty is a defeasible duty, which means that it can be overridden or suspended in light of other considerations. It is in contrast to absolute moral duties, such as our moral duty to refrain from murdering other beings.
3. Christine Overall, *Why Have Children? The Ethical Debate* (Cambridge, MA: MIT Press, 2012), 217.
4. Rosalind Hursthouse, *Beginning Lives* (Oxford: Blackwell, 1987), 241.

a distinctive contribution to well-being."[5] Given these observations, the argument for a right to become a parent is straightforward: we have a right to what is foundational and integral to our well-being, and parenting is foundational and integral to our well-being. Therefore, we have a right to become parents.[6]

The right to become a parent is distinct from the right to procreate, and so the case can be made that would-be parents should pursue adoption. In other words, the goods of parenthood may be achieved by adoption, not necessarily procreation, and there are ethical reasons to consider adoption over procreation. I offer two arguments from the broader philosophical literature for positing a pro tanto obligation to adopt foster children. To be clear, this obligation is defeasible, and its existence may well be compatible with ethical procreation. Still, to think well about embryonic adoption, we need to examine the case for adoption simpliciter.

The first argument for adoption begins by noting the harms that foster children suffer from not having a loving, stable home. Tina Rulli writes that "only in adopting do you alleviate an extant harm or prevent one from occurring."[7] She observes in a different article that adoption is critical for the adopted child, benefitting the child in significant ways, and many harms befall children who are in need of a new family and lack parental love and care: "Many [children without stable parents] lack basic nutrition and medical care. They are the helpless victims of neglect and abuse."[8] Unfortunately, there is compelling evidence that Rulli is correct. There are high rates of sexual and physical abuse in foster care, and children in foster care experience

---

5. Harry Brighouse and Adam Swift, "The Goods of Parenting," in *Family-Making: Contemporary Ethical Challenges*, ed. Françoise Baylis and Carolyn McLeod (New York: Oxford University Press, 2014), 18.
6. For defense of this conception of rights, see S. Matthew Liao, *The Right to Be Loved* (New York: Oxford University Press, 2015), chap. 2.
7. Tina Rulli, "The Unique Value of Adoption," in Baylis and McLeod, *Family-Making*, 109–130, 113.
8. Tina Rulli, "Preferring a Genetically-Related Child," in "New Developments in Family Ethics," ed. Monika Betzler and Jörg Löschke, special issue, *Journal of Moral Philosophy* 13.6 (November 2016): 674.

delays in emotional and cognitive development.⁹ A significant number of foster children never earn a college degree or enjoy gainful employment, but many experience post-traumatic stress disorder and homelessness.¹⁰ By contrast, studies show that adopting foster children mitigates many of the adverse effects of living in foster care and that adopted children catch up on many of the measures of well-being.¹¹ To become a parent to an orphan is to offer that child what he or she so desperately needs.

With the harms of foster care before us, the first argument can be set out as follows: We have a prima facie moral duty to help those in need.¹² For example, you cannot ethically ignore a child in danger when helping that

---

9. Saskia Euser et al., "The Prevalence of Child Sexual Abuse in Out-of-Home Care: A Comparison between Abuse in Residential and in Foster Care," *Child Maltreatment* 18.4 (November 2013): 221–231, doi: 10.1177/1077559513489848; Sasika Euser et al., "The Prevalence of Child Sexual Abuse in Out-of-Home Care: Increased Risk for Children with a Mild Intellectual Disability," *Journal of Applied Research in Intellectual Disabilities* 29.1 (January 2016): 83–92, doi: 10.1111/jar.12160; Laurel K. Leslie et al., "Addressing the Developmental and Mental Health Needs of Young Children in Foster Care," *Journal of Developmental and Behavioral Pediatrics* 26.2 (April 2005): 140, doi: 10.1097/00004703-200504000-00011; and Jessie C. Krier et al., "Youths in Foster Care with Language Delays: Prevalence, Causes, and Interventions," *Psychology in the Schools* 55.5 (May 2018): 523–538, doi: 10.1002/pits.22129.
10. Angelique Day et al., "An Examination of Post-Secondary Retention and Graduation among Foster Care Youth Enrolled in a Four-Year University," *Children and Youth Services Review* 33.11 (2011): 2335–2341, doi: 10/1016/j.childyouth.2011.08.004; Amy Dworsky et al., "Homelessness during the Transition from Foster Care to Adulthood," *American Journal of Public Health* 103 suppl 2 (December 2013): S318–S323, doi: 10.2105/AJPH.2013.301455; and Amy Dworsky and Mark E. Courtney, "Homelessness and the Transition from Foster Care to Adulthood," *Child Welfare* 88.4 (2009): 23–56.
11. Marinus H. Van Ljzendoorn and Femmie Juffer, "The Emanuel Miller Memorial Lecture 2006: Adoption as Intervention. Meta-Analytic Evidence for Massive Catch-Up and Plasticity in Physical, Socio-Emotional, and Cognitive Development," *Journal of Child Psychology and Psychiatry* 47.12 (December 2006): 1228–1245, doi: 10.1111/j.1469-7610.2006.01675.x.
12. For extended defense of this argument, see Daniel Friedrich, "A Duty to Adopt?," *Journal of Applied Philosophy* 30.1 (January 2013): 25–39, doi: 10.1111/japp.12003.

child does not place you in comparable danger. If the child is drowning, you should jump in to help, even if doing so ruins your clothes and makes you miss an important work meeting. The child's death is worse than your inconvenience. Foster children are in need of a stable, loving home, and until they receive parental love, they are vulnerable and subject to immense harm. A would-be parent's desire to have a biological child does not override the significant harms that befall a child in foster care, just as the desire to not get wet does not override the harm of drowning. Would-be parents, therefore, have a strong reason to pursue adoption rather than procreation.

The second argument in favor of adoption appeals to the praiseworthiness of love that is present in adoption. Love is the virtue that disposes one to will the good of the other person. As Ryan West explains, the virtue of love "orients the heart of the self-respecting person beyond the protection of her own dignity, placing her will squarely on the well-being of others."[13] Christians are called to manifest selfless love toward others, including and especially orphans (see James 1:27). As noted already, the parent-child relationship is among the most intimate relationships one can enter into, for it is one of vulnerability, care, and sacrifice. To let such others-focused concern be the starting point of a lifetime of love, especially when directed to a vulnerable person, is paradigmatic of sacrificial love—parenting can be emotionally, financially, spiritually, and physically taxing. As Rulli highlights, to "willingly share this deeply intimate connection with a stranger is morally exemplary."[14] This is not to say that creating a child is not exemplary but merely to observe that adopting a child as one's own is an act of sacrificial love, since it sacrifices the biological connectedness present in procreation in addition to all of the other sacrifices involved in procreative parenting. Adoptive parenting requires more sacrifice than procreative parenting. Since Christians are called to love sacrificially, and adoption is an act of sacrificial love, would-be Christian parents have a strong reason to adopt. Pope St. John Paul II affirms, "The existence of so many children without families suggests *adoption as a concrete way of love*."[15]

---

13. Ryan West, "Anger and the Virtues: A Critical Study in Virtue Individuation," *Canadian Journal of Philosophy* 46.6 (June 24, 2016): 883–884, doi: 10.1080/00455091.2016.1199232.
14. Rulli, "Unique Value of Adoption," 119.
15. John Paul II, Address to the Meeting of the Adoptive Families Organized by the Missionaries of Charity (September 5, 2000), n. 3, emphasis original.

PART 2: OBJECTIONS TO EMBRYO ADOPTION

Children's Rights

We can examine the issue from the perspective of children as well. I think the most compelling argument is given by S. Matthew Liao, who argues that children have a right to be loved.[16] His argument begins by noting that people "have rights to the primary essential conditions for a good life because having these conditions is of primary importance to human beings."[17] Food, water, and security are basic goods that enable human beings to sustain themselves in their pursuit of a good life—they are fundamental conditions for pursuing what one considers to be a life worth living. Life, for example, is necessary to pursuing everything else, which is one reason why we have a right to life. Food, water, and shelter are also integral and foundational to pursuing a good life, for it is difficult to live a good life if you are constantly hungry, thirsty, and cold. We, therefore, have a right to these things as well.

Liao argues that physical and psychological closeness is good for children in this basic sort of way, as evidenced by the effects of its lack in institutionalized children: "Studies of children in institutions found, for example, that children who did not receive love but only adequate care became ill more frequently; their learning capacities deteriorated significantly; they became decreasingly interested in their environment; ... they suffered insomnia; they were constantly depressed; and they eventually developed severe learning disabilities."[18]

Children in institutional settings lack parental love, which is the kind of love that involves valuing the child for the child's sake and seeking closeness and intimacy with the child. All this and more are directed toward the well-being of the child. Children who lack parental love suffer profound harm as a result. Love is integral to trust; love promotes positive self-conception; love helps one know how to love others; love encourages development. Conversely, a lack of parental love promotes psychosocial dwarfism, emotional

---

16. S. Matthew Liao, *The Right to be Loved* (New York: Oxford University Press, 2015); and S. Matthew Liao, "The Right of Children to Be Loved," *Journal of Political Philosophy* 14.4 (November 2006): 420–440, doi: 10.1111/j.1467-9760.2006.00262.x.
17. Liao, "Right of Children to Be Loved," 424.
18. Liao, "Right of Children to Be Loved," 423.

trauma, cognitive delay, and so on.[19] Since being loved by a parent is integral to human flourishing, children have a compelling interest in parental love just as much as they have compelling interests in food, shelter, and water. Because rights protect our basic interests, and because of the role of parental love in the child's well-being, children have a right to parental love.

Liao's position has clear implications for children in foster care: everyone has a moral duty to promote parental love, and since children in the foster care system lack parental love, those who are able to adopt and provide parental love should do so. Liao concludes that "all able human beings in appropriate circumstances have a duty to promote every child's being loved."[20] Biological parents incur the primary duty to provide parental love to their children, but the right to parental love is not tethered to biological parents: if biological parents die, a child still has a right to parental love. Still, though, it is ordinarily the case that biological parents have the primary duty or obligation to love their children, while everyone else has associate duties to help the parents achieve their duty. When biological parents are missing, everyone else now has a primary duty, or obligation, to give the child parental love: "Someone else has the duty to step in and become the primary dutybearer" for parentless children.[21] Consequently, individuals who are able to offer parental love to children have an obligation to adopt children who lack parental love. Not to adopt a child when one is able and ready to become a parent is to violate that child's right to parental love.

Considerations in Favor of Traditional Adoption

All agree that adoption is morally permissible, and all agree that it is praiseworthy. Catholic teaching affirms adoption to be good, praiseworthy, and in no way inferior to biological procreation. John Paul II, for example, writes that the adoptive parent-child relationship "is in no way inferior to one based on a biological connection."[22] The arguments offered in the preceding sections, however, seek to show more than that: adoption is morally preferable, if not obligatory. Each of the arguments is subject to criticism,

---

19. For a comprehensive defense, see Laio, *Right to be Loved*, chap. 3.
20. Laio, "Right of Children to Be Loved," 431.
21. Laio, *Right to Be Loved*, 190.
22. John Paul II, Address to the Meeting of the Adoptive Families, n. 4.

and there are other arguments not explored here. Importantly for purposes of this chapter, many of the arguments of the preceding sections extend to embryo adoption. All children, embryonic and non-embryonic, are entitled to parental love and rescue when abandoned. Embryo adoption, therefore, would seem to be not only morally permissible but even obligatory, inasmuch as it is a form of adoption.

But the case in favor of embryonic adoption is not as compelling as I have made it out to be. There are clear differences between traditional adoption and embryonic adoption—differences that may undermine the extension of pro-adoption arguments to embryonic adoption. For example, traditional adoption does not require adoptive mothers to gestate and then birth a child. Traditional adoption does not require the adoptive mother to become impregnated by someone other than her husband. Traditional adoption does not involve the biological connection that results from gestation. Differences such as these complicate the extension of pro-adoption arguments to embryonic adoption. To see why, and for the sake of argument, let us consider a married couple who are motivated by love to adopt a child who is in need of a stable, loving home. Let us stipulate that the couple is not motivated by selfish reasons but is in a life stage in which it is appropriate for them to adopt. In a previous publication, I gave the example of Javier and Marissa, devout Catholics with biological children, who are moved by love to adopt another child as their own.[23] There are many children in need of adoption, so Javier and Marissa have a choice to make: adopt a child from the foster care system or adopt a frozen embryonic child. Let us assume there is no significant financial cost difference. In the following sections, I offer three considerations in favor of adopting a child from the foster care system.

Moral Ambiguity

The first consideration for adopting a child from the foster care system appeals to precaution in response to Javier and Marissa's moral uncertainty about the practice of embryonic adoption. Some Catholic scholars argue that participating in embryo adoption is illicit, for embryo adoption

---

23. Christopher Bobier, "A Practical Problem for Proponents of Heterologous Embryo Transfer," *National Catholic Bioethics Quarterly* 22.3 (Autumn 2022): 455–462, doi: 10.5840/ncbq202222342.

requires that the woman participate in in vitro fertilization, which undermines the rights of spouses and betrays the rights of children. The extended inseparability argument posits that we cannot meaningfully distinguish procreation from gestation and birth, and procreative parenting should occur only through marital intercourse. Rev. Tadeusz Pacholczyk, among others, argues that embryonic adoption is intrinsically evil, as it is "an instrumentalization and misuse of goods proper to procreation and marriage," because it makes the woman pregnant apart from her spouse.[24] Support for this is drawn from the *Catechism of the Catholic Church*, which states, "Techniques that entail the dissociation of husband and wife, by the intrusion of a person other than the couple (donation of sperm or ovum, surrogate uterus), are gravely immoral. These techniques (heterologous artificial insemination and fertilization) infringe the child's right to be born of a father and mother known to him and bound to each other by marriage."[25] Embryo adoption partially uses the woman's body as a gestational surrogate, unlike conventional forms of adoption, which is perhaps why the Congregation for the Doctrine of the Faith's *Dignitas personae* states that abandoned embryos "represent a *situation of injustice which in fact cannot be resolved.*"[26]

Other scholars defend the practice as morally licit, even praiseworthy. Christopher Reilly, for example, argues that there is nothing wrong with "defending and caring for" a vulnerable person in need of saving, especially

---

24. Tadeusz Pacholczyk, "On the Moral Objectionability of Human Embryo Adoption," in *The Ethics of Embryo Adoption and the Catholic Tradition: Moral Arguments, Economic Reality and Social Analysis*, ed. Sarah-Vaughn Brakman and Darlene Fozard Weaver (New York: Springer 2007), 80. See also Nicanor Austriaco, "Embryo Adoption and the Extended Inseparability Argument," *National Catholic Bioethics Quarterly* 21.1 (Spring 2021): 29–35, doi: 10.5840/ncbq20212114; and Christopher Oleson, "The Nuptial Womb: On the Moral Significance of Being with Child," in *Human Embryo Adoption: Biotechnology, Marriage and the Right to Life*, ed. Thomas V. Berg and Edward J. Furton (Philadelphia: National Catholic Bioethics Center, 2006), 169–172.
25. *Catechism of the Catholic Church*, 2nd ed. (Washington, DC: US Conference of Catholic Bishops / Libreria Editrice Vaticana, 2018 update), n. 2376. All subsequent citations appear in the text.
26. Congregation for the Doctrine of the Faith (CDF), *Dignitas personae* (December 12, 2008), n. 19, emphasis original.

a person who is subject to harm and injustice. He argues that the evils of in vitro fertilization do not apply to embryonic transfer for the sake of adoption, for embryonic transfer "is not in itself a conjugal act or a form of procreation, insemination, or impregnation."[27] Rob Lovering, likewise, argues that since death is a very bad harm and it is in our power to prevent such significant harm, we have a moral duty to prevent embryonic death.[28] Support for this position can be drawn from the *Catechism*'s statements that human life "must be respected and protected absolutely from the moment of conception," and "the embryo must be defended in its integrity, cared for, and healed, as far as possible, like any other human being." To protect another human person involves protecting that person from death when one is able to do so, for the moral law prohibits "refusing assistance to a person in danger" (nn. 2265, 2270, 2274). Another line of argument posits that parenting is a moral commitment, not so much a biological category, as evidenced by adoptive parents' being parents. John Paul II writes that adoptive parents are "truly parents" and that there is a form of procreation "which occurs through acceptance, concern and devotion."[29]

For those like Javier and Marissa, the disagreement among scholars can be unsettling, but practical advice can be given in the form of a precautionary argument. If embryonic adoption is morally problematic, then Javier and Marissa commit a morally illicit act by adopting an embryonic child. Embryonic adoption is, therefore, morally risky, and for this reason, some scholars have advised a cautious approach. Michel Accad writes that "unless the Church explicitly indicates otherwise, it would be prudent to refrain from" embryonic adoption.[30] Support for a practically cautious approach can be drawn from the literature on what the rational response for a nonexpert should be after learning of entrenched disagreement among

---

27. Christopher M. Reilly, "Rescuing the Good Samaritan in Embryo Adoption and Beyond," *National Catholic Bioethics Quarterly* 20.3 (Autumn 2020): 491, 493, doi: 10.5840/ncbq202020345.
28. Rob Lovering, "A Moral Argument for Frozen Human Embryo Adoption," *Bioethics* 34.3 (March 2020): 242–251, doi: 10.1111/bioe.12671.
29. John Paul II, Address to the Meeting of the Adoptive Families, n. 4.
30. Michel Accad, "Heterologous Embryo Transfer: Magisterial Answers and Metaphysical Questions," *Linacre Quarterly* 81.1 (February 2014): 44, doi: 10.1179/2050854913Y.0000000016.

thoughtful, equally informed experts. Jonathan Matheson explains that "once we are aware of the widespread disagreement among the experts on moral matters, we should be skeptical about the relevant moral propositions as well."[31] Nonexperts who are aware of entrenched expert disagreement should not hold a position with confidence, especially if the disagreement is about the moral wrongness of an action, and practically speaking, it is better to err on the side of caution and refrain from performing a morally risky action. This is especially the case if the alternative course of action is agreed to be morally permissible or praiseworthy. As noted already, everyone agrees that it is morally permissible, even praiseworthy, to adopt a child from the foster care system. There is no concern that traditional adoption is morally illicit. In light of both the disagreement and uncertainty surrounding the moral permissibility of embryonic adoption and the moral praiseworthiness of traditional adoption, the best course of action for would-be adoptive parents is to adopt a child from the foster care system.

Harm Imprint

The preceding argument is conditional, relying as it does on our current uncertainty, and can be resolved by a clear resolution by the Church. The next two arguments seek to show that, even if the Catholic Church clarifies embryonic adoption to be licit, Javier and Marissa should still pursue traditional adoption. I will first argue that embryonic adoption contributes significant harm to others, because it increases carbon emissions and overconsumption of natural resources, whereas traditional adoption does not. Underlying this argument is the observation that adding more people, especially people with high carbon footprints, via gestation and birth contributes to environmental degradation and climate change, which in turn contributes to harm suffered by others: "Average patterns of consumption in wealthy nations," Sam Shpall writes, "seem unfair by the standards of global and historical justice; and, independently of this, such consumption patterns cause harm" to future people.[32]

---

31. Jonathan Matheson, "Moral Caution and the Epistemology of Disagreement," *Journal of Social Philosophy* 47.2 (Summer 2016): 125–126, doi: 10.1111/josp.12145.
32. Sam Shpall, "Parental Love and Procreation," *Philosophical Quarterly* 73.1 (January 2023): 206, doi: 10.1093/pq/pqac017.

Part 2: Objections to Embryo Adoption

In his encyclical letter *Laudato si'*, Pope Francis highlights how excessive consumerism and climate change are fundamentally issues of social justice, because "the earth is essentially a shared inheritance." He explains, "Intergenerational solidarity is not optional, but rather a basic question of justice, since the world we have received also belongs to those who will follow us"; "Furthermore, our inability to think seriously about future generations is linked to our inability to broaden the scope of our present interests and to give consideration to those who remain excluded from development."[33] Evidence is debatable, but according to John Nolt, one individual from a wealthy country such as the United States of America produces emissions sufficient to harm one to two future people.[34] Devout Catholics such as Javier and Marissa ought to be attentive to the common good and social justice, both present and future. Accordingly, they may observe that embryonic adoption involves bringing a person into the world who will consume and emit a lot. Traditional adoption, by contrast, involves a postnatal child who already has an existing carbon footprint.

The Harmfulness of Embryonic Death

At this juncture, it may be replied that there is compelling reason to pursue embryonic adoption. If Javier and Marissa do not pursue embryonic adoption, the child they would have otherwise adopted will probably die. On the other hand, if Javier and Marissa do not pursue traditional adoption, the child they would have otherwise adopted will not die. Thus, it might be argued, the decision is clear: all things considered, embryonic adoption offers a greater good than traditional adoption on the grounds that death is a great harm. Even if embryonic adoption is illicit and promises greater environmental harm, the wrongness of death is so significant that it trumps these other considerations.

This argument gets its strength from the claim that death is a great harm for a person. In his argument for embryo adoption, Lovering sets out as a premise the claim that the death of a frozen embryo "is a very

---

33. Francis, *Laudato si'* (May 24, 2015), nn. 93, 159, 162.
34. John Nolt, "How Harmful Are the Average American's Greenhouse Gas Emissions?," *Ethics, Policy and the Environment* 14.1 (May 2011): 3–10, doi: 10.1080/21550085.2011.561584.

bad thing."[35] It is interesting that he does not seek to defend this claim; instead, he takes it for granted that death is a great harm for a person. This idea rings true: all people have a right to life, that fundamental good that makes possible all other goods that this life has to offer. A prevailing view in the anti-abortion literature is that death harms a person by depriving him or her of a valuable future. Don Marquis, for instance, argues that it is typically seriously wrong to kill a mature human being, because death "deprives us not only of what we value now and would have, given our current predilections, valued later, but also of what we would have come to value."[36] Alexander Pruss more recently identifies the harm of death as a deprivation: "What would make killing me now wrong is the harm it would do to me: it would deprive me, who am juridically innocent, of life, indeed of the rest of my life."[37] The deprivation view makes sense of the strong intuition that it is, all things considered, worse for someone to die young rather than old. Death harms embryonic children by depriving them of the rest of their lives, and this is a significant harm.

I want to resist the claim that death is such a great harm, at least for embryonic children. Because this is a not a popular position, allow me to explain my reasoning with three propositions. First, Christians do not believe that death is the end of the person altogether. A central tenet of Christian teaching is that we live in the hope of an afterlife in heaven, and death is the end of our earthly life but not the end of our life simpliciter. We live on, by God's grace and power, after the death of our earthly bodies. Moreover, life after death promises complete happiness for those who love God. St. Thomas Aquinas, following St. Augustine of Hippo and others, posits that complete human happiness cannot be found in anything created. Rather, complete human happiness can be found only in him who can fully satisfy our infinite desires: "God, Who alone by His infinite goodness, can

---

35. Lovering, "Moral Argument for Frozen Human Embryo Adoption," 244.
36. Don Marquis, "Why Abortion Is Immoral," *Journal of Philosophy* 86.4 (April 1989): 190, doi: 10.2307/2026961.
37. Alexander R. Pruss, "I Was Once a Fetus: That Is Why Abortion Is Wrong," in *Persons, Moral Worth, and Embryos: A Critical Analysis of Pro-Choice Arguments*, ed. Stephen Napier (New York: Springer, 2011), 30.

perfectly satisfy man's will."[38] Because we can enter God's presence only after the death of our body, we can attain complete happiness only after death. For this reason, Christians live in the hope of an afterlife. The *Catechism* states that Jesus "has transformed the curse of death into a blessing," and "death has a positive meaning" for those who enjoy God's grace and are in communion with him (nn. 1009, 1010). Indeed, a Christian can even come to desire death, as St. Paul did (Phil. 1:23–24), precisely because death is necessary to reach heaven, that perfect life in communion of love with the Trinity and the blessed. Heaven, not this life, is our ultimate end and fulfillment.

The second proposition is that our life here and now is ordinarily integral to attaining perfect happiness in the life to come. This side of eternity presents us with the wonderful yet mysterious opportunity to either accept or reject God's love and grace. Through proper development in a moral and faithful community, along with divinely infused grace and gifts, individuals grow in relationship with God and others: they grow in theological, moral, and intellectual virtue and in exercise of the gifts of the Spirit as they use their grace-infused free will properly. Along the way, of course, this life offers many opportunities for pleasure (e.g., marital intercourse, food, friendship) as well as a kind of earthly happiness. For example, virtuous activity is intrinsically enjoyable, while growing in relationship with God in this life enables a certain foretaste of perfect happiness; but perfect happiness remains unattainable this side of eternity, and all of the goods in this life should be ordered toward our ultimate good: relationship with God. The pleasures of this life pale in comparison to perfect happiness, which is part of the reason that Jesus exhorts the disciples to pursue treasures of the Kingdom of God (Matt. 6:33). Everything we do and enjoy should be properly ordered toward God. Death ends a person's opportunity to accept or reject God, and as the *Catechism* teaches, each "receives his eternal retribution in his immortal soul at the very moment of his death" (n. 1022). It is for this reason that St. Therese of Lisieux can write on her deathbed, "I am not dying. I am entering life."[39]

---

38. Thomas Aquinas, *Summa theologiae*, trans. Fathers of the English Dominican Province (Benziger, 1947; Thomistic Institute, 2017), I-II.3.1 corpus, https://aquinas101.thomisticinstitute.org/st-iaiiae-q-3#FSQ3OUTP1.
39. James McTavish, "Suffering, Death, and Eternal Life," *Linacre Quarterly* 83.2 (May 2016): 139, doi: 10.1080/00243639.2016.1166338.

With this in mind, let us revisit the harmfulness of embryonic death and investigate the fate of deceased embryonic children. The third proposition I wish to defend is that there is strong reason to hope that terminated embryonic children enjoy complete happiness with God. The *Catechism* is clear that "God has bound salvation to the sacrament of Baptism, but he himself is not bound by his sacraments" (n. 1257), meaning that God can save an individual apart from Baptism and that unbaptized children who die are entrusted "to the mercy of God" (n. 1261), a trust that is grounded in hope that God desires all to be saved and that Jesus manifests tenderness and love to children. Addressing women who have had an abortion, John Paul II writes in *Evangelium vitae*, "To the same Father and his mercy you can with sure hope entrust your child."[40] The Feast of Holy Innocents, which is celebrated on December 28, honors the children who were slaughtered instead of Jesus Christ by Herod the Great. It is curious to note that the children are described as innocent and holy, innocent of personal sin and suffering a martyr's death. In *Instruction on Children's Baptism*, the Congregation for the Doctrine of Faith affirms that, "as for children who die without Baptism, the Church can only entrust them to God's mercy, as she does in the funeral rite provided for them."[41]

The clearest expression of the hope that unbaptized infants who die enjoy the beatific vision is provided by the International Theological Commission, which concludes that there are "strong grounds for hope that God will save infants" who die without having been baptized. The commission offers at least five considerations for this position. First, "the idea of Limbo, which the Church has used for many centuries to designate the destiny of infants who die without Baptism, has no clear foundation in revelation," and there is no mention of Limbo in the liturgy. Second, while Scripture is silent about the fate of unbaptized infants, it is clear that God wills the salvation of all people: the "universal salvific will of God through Jesus Christ ... is directed to all humans." Third, as noted above, the liturgy contains a feast of the Holy Innocents, who were martyred without having

---

40. John Paul II, *Evangelium vitae* (March 15, 1995), n. 99.
41. CDF, *Pastoralis actio* (October 20, 1980), n. 13.

received Baptism.[42] Fourth, God does not demand the impossible from us, but it is impossible for unbaptized infants to pursue Baptism on their own. Finally, God can give the grace of Baptism without the sacrament of Baptism being conferred. His power is not "restricted to the sacraments." For example, it is possible "that God simply acts to give the gift of salvation to unbaptized infants by analogy with the gift of salvation given sacramentally to baptized infants."[43]

Let us take stock of the argument thus far: (1) Perfect union with God is our ultimate end, and it requires the death of the body as a result of the curse of sin. (2) This life offers many goods but not complete happiness, and all the goods of this life should be ordered to our ultimate end. (3) An embryonic child that dies, we confidently hope, enjoys the love of God.

What, then, is the harm of death for an embryonic child? The embryonic child will not suffer any pain involved in dying, but she will also not enjoy future experiences that this side of eternity promises, and this is a tragedy. Although the child loses out on the many opportunities and experiences on this side of eternity, we confidently hope she attains her ultimate end. If, as Christians maintain, the goods of this life pale in comparison with perfect union with God, then a deceased embryonic child who subsequently enjoys perfect union with God is not significantly harmed by losing out on goods that are trivial by comparison. The harm of death is not so significant in light of the perfect union of God that is hoped for. Death has lost its sting, after all, for those whom we confidently hope enjoy God after death.

That embryonic death is not a significant harm does not license the killing of embryonic children. It is not in our power to take a life that God has created. But when it comes to deciding who to adopt, the realization that embryonic death is not a significant harm strengthens the case for would-be adoptive parents to pursue traditional adoption. The foster child, if not adopted by Javier and Marissa, may remain in the foster system for a time,

---

42. It might be pointed out that the Holy Innocents received a Baptism of blood and, therefore, are a weak analogy to cryopreserved embryos who die. This observation is well taken, although the International Theological Commission notes that such a Baptism is not without "difficulties" (*The Hope of Salvation for Infants Who Die without Being Baptized* [January 19, 2007], n. 29).
43. International Theological Commission, *Infants Who Die without Being Baptized*, nn. 3, 5, 53, 82, 87, 103.

and then, if the child is lucky, she will be adopted by another family. There are many unknowns, however. Hopefully, the adoptive family will provide her a loving, stable home, but she may be adopted into an abusive or otherwise unideal home setting.[44] Hopefully, she will be able to process adoption and foster care traumas in a healthy manner, but this may not happen, and she may develop post-traumatic stress disorder. While she probably will not die, she may not be adopted by a Christian family and baptized into the faith. She may be adopted by avowed atheists or pagans who teach her to deny the salvific work of Jesus Christ. While not discounting divine providence, parental religious affiliation has a profound effect on child religiosity.

This is not presumptuous, but grounded in the received wisdom that parents have a significant role in the religious formation of their children. A 2020 Pew Research Center study found that "most U.S. teens (ages 13 to 17) share the religious affiliation of their parents or legal guardians" and that "U.S. teens attend religious services about as often as their parents do."[45] By contrast, the embryonic child, if not adopted by Javier and Marissa, may remain frozen for a time before being killed. This is the most probable outcome, given a lack of embryonic adoption and the standard practice of discarding embryos. If this is the case, the embryonic child will not suffer, but she will also not enjoy future experiences that this side of eternity promises. This is a tragedy. However, we have strong reason to hope that the child will enjoy God's presence.

The trade-off, then, is between a completely painless, unaware death followed by confidently hoped-for eternal happiness and a life lived with an uncertain eternal outcome and uncertain traumas. The choice to adopt

---

44. Ashley L. Landers et al., "Abuse after Abuse: The Recurrent Maltreatment of American Indian Children in Foster Care and Adoption," *Child Abuse and Neglect* 111 (January 2021), 104805, doi: 10.1016/j.chiabu.2020.104805. See also Marinus H. van Ijzendoorn et al., "Elevated Risk of Child Maltreatment in Families with Stepparents but Not with Adoptive Parents," *Child Maltreatment* 14.4 (November 2009): 375, doi:10.1177/1077559509342125.
45. Elizabeth Podrebarac Sciupac et al., "U.S. Teens Take after Their Parents Religiously, Attend Services Together and Enjoy Family Rituals," Pew Research Center, September 10, 2020, https://www.pewresearch.org/religion/2020/09/10/u-s-teens-take-after-their-parents-religiously-attend-services-together-and-enjoy-family-rituals/.

is ideally motivated by love, with the adopted child's physical, emotional, and spiritual well-being in mind. Recognizing that suffering and death are not harms to be avoided at all cost—but hell is—there is, therefore, good reason for Javier and Marissa to adopt from foster care in the hopes of providing that child a life that provides for her physical, emotional, and spiritual well-being.[46]

Traditional Adoption First

The case for adoption is compelling. Considerations of sacrificial love, helping those in need, and fulfilling obligations of environmental justice and parental love—individually and collectively—support the pursuit of adoption. While many of these considerations support embryonic adoption as well, I have argued that other considerations practically favor traditional adoption. In other words, would-be adoptive parents have good reason to favor traditional adoption, even if embryo adoption is morally licit.

It is important to close by mentioning that critics of embryonic adoption do not consider this to be a conclusion worth celebrating. Children in the foster care system are subject to significant harms, while embryonic children are subject to immense injustice. Proponents of the argument sketched in this chapter agree that the situation is a moral tragedy, a situation in which would-be adoptive parents have to make a morally difficult, if not objectionable, decision. There are good concerns on both sides of the debate, precisely because the situation is tragic. Defenders and critics can agree on this much: we should work together to ensure the justice and well-being of all children.

---

46. It might be argued that human beings are morally obligated to use ordinary means to preserve life and to use their lives here on earth as stewards. This arguably applies to embryos (as human persons), and gestation seems to represent an ordinary (or common) means of preserving life for humans at that developmental stage. This consideration can be doubted, for there is nothing ordinary about in vitro fertilization involved in embryonic adoption.

6

Embryo Adoption and Becoming a Parent
Charles Robertson

A recurring theme in the embryo adoption-rescue debate is the question of the applicability of the principle, enunciated by the Congregation for the Doctrine of the Faith in *Donum vitae*, that spouses ought to become parents only through each other. In that document, the CDF insists that procreation must be the fruit of marriage, from the standpoints of both the moral obligation of the spouses and the rights of the child:

> For human procreation is entirely distinguished from others by its proper notes on account of the dignity both of the parents and the children: for the procreation of a new person, in which a man and his wife associate their work with the power of the Creator, ought to be at the same time the fruit and the sign of the mutual gift of the spouses, likewise of their love and fidelity. *But the fidelity of the spouses, in the unity of matrimony, bears with it the mutual observance towards the rights of each, such that one becomes a father or a mother only through the other.* The child has the right that it be conceived, contained in the womb, born and educated in matrimony: it can only know its identity, with certain and public reason, by referring to its parents and so proceed to its formation to maturity as a man.[1]

---

1. Congregation for the Doctrine of the Faith (CDF), *Donum vitae* (February 22, 1987), II.A.1, emphasis original. All translations are by the author.

Part 2: Objections to Embryo Adoption

Consequently, the CDF made the judgment that heterologous artificial fertilization and embryo transfer (ET) "clearly contradicts the unity of matrimony, the dignity of the spouses, the proper vocation of the parents as well as the right of the child with a view to which it should both be conceived and brought forth in marriage and through marriage," giving as its reason that "the bond which comes to be between the spouses gives to them the objective and inalienable exclusive right that each become a father and mother only through each other."[2]

In light of this principle that spouses have "the objective and inalienable exclusive right that each become a father and mother only through each other," many opponents of embryo adoption-rescue consider at least heterologous ET to be morally disordered on account of its making a woman to be a mother apart from her spouse. These argue in favor of some version of what Rev. Nicanor Austriaco calls the extended inseparability argument.[3] Advocates of embryo adoption agree with some of their opponents that ET makes a woman to be a mother, but they argue that, on the adoption model, this becoming a mother sufficiently respects the principle that spouses ought to become parents only through each other. In what follows, we will examine the arguments employing the premise that by means of embryo transfer, a woman becomes a mother. Then I will argue that ET does not in fact make a woman a mother, but this by no means entails that ET is morally licit. I conclude that a successful version of the extended inseparability argument is possible and outline the criteria that need to be met for its success.

---

2. CDF, *Donum vitae*, II.A.2.
3. See Nicanor Austriaco, "Embryo Adoption and the Extended Inseparability Argument," *National Catholic Bioethics Quarterly* 21.1 (Spring 2021): 29–35, doi: 10.5840/ncbq20212114. This argument also finds a foundation in the above text of *Donum vitae*, particularly in its assertion that "the child has the right that it be conceived, contained in the womb, born and educated in matrimony: it can only know its identity, with certain and public reason, by referring to its parents and so proceed to its formation to maturity as a man" (II.A.2).

Embryo Transfer Is Wrong Because It Makes a Woman to Be a Mother Apart from Her Spouse

Nicholas Tonti-Filippini argues that the fundamental aspect of ET that vitiates the project is the fact that the father is excluded from the whole process. In that connection, ET is seen as a violation of the marital bond, a kind of infidelity to the husband. This is because the woman who receives a child into her womb by that fact becomes a mother but not through her husband. This is contrary to the principled assertion of the CDF that a husband and wife should become a father and mother only through each other. The justification of the CDF's judgment is that the generative capacity of the spouses are to be ordered to each other. This capacity "includes or is at least so linked to her capacity to become pregnant and to bear a child in her womb, and is not merely her capacity to produce ova and to express her love in the conjugal act."[4] The right use of this capacity belongs exclusively to the marital union.

Consequently, the physician who impregnates a woman by means of ET does what only the husband has the moral right to do: "For a woman to request such assistance would be to will the clinician to perform an act of making her pregnant. That would seem to be an infidelity to her marriage—although I am a little uncomfortable with the language in that respect. 'Infidelity' has so many other connotations. By 'infidelity' I mean only that she is inviting the clinician to bring about pregnancy in her when she has already willed that power exclusively to her relationship with her husband and within their marriage." Moreover, to impregnate a woman by clinical means is to reduce her to being an object subject to undignified manipulations of her generative potential: "Non-conjugal impregnation would appear to be a violation of her bodily integrity, a use of her as an object, because it lacks the meaning and character of marriage that dignifies being impregnated, because the latter happens in marriage as part of the

---

4. Nicholas Tonti-Filippini, "The Embryo Rescue Debate: Impregnating Women, Ectogenesis, and Restoration from Suspended Animation," in *Human Embryo Adoption: Biotechnology, Marriage, and the Right to Life*, ed. Thomas V. Berg and Edward J. Furton (Philadelphia: National Catholic Bioethics Center, 2006), 91.

meaning of the expression of the conjugal act, which itself is the expression of the communion of persons."[5]

Christopher Oleson offers a version of the extended inseparability argument to establish that procreation includes conception, gestation, and birth. He accepts as an indemonstrable first principle *Donum vitae*'s assertion that spouses "have the exclusive right to become father and mother solely through each other." Consequently, the proper evaluation of ET must be carried out by discovering what is essential to becoming a mother or father, and thus the question of its liceity hinges on whether becoming a mother encompasses conception, gestation, and birth or is limited to conception. Oleson argues that heterologous ET "intrudes into the unity of parenthood that is at the heart of the marriage covenant" by giving rise to a situation in which a woman becomes a mother without her husband, at the same time, becoming a father. Because the child conceived naturally is the fruit of their marriage union, it embodies the common good of the spouses and enables each "to see the other's fatherhood or motherhood as intrinsically linked to their own."[6] This connection is simply not present when a woman becomes a mother to a child that is not genetically related to her husband. A woman who chooses to become pregnant by ET chooses to become a mother "in a radically more intimate way than a woman legally adopting a born child does." By dint of becoming the gestational mother of the abandoned embryo, she actualizes "an essential element of natural motherhood" apart from her husband, which is contrary to that first, indemonstrable principle enunciated in *Donum vitae*.[7]

---

5. Tonti-Filippini, "Embryo Rescue Debate," 94, 105.
6. Cristopher Oleson, "The Nuptial Womb: On the Moral Significance of Being 'with Child,'" in Berg and Furton, *Human Embryo Adoption*, 174, 175. This point implicitly opens the door to homologous ET, though Oleson does not explicitly make that connection. Since the embryo is genetically related to both mother and father in the case of homologous transfer, the implantation of the embryo does not take place apart from the husband, and so they can still see their motherhood and fatherhood as intrinsically linked.
7. Oleson, "Nuptial Womb," 181, 182.

Two Objections: Procreation as Terminating at Conception and the Moral Equivalence of Natural and Adoptive Parenthood

E. Christian Brugger, in responding to Tonti-Filippini's arguments, includes Oleson's position within the scope of his objections. Recognizing that gestational motherhood is somehow special, Brugger does not think that it has the moral significance attributed to it by Tonti-Filippini and Oleson. Brugger summarizes the argument as follows: "Becoming pregnant means becoming a gestational mother; becoming a gestational mother by means other than one's husband through marital intercourse is always wrong; a woman who becomes pregnant through HET [heterologous ET] becomes a gestational mother by means other than by her husband through marital intercourse; therefore, HET is always wrong (i.e., intrinsically evil)."[8] He then points out that the section of *Donum vitae* containing the principle that a husband and wife should become a mother and father only through each other is dealing with procreation, and so this principle should be understood within that context. In other words, a husband and wife should become a mother and father through each other only when they procreate, which Brugger understands as the process leading up to and including the fertilization of the ovum. Hence, *Donum vitae* should not be seen as condemning ET in itself.

Moreover, Brugger identifies a certain incongruity in the positions of Tonti-Filippini and Oleson vis-à-vis traditional adoption. Tonti-Filippini and Oleson hold that a woman should not become a mother through ET, but they agree that it is acceptable for her to adopt a baby that has already been born. But if we are to take that principle of *Donum vitae* at face value, should we not also condemn traditional adoption? After all, traditional adoption is a case of a husband and wife becoming a father and mother but not through each other. Tonti-Filippini and Oleson consider there to be a vast difference between becoming a gestational mother and becoming an adoptive mother, but, asks Brugger, are not the moral duties of prenatal adoptive parents and postnatal adoptive parents the same? Even if there is a biological and psychological difference between the two ways of becoming

---

8. E. Christian Brugger, "A Defense by Analogy of Heterologous Embryo Transfer," in Berg and Furton, *Human Embryo Adoption*, 203.

a mother, there is little reason to suppose that the moral bonds between mother and child differ essentially. Further, the moral bond between an adoptive parent and her adopted child is often far greater than the bond that exists between that child and his natural parents. In fine, Tonti-Filippini and Oleson offer "no practical principles explaining why becoming an adoptive mother (of a gestated child, not an embryo) outside the marital act—in every sense a *mother* except biologically and gestationally—is morally legitimate while becoming a gestational mother is not, except to say 'an adoptive parent is not a parent in the same sense that a child's natural parents are parents.'"[9]

Embryo Adoption Makes Spouses Parents through Each Other

Those who argue in favor of embryo adoption press that point further and even go so far as to maintain that there is no significant sense in which natural and adoptive parents differ. The moral theologians in this group maintain that ET is licit only when a married woman together with her spouse choose to adopt the embryo to be implanted and raise it as their own. In this way, they believe that they can maintain the principle that spouses can become parents only through each other, while providing concrete means whereby frozen embryos can enjoy a life befitting their human dignity. The advocates of embryo adoption consider homologous ET to be morally licit and perhaps even obligatory but recognize that, practically speaking, many cryopreserved embryos will in fact be abandoned by those who ordered their production; consequently, adoption is the next best available option to ensure the survival of these tiny human beings. Although these authors largely focus on arguments against those who think ET is always illicit, they are not devoid of positive argumentation buttressing the claim that embryo adoption is morally licit. These positive arguments seek to elaborate on the meaning of becoming a mother or a father, and they emphasize that adoption corresponds to that meaning. In examining these contributions, we will privilege the articles of the authors who present the most robust accounts of adoption as a means of becoming a parent.

---

9. Brugger, "Defense by Analogy of Heterologous Embryo Transfer," 207, emphasis original.

John Berkman frames his treatment of embryo adoption with reference to the practice of virtuous parenthood. He chooses this frame of reference, because he considers that "the most adequate description of the moral issue is that of the proper response to an orphan." The principle that governs our response to orphans is a commitment to *parent*, which is "a moral practice fundamental to the human good of children and the common good of our society."[10] Only by understanding this practice of responsible Christian parenthood can we properly evaluate what our response to these orphaned embryos can and should be. Although parenthood does admit of a biological description, it is much more important to see parenting as a moral commitment. This is evidenced by the way the state may intervene to find suitable adoptive parents or guardians for the good of the child.

Moreover, the Church herself "employs familial language to point to a set of relationships even more fundamentally important than those in earthly families, when it points, for example, to the new identity given to a Christian at baptism." Even legal adoption gives rise to a new identity for adopted children, who will consider their adoptive parents simply parents, since "their parents have lived out the long-term commitment to parent them." In moral terms, then, what makes one a parent "is the *permanent* commitment to unconditionally love one's child."[11] Permanent commitment is fundamental to the practice of parenting, and the proposal to give up the neonate after birth directly contradicts the permanence of that commitment.[12]

Sarah-Vaughan Brakman frames her approach to embryo adoption by viewing adoption from the standpoint of responsible stewardship. She notes that those who advocate for embryo adoption share two important principles with those who reject it, namely, (1) that adopting an embryo makes a woman its mother, and (2) *Donum vitae*'s principle that only spouses have the mutual right to become mother and father through each other. The point on which disagreement with the opponents of embryo adoption arises is with respect to the claim that it is only by means of sexual intercourse that couples can exercise this right. After all, becoming a mother can occur by

---

10. John Berkman, "Virtuous Parenting and Orphaned Embryos," in Berg and Furton, *Human Embryo Adoption*, 13, 15.
11. Berkman, "Virtuous Parenting," 22–23, 24, emphasis original.
12. Berkman, "Virtuous Parenting," 28.

means of adoption, and the Church has historically approved and encouraged the practice of adoption. Now, the choice to become a mother includes a permanent commitment to the child, so if a woman chooses to become a mother by means of ET, she must also have a permanent commitment to that child.

Brakman is astonished that those who oppose embryo adoption object that "adoptive motherhood offers a less genuine form of parenthood," and she thus argues that "post-natal adoption of abandoned children is a noble gesture that causes no problem to conjugal unity because it does not disturb the vocational significance of true (i.e. embodied) motherhood."[13] According to Brakman, the view that "adoptive motherhood offers a less genuine form of parenthood" is problematic, because no Church teaching claims that adoptive parenthood is less categorical or real than natural parenthood. In fact, the way Pope St. John Paul II speaks of adoptive parenthood in his encyclical *Evangelium vitae* leads us to see that adoptive couples are just as "truly parents" as those whose children are the fruit of intercourse.[14] Moreover, the late Pontiff even speaks of a type of procreation exercised by adoptive parents: "There is a form of 'procreation' which occurs through acceptance, concern and devotion. The resulting relationship is so intimate and enduring that it is in no way inferior to one based on a biological connection."[15]

Like Berkman and Brakman, John Grabowski and Christopher Gross insist that parenting is more fundamentally a moral practice than a natural category, and so by adoption, spouses truly become parents: "Surely couples who adopt children whom they did not conceive through a conjugal act and whom the women did not carry through pregnancy become fathers and mothers to these children. And if this is true of infants and adolescents, why

---

13. Sarah-Vaughan Brakman, "Real Mothers and Good Stewards: The Ethics of Embryo Adoption," in *The Ethics of Embryo Adoption and the Catholic Tradition: Moral Arguments, Economic Reality, and Social Analysis*, ed. Sarah-Vaughan Brakman and Darlene Fozard Weaver (New York: Springer, 2007), 122.
14. John Paul II, *Evangelium vitae* (March 25, 1995), n. 93.
15. John Paul II, Address to the Meeting of the Adoptive Families Organized by the Missionaries of Charity (September 5, 2000), n. 4, cited in Brakman, "Real Mothers," 123.

is it not also true of embryos 'who have the dignity of persons' albeit at an earlier stage of development?"[16]

Those who distinguish between adoptive and biological parents, they say, "do so apart from any theology or definition of parenthood. If, as Germain Grisez suggests, parenthood is 'far more a moral than a biological relationship' and if 'its essence is not so much in begetting and giving birth as in readiness to accept the gift of life, commitment to nurture it, and a faithful fulfillment of that commitment through many years,' then any attempt to draw a distinction between adoptive and biological parents who care for their children is not only invalid but also misleading."[17] Grabowski and Gross emphasize the covenantal nature of adoption, indicating that the "relationships that are formed through adoption are equal to or transcend biological ties," and so "once HET is considered in light of the Christian tradition's theology of adoption, the biological aspects of the procedure become much less relevant, and it becomes clear that embryo adoption is at least potentially a morally licit and even praiseworthy practice—and not merely in the intentions of those who engage in it."[18]

Christopher Tollefsen, by considering the nature of divine adoption and drawing out parallels between it and human adoption, seeks to discover what adoption should be and how it ontologically changes the adoptive parents. Understanding divine adoption will help us to know what human adoption can and should be. The first parallel he considers is the gratuity of divine adoption as a model for human adoption. Although some people need to adopt in order to have children, adoption is perhaps better understood as arising not so much from need, that is, a lack on the part of the adoptive couple, as from an abundance of love the couple wishes to share with a child who is himself in need. This approach to human adoption brings it more in line with divine adoption and serves to prevent the adoptive couple from seeing the child as a remedy for a feeling of being

---

16. John S. Grabowski and Christopher Gross, "*Dignitas Personae* and the Adoption of Frozen Embryos: A New Chill Factor?," *National Catholic Bioethics Quarterly* 10.2 (Summer 2010): 317, doi: 10.5840/ncbq201010255.
17. Grabowski and Gross, "Adoption of Frozen Embryos," 317–318, citing Germain Grisez, *The Way of the Lord Jesus*, vol. 2, *Living a Christian Life* (Chicago: Franciscan Press, 1997), 689.
18. Grabowski and Gross, "Adoption of Frozen Embryos," 321.

incomplete or unfulfilled in their married life: "By adopting as an expression and outpouring of their mutual love, they mirror God more adequately than if they adopted to complete or to satisfy themselves."[19]

A second parallel is in the notion of responding to the call of God. When He calls us to be a part of his family, we must respond and accept or reject that gift. God's patience with us in our struggles to say yes to him should be the model for adoptive parents as they wait for their child's "reciprocal act of the will, required of the adoptee at some point, in order for him or her to genuinely, rather than simply legally and conventionally, become a part of their adoptive family."[20] A third parallel is that adopted children take on a second identity, the new identity of the adoptive family. In giving us a new identity as his children, God does not destroy our human identities; so also, an adoptee retains the biological and perhaps even cultural identity of his birth parents even as he becomes a member of another family. The adoptive parents, then, together with their child, "must work to maintain both in an 'absurd' unity." The fourth and final parallel is that both divine adoption and human adoption are a kind of rescue; God rescues us "from our profound alienation from Him," while human adoptive parents rescue a child from "the condition of being without a human family."[21]

Tollefsen considers the foregoing considerations to imply that "embryo adoption would need to be a practice pursued by married couples as an expression and realization of their marital love, in which the offer of a family is freely made to the child, to be accepted or rejected, and in which not only does the child enter into the parental family unity, but the parents too take on a share of the child's previous familial reality." In this way, embryo adoption can be seen to be in harmony with marital unity and would not be "an effort to *make* a child be one's own, or to *make* oneself, unilaterally or with another, to be a parent."[22] Also, embryo adoption should not be undertaken as a treatment for infertility, for that would make it not so much a sharing of the abundance of love as the fulfilling of a need. Therefore, the

---

19. Christopher Tollefsen, "Divine, Human, and Embryo Adoption: Some Criticisms of *Dignitas Personae*," *National Catholic Bioethics Quarterly* 10.1 (Spring 2010): 80, doi: 10.5840/ncbq201010173.
20. Tollefsen, "Divine, Human, and Embryo Adoption," 81.
21. Tollefsen, "Divine, Human, and Embryo Adoption," 82, 83.
22. Tollefsen, "Divine, Human, and Embryo Adoption," 84, emphasis original.

intention of the couple who chooses embryo adoption should be purified so that they may conform their adoption of a human child to the model of divine adoption.

In summary, Tollefsen directs us to consider divine adoption as the model that will answer the questions, "What, normatively, is [adoption] to be, and, when it is rightly pursued, what is the ontological relationship that thereby obtains between parents and children through adoption?"[23] He emphasizes the *gratuitous* nature of adoption undertaken as a *response to God's call*, which then changes the adoptee by giving him *two identities* and *rescuing* him from potential harm. In light of these considerations, he concludes that, if pursued with the correct motives, "embryo adoption would be, like both conventional adoption and procreation in the context of marital sexuality, normatively a matter of gift as expression and realization of marital love."[24]

The fundamental claims above are that parenting is more fundamentally a moral commitment than it is a natural category, and so adoptive parenthood is just as real a parenthood as natural parenthood. Further, there is no theological evidence that adoptive parenthood differs essentially from natural parenthood. Tollefsen and Brakman seek to fill in a purported theological lacuna by giving an account of how the practice of adoption should be modeled on divine adoption, pursued as the outpouring of spousal love in response to God's call that imparts on the adoptee a new identity and rescues him or her from orphanhood.

Embryo Transfer Does Not Make a Woman to Be a Mother

The claim that no theological evidence supports an essential distinction between natural and adoptive parenthood is manifestly false.[25] The Church has condemned the various forms of the doctrine that Christ is the Son of God by adoption and not by nature (advocated by Apollinaris, Theodotus of Byzantium, Paul of Samosata, Theodore of Mopsuestia, and others) as

---

23. Tollefsen, "Divine, Human, and Embryo Adoption," 78.
24. Tollefsen, "Divine, Human, and Embryo Adoption," 84.
25. This section is largely taken from my paper "A Thomistic Analysis of Embryo Adoption," *National Catholic Bioethics Quarterly* 14.4 (Winter 2014): 673–695, doi: 10.5840/ncbq201414470.

denials of Jesus's full divinity. The forceful condemnation of the version held by certain eighth-century theologians is quite instructive.[26] The basic conviction underlying that condemnation was that the proper term of natural filiation is the Person of the Word, and that if Jesus the man is the Son of God by adoption and not by nature, then He is not truly God. This suggests that the distinction between biological and adoptive parenthood, far from being invalid or misleading, is in fact fundamental for understanding not only the Incarnation but also, on the one hand, human paternity and maternity and, on the other hand, the revelation of God as Father, "of whom all paternity in heaven and earth is named" (Eph. 3:15 DRC).

I mentioned above that opponents of embryo adoption-rescue advance some version of the extended inseparability argument in order to show that ET is itself illicit. One version of that argument that will help introduce the analysis of the distinction between adoptive and biological parenthood is advanced by Rev. Tadeusz Pacholczyk, who suggests that to "understand the fissure in parenthood that embryo adoption effects, it may be helpful to dissociate motherhood into three categories: *genetic, gestational,* and *social* motherhood."[27] He exploits this division to show that motherhood, in its full sense, includes all three elements, whereas other ways of being a mother might not.

This approach, however, has certain problems. First, genetic, gestational, and social motherhood admit of various permutations, making the comparison between the various forms it can take overly burdensome. First, in normal motherhood and homologous in vitro fertilization (IVF) and ET, the three coincide, but in heterologous IVF and ET, it is also possible for all three to coincide, provided that the ovum used is that of the mother. Second, this division is not very helpful in determining the difference between social motherhood proceeding from natural motherhood and that proceeding from adoption. Third, genetic and gestational motherhood have more

---

26. See Heinrich Denzinger and Adolf Schönmetzer, eds., *Enchiridion symbolorum definitionum et declarationum de rebus fidei et morum*, 36th ed. (Barcelona: Herder, 1976), n. 611. "He (Jesus) manifested the paternal name when he made himself known to be the true, not the putative, the proper, not the adoptive, Son of the Father" (translation by the author).
27. Tadeusz Pacholczyk, "Some Moral Contraindications to Embryo Adoption," in Berg and Furton, *Human Embryo Adoption*, 46.

to do with some attribute of the child, namely, its material constitution and location, whereas social motherhood has more to do with the social relationship which obtains between mother and child. Hence, Pacholczyk's division does not adequately divide a generic notion of motherhood into its various species.

In order to have a true comparison between kinds of motherhood, we must divide the generic notion of motherhood, or rather, parenthood, into its various species. To make a proper division, the parts must be less universal, exhaustive, formally opposed one to another, and made on the same basis.[28] Now, since parenthood is effected by an activity on the part of the parent, the basis of the division should be the efficient cause of filiation, that is, that which makes a child to be one's own. In this way, human parenthood can be brought into direct comparison with God's fatherhood, and we will be able to highlight the similarities and differences between the two. This is in fact the way in which St. Thomas Aquinas proceeds in defining adoption and determining the differences between parenthood by adoption and natural parenthood.

In his *Commentary on the Sentences*, St. Thomas determines the essence of adoption, which is there defined as "the legitimate assumption of a person not of one's family as a son, grandson, or heir." In his defense of this definition, he distinguishes between filiation proceeding from nature, on the one hand, and from art, on the other hand: "I respond, it ought to be said that art imitates nature and supplies for a defect of nature in those things in which nature is defective; whence just as someone produces a son by natural generation, so also can someone, by positive law, which is the art of the just and good, assume someone as a son to the likeness of a natural son, and to supply for the defect of the aforesaid sons for which sake especially adoption was introduced."[29]

---

28. John Oesterle, *Logic: The Art of Defining and Reasoning*, 2nd ed. (Upper Saddle River, NJ: Prentice Hall, 1963), 49–53.
29. Thomas Aquinas, *Commentary on the "Sentences,"* lib. IV, dist. 42, q. 2, art. 1. Citations are from Thomas Aquinas, *Scriptum super "Sententiis,"* ed. Pierre Mandonnet and Maria Fabianus Moos (Paris: Lethielleux, 1929–1947); and Thomas Aquinas, *Commentum in quartum librum "Sententiarum" magistri Petri Lombardi* vol. 7/2 (Parma: Peter Fiaccadori, 1858), available as *Scritpum super "Sententiis,"* transcribed by Robert Busa and Enrique Alarcón, Corpus Thomisticum,

Part 2: Objections to Embryo Adoption

Hence, the first division of parenthood should be made on the basis of the agency of nature versus the agency of art. Nature is understood as an internal principle of motion and rest; hence, *natural generation* is the first category. In contrast, art is understood here as the principle governing things to be done according to positive law (governed by prudence); hence, *legal generation* is the second category. In comparing the two and clarifying the differences, St. Thomas focuses on the notion of generation as a kind of motion. Every motion has a mover and a moved. Although a motion is one in being, it is diverse in relation; it is *from* the mover but *in* the moved. Consequently, the motion of generation, although itself one, gives rise to the parent-child relation. The mover is the parent, the moved is the child: "Therefore, just as natural generation has a term to which, namely the form which is the end of generation, and a term from which, namely the contrary form, so also legal generation has a term to which, son or grandson, and a term from which, a person not of one's family."[30] Hence the *term from which*—the principles of nature on the one hand, an already constituted nature on the other—is the primary difference between natural generation and legal generation.

But there is a difference also in the *term to which*. In the case of natural generation, it is the form of a new human being. This new person, by nature, has a right to a share in his parents' goods. He has, then, the right to be nourished and educated by his parents and the right to be an heir to the family's material goods. The adopted child, on the other hand, already has the form aimed at by natural generation. The *term to which* of legal generation is a legal relation; by nature the adoptee does not have a natural right to be educated and nourished by the adoptive parents nor to be an heir to the family's material goods, but by the legal act of adoption, the child acquires the legal right to what belongs by nature to the child born by natural generation. Quite clearly, then, embryo adoption, even though it entails gestation on the part of the woman, must be placed in the category of legal generation, because it does not have a contrary nature as its *term from which*, and it has a legal relation as its *term to which*. Consequently, whether the adoption

---

Fundación Tomás de Aquino, 2019, lib. IV, dist. 23ff, https://www.corpus thomisticum.org/iopera.html. All translations are by the author.
30. Aquinas, *Commentary on the Sentences*, lib. IV, dist. 42, q. 2, art.1.

is effected before the child's birth or after, the adopted child is directed to the same end as the child who is generated by nature; namely, the child becomes an heir to the family's goods and shares in the society of the family.

In light of these considerations, we may address Tollefsen's treatment of divine adoption. It is clear that the inner life of the Trinity is analogous to natural generation. God the Father, in eternally begetting the Son, is conceived of as the subject of a real relation of paternity. (Of course, in St. Thomas's language, the Father simply is that relation.) As human parents, by their own activity, beget a child who shares their nature, so God, by his immanent activity, begets a Son who shares his nature. Legal adoption, on the other hand, is analogous to divine adoption. For God, in adopting us as his children, makes us heirs and shares with us the good of his being through the beatific vision. Now, as rational creatures, we can be considered the children of God in two ways: by virtue of creation and by virtue of grace. We are children by virtue of creation, because we are created in God's image, and children by grace by becoming heirs:

> It pertains to the essence of filiation that the son is produced in the likeness of the species of the generator himself. But man, insofar as he is produced in a sharing of intellect by creation, is produced as it were in the likeness of the species of God himself because the highest of those things according to which a created nature participates in the likeness of the uncreated nature is intellectuality, and therefore only the rational creature is said to be to the image (of God) ... whence only the rational creature attains the name of filiation by creation. But adoption, as has been said, requires that the one adopted acquires the right to the heredity of the adopter. But the heredity of God himself is his very beatitude, of which only the rational creature is capable. Nor is this acquired from creation itself, but from the gift of the Holy Spirit as has been said.[31]

We can see, then, that there is a great similarity between human adoption and divine adoption. The *term from which* is a person who is not of one's family. In human adoption, it is another human being who is equal to his adoptive parents in nature, whereas in divine adoption, it is a creature

---

31. Aquinas, *Commentary on the Sentences*, lib. III, dist. 10, q. 2, art. 2, qc. 1.

who does not belong to the divine family of the Trinity in virtue of creation. The *term to which* is the right to the heredity of the parents: in legal adoption these are the riches of the family, whereas in divine adoption, it is the riches of the Godhead:

> It ought to be said ... that adoption is transferred to the divine from a likeness of human acts. For a man is said to adopt one as a son according to which he gives (the son), out of good will, the right to secure his heredity to which he is not adequate by nature. But the heredity of a man is said to be that by which a man is wealthy; but that by which God is wealthy is his enjoyment of himself since he is blessed on account of this, and so this is his heredity. Whence insofar as he gives to men, who are not able to attain to that enjoyment by his natural powers, the grace by which man can merit that beatitude so that thus the right to that heredity will be adequate to him, according to this is he said to adopt someone as a son.[32]

As human adoption is effected by human law, so divine adoption is effected by divine law, that is, the law of grace, the gift of the Spirit: "For you have not received the spirit of bondage again in fear; but have received the spirit of adoption of sons, whereby we cry: Abba (Father)" (Rom. 8:15 DRC).

Having highlighted the similarities and differences between legal generation and natural generation, we are in a position to determine the ontological status of the relationship between natural parents and their children, on the one hand, and adoptive parents and their children, on the other hand. St. Thomas holds that there is a difference here, because the *cause* of filiation is different in each case:

> For the unity of relation or its plurality is not considered according to its termini, but according to its cause or subject. For if it is considered according to its termini, it would be necessary that every man would have two filiations in himself, one by which he is referred to his father and another by which he is referred to his mother. But to those considering the case rightly, it is clear that each and every one is referred to his father and mother by the same relation on account of the unity of the cause. For a man is

---

32. Aquinas, *Commentary on the Sentences*, lib. III, dist. 10, q. 2, art. 2, qc. 1.

> born from the father and mother by the same nativity, whence he is referred to each by the same relation. ... But it sometimes happens that someone has a relation to several things according to diverse causes, nevertheless of the same species, as when someone is the father of diverse sons according to diverse acts of generation. Whence paternity cannot differ in species since the acts of generation are of the same species. And since several forms of the same species cannot be in the same subject at one time, it is not possible that there be several paternities in him who is the father of several sons by natural generation. But in a different way, there could be, if he were the father of one by natural generation and of another by adoption.[33]

In other words, although legal generation and natural generation differ in definition because of the *term from which*, that is, whether the child is one's own or not, the relation is established in the parent by virtue of what the parent does in order to cause filiation, which is thus the basis, foundation, or cause of the relation. The cause of the relationship determines the nature of the relationship. Consequently, there is a difference in the parenthood one has by natural generation and that which one has by adoption; they are specifically different parenthoods. And since the specific difference is due to the agent of generation in virtue of the kind of act he performs, *natural generation* establishes a *real relation* by proceeding from a natural motion, whereas *adoption* establishes a *relation of reason* by proceeding from law as an ordinance of reason. The child by natural generation is the subject of a real relation to his parents; the adopted child is the subject of a relation of reason to his adopted parents. We can see that this is necessarily the case, since the adopted child retains a real relation to his natural parents, and so he could not possibly be the subject of an identical real relation to his adoptive parents. However, the same reasoning does not hold in the case of divine adoption; creatures are the subjects of real relations to God, but there is no real relation of God to creatures. The only real relations in God are between the divine Persons. Hence, the relation that is created by divine adoption exists only in his adopted children, who become heirs of the divine riches. We give God the name of Father by creation and adoption, then, by

---

33. Thomas Aquinas, *Summa theologiae* (*ST*), Collana reprint, 3rd ed. (Turin: Edizione San Paolo, 1999), III.35.5 corpus. All translation are by the author.

referring the real relation that exists in us to its cause; the relation of paternity exists in God only as a relation of reason.[34]

The charge of the objectors—that those who distinguish between adoptive and biological parenthood "do so apart from any theology or definition of parenthood"—is not well founded. We come to understand divine adoption by means of knowing what human adoption is directed to, namely, a share in the inheritance of the parents. Comparing human adoption to divine adoption enables us to understand not so much what human adoption "is and should be" but rather what divine adoption "is and should be," for the essence of human adoption is more known to us than the essence of divine adoption, and so the latter is understood by analogy with the former. As we have shown, there are significant differences between the *term from which* generation proceeds, the acts in virtue of which the relation is established, and the ontological status of the relationship itself. Since the basis of the relation of paternity-filiation is the action by means of which the relation is generated, there is an essential difference between legal filiation or adoption effected by a legal act, on the one hand, and natural filiation effected by natural generation, on the other hand.

Now, the change of natural generation is considered to be complete when a new substance comes to be from the contributions of the man and the woman. Usually this occurs within the body of the woman, but it can also be accomplished in vitro. It seems, then, that the parent-child relation is established at the moment of generation, whether that generation occurs in the body of the woman, thus making her to be pregnant, or outside the body of the woman.[35] Impregnating a woman with a thawed embryo, then, is not

---

34. Aquinas, *ST* I.13.7, I.28.1 and 3.
35. The argument could be made that an act of coitus is necessary to found the relation of paternity-maternity and, consequently, that children conceived in vitro lack parents. This seems to be Rev. Thomas Williams's thinking on the matter. See his "Heterologous Embryo Transfer and the Meaning of 'Becoming a Mother,'" in Berg and Furton, *Human Embryo Adoption*, 248. However, St. Thomas considers a man who begets a child by means of nocturnal pollution to be a father. See *Questiones de quolibet*, ed. R. A. Gauthier, *Opera omnia iussu Leonis XIII P. M. edita*, vol. 25.2 (Paris, Commissio Leonina, Éditions du Cerf, 1996), VI.10, 312b–314a. The rationale may be that the action of the male and female principles are instrumental, and so their proper activity is essentially referred to the agents to whom they belong (the male and the female), even if their coming together is effected by art.

an act fit to establish a real relation of maternity, for that relation already exists in the man and woman who contributed the gametes of the conceptus.

Is the Parenthood Principle Irrelevant or Misapplied?

What are we to conclude from the above observations? On the one hand, the conclusion of the advocates of embryo adoption—that the spouses' decision to adopt the child truly makes them parents through each other—rests on an equivocal use of the term *parenthood*. Since legal generation is called generation with respect to a likeness to natural generation but is not a *real* generation, the analogy is one of proportion, and so, from the logical point of view, generation is said equivocally of legal and natural. Similar moral requirements are incumbent on both natural and adoptive parents, but the moral responsibilities of the former are rooted in nature, while those of the latter are rooted in law. While both have *real* moral obligations, the natural parental relation is a *real* relation, while the adoptive parental relation is *non-real*, that is, a relation of reason. Further, when the CDF says that spouses may become parents only through each other, adverting to the fact that the Church has always recognized the legitimacy of becoming parents through adoption is beside the point, for the document is explicitly addressing the use of technology to bring about biological parenthood. The fact that spouses may morally become adoptive parents through each other, then, is completely irrelevant to the point at hand, which is whether it is morally licit to effect a pregnancy by means other than natural coitus.

On the other hand, embryo adoption cannot be seen as violating the principle that spouses may become parents only through each other, for ET does not in fact make a woman a mother. It seems, then, that some opponents of embryo adoption have also appealed to an irrelevant principle in determining the morality of the act. But perhaps that overstates the issue. It may merely be the case of a misapplication of a relevant principle. For even if it is not the case that embryo transfer makes a woman to be a mother apart from her spouse, it could still be the case that the principle according to which spouses should become parents only through each other forbids artificial impregnation through ET, just as it forbids artificial insemination. Perhaps the principle is one way of saying that we rightly order ourselves to the human good of begetting offspring only by means of marital coitus, and so the only means by which a woman can be ordered to birth is by means of the marriage act. This understanding of the principle is far broader than advocates of embryo adoption are willing to accept, and so we will conclude with a brief look at how those advocates of embryo rescue, who rightly deny that gestation alone makes a woman to be a mother, argue for an understanding of the principle that would allow for the liceity of ET. This will, in turn, show what criteria need to be met for a successful defense of the extended inseparability argument.

Criteria for a Successful Defense of Extended Inseparability

As we have already seen, some advocates of embryo rescue argue that, by enjoining that spouses may become parents only though each other, this section of *Donum vitae* rules out the *procreation* of the child by means of IVF or the combined project of IVF-ET, while leaving the proposal to undergo ET alone as a separate moral project untouched. Some embryo rescue advocates, such as Thomas Williams, Melissa Moschella, and Elizabeth Rex, defend that position while denying that ET, just by itself, makes a woman to be a mother apart from her spouse. Williams points out that the nomenclature employed to divide motherhood into various kinds (genetic, birth, gestational, adoptive, and social) is analogical, and that "adoptive motherhood, be it gestational or social, will never make a woman the mother of the child in a strict sense, since she did not beget the child but rather assumes responsibility for and nourishes a preexisting human being."[36]

Moschella expands on this line of thinking by pointing out that, whereas "gestation is certainly identity-*influencing*," it is the genetic relationship of parents to their child that permanently *defines* the personal identity of the child: "Assuming that humans are a psychophysical unity, and that our identity as human organisms is an intrinsic and essential aspect of our identity as human persons, genetic parents and their genetic children have, beginning at conception, an intimate and permanent personal relationship at the bodily dimension of their being. ... Your relationship to your progenitors is not only identity-defining but also permanent in a

---

36. Williams, "Heterologous Embryo Transfer," 247. He goes on: "Since becoming a mother and becoming a father refers specifically to a generative act resulting in the existence of a new human being, I would tentatively suggest that a child manufactured by IVF in a sense *has no mother and father*" (emphasis original).

way that non-genetic relationships are not."[37] Rex, though an advocate of embryo adoption, maintains that impregnation and motherhood are concurrent with the fertilization of the ovum, and "since impregnation and motherhood both occur *prior* to ET, then ET cannot be 'per se ordered to the motherhood of the woman.'"[38] Since motherhood and pregnancy are established at fertilization, it is not the case that ET by itself makes a woman to be a mother. In fact, since the fertilization of the ovum simply is the same thing as impregnation, ET does not even effect a pregnancy.[39]

Since these authors deny that ET alone makes a woman to be a mother, they base their advocacy of embryo rescue on other principles. Rex sees herself to have defeated the extended inseparability argument by her denial that the woman on the receiving end of ET has thereby been impregnated. She thus emphasizes the right of the child to life and the liceity of technical interventions on the embryo mentioned in *Donum vitae* I.3.[40] This raises the question of how the defenders of the extended inseparability argument will harmonize this passage with their disapproval of ET.[41] Against

---

37. Melissa Moschella, "Gestation Does Not Necessarily Imply Parenthood: Implications for the Morality of Embryo Adoption and Embryo Rescue," *American Catholic Philosophical Quarterly* 92.1 (Winter 2018): 26, 29, 33, doi: 10.5840/acpq20171130137, emphasis original.
38. Elizabeth Rex, "IVF, Embryo Transfer, and Embryo Adoption: A Response to Repenshek and Delaquil," *National Catholic Bioethics Quarterly* 14.2 (Summer 2014): 232, doi: 10.5840/ncbq201414226, emphasis original.
39. See Elizabeth Rex, "Impregnation versus Implantation in the Embryo Adoption Debate," colloquy, *National Catholic Bioethics Quarterly* 17.3 (Autumn 2017): 385, doi: 10.5840/ncbq201717339.
40. That paragraph reads, "Just like all interventions of the medical art on the sick, *so also those interventions on the human embryo are to be held licit on this condition, namely, that they preserve the embryos' life and integrity such that they do not bear with them disproportionate dangers, but look to the healing of disease, to changing the state of health for the better, and to placing the surviving life of the singular fetus itself in safety*" (emphasis original).
41. Rex and I debated both her view of impregnation and the applicability of *Donum vitae* I.3 to the embryo adoption debate in Robertson, "Thomistic Analysis of Embryo Adoption," 673–695; Rex, "The Magisterial Liceity of Embryo Transfer: A Response to Charles Robertson," *National Catholic Bioethics Quarterly* 15.4 (Winter 2015): 701–722, doi: 10.5840/ncbq201515471;

the extended inseparability argument, Williams maintains that *procreation* is properly defined as the "punctual moment" when a new human being is generated.[42] Like Rex, Williams sees the right of the child to life as determinative and adds a further more tentative argument in favor of embryo rescue on an analogy with heterologous organ transplantation.[43] He thus suggests that the use of the uterus in ET could be viewed along the lines of a temporary organ donation, which raises the question of whether there are some identifiable limits placed upon the use of that organ by the natural law.

Although Moschella sees her arguments against ET as "making a woman a mother apart from her spouse" as directly responding to Oleson's and Tonti-Filippini's versions of the extended inseparability argument, she recognizes other ways to defeat that argument. First, by showing that motherhood is established at conception, she believes herself to have shown that "there is no essential difference in kind" between wet-nursing and gestation. This raises a question akin to that raised by the analogy with organ donation, namely, whether there is some limit that restricts a woman from using her uterus to nourish another person's child while not restricting use of the breasts for the same purpose.[44] Second, she mentions the new natural law theorists' argument advanced by Tollefsen, which concludes that "pregnancy, and how it proceeds, does not enter *at all* into an account of what, biologically, renders two individuals one, biologically, in performing a generative type of act."[45] Consequently, to impregnate a woman by ET cannot be an offense against marriage. Tollefsen's argument is based on the

---

Robertson, "Navigating an Impasse in the Embryo Adoption Debate: A Response to Elizabeth Rex," *National Catholic Bioethics Quarterly* 16.3 (Autumn 2016): 409–417, doi: 10.5840/ncbq201616339.

42. Williams, "Heterologous Embryo Transfer," 241ff. I argue against understanding *procreation* in such punctual terms in "Generation, Gestation, and Birth: An Important Element in the Embryo Adoption Debate," *Linacre Quarterly* 85.1 (February 2018): 35–48, doi: 10.1177/0024363918756388.

43. Williams, "Heterologous Embryo Transfer," 235–236, 238–241.

44. I address that question in "Generation, Gestation, and Birth," 36–37.

45. Christopher Tollefsen, "Could Embryo Transfer Be Intrinsically Immoral?," in Brakman and Weaver, *Ethics of Embryo Adoption*, 93, emphasis original. See also Moschella, "Gestation Does Not Necessarily Imply Parenthood," 23n5.

new natural law theory's conception of marriage as a basic good.[46] This raises the question of whether that theory has rightly identified marriage as a basic good, together with the question of whether proponents of that theory have proceeded rightly in identifying the moral object of the act of ET.[47]

From the foregoing, it should be clear that if some version of the extended inseparability argument is to be successful, it needs to be able to (1) offer an alternative to the new natural law theorists' claims about marriage as a basic good and their identification of the object of the act, (2) show why the use of the uterus in ET is not like the use of the breasts in wet-nursing or like the use of organs we can licitly donate for the use of others, (3) harmonize the child's right to medical assistance with our inability to help it by precisely these means, and (4) correctly state that a woman who gestates a child is indeed pregnant.

It will need to show that *Donum vitae*'s statement that "the child has the right that it be conceived, contained in the womb, born and educated in matrimony: it can only know its identity, with certain and public reason, by referring to its parents and so proceed to its formation to maturity as a man" entails a complement like "parents have the duty to bring children into this world only by means of a definite act of marital intercourse from which proceeds the conception, gestation, and birth of the child born to them, which also serves as the basis for the certain and public reason of the child's identity and his growth to maturity as a man." It is my conviction that the traditional natural law thought of St. Thomas Aquinas, together with the philosophy of nature it necessarily presupposes, is capable of providing such an argument, but that is beyond the scope of this chapter.

---

46. Moschella herself also defends the new natural law conception of marriage as a basic good in "Sexual Ethics, Human Nature, and the 'New' and 'Old' Natural Law Theories," *National Catholic Bioethics Quarterly* 19.2 (Summer 2019): 251–278, doi: 10.5840/ncbq201919218.
47. I argue that the new natural law view of marriage as a basic good is untenable in "Is Marriage a Basic Good?," *Proceedings of the American Catholic Philosophical Association* 90 (2016): 163–173, doi: 10.5840/acpaproc20182871. I offer an alternative account of identifying the goods of nature, which implies a different way of analyzing the morality of an act, in "Lawrence Dewan, Legal Obligation, and the New Natural Law," *Thomist* 83.3 (July 2019): 437–459, doi: 10.1353/tho.2019.0027.

7

The Feminine Act of Admission
Mary Gormally

I am going to argue here that for a woman to allow an intromission of impregnating kind is for her to imitate the marriage act in respect of unitively significant function, and that this is contrary to the reproductive integrity which forms a part of the virtue of chastity. This virtue is different in men and in women, as the female marriage act is different from the male marriage act. Some may argue that Mary's fiat is a counterexample to my general contentions. The act whereby Mary allowed herself to be impregnated was not an act of admission allowing an intromission of impregnating kind, since nothing was put into her from outside. She was not imitating the female marriage act, since her relationship with God was more profound than marriage: the marriage relation is a copy of the more profound reality of which Mary's fiat was the central expression.

Mary's Act at the Annunciation

The salvation of the human race was made possible by the action of a woman, Mary our mother, when she said to the angel Gabriel, "Be it done to me according to thy word" (Luke 1:38 DRC). This action of hers was the central expression of her already-existing relationship with God. When she asked the angel how she could bear this son, since, as she put it, "I know not man" (Luke 1:34 DRC), she was averting to the fact that she was committed to being forever a virgin. The question would not have made sense otherwise, coming from a woman who was already betrothed to a man. Between her and her Creator there already existed, she did not know what for, a bond which was inconsistent with loss of her virginity. How she and Joseph had come to an understanding about this, we do not know. Having been told how this conception was not going to come between her and the virginity she was conserving for her Master, Mary did as God asked and gave permission for the act whereby God made her pregnant.

The Incarnation took place by Mary's free choice. God did not force her: she had with him already a bond of love, and her fiat was the central expression of this profound and permanent bond, both more profound and more permanent than marriage. Because of this, she has been called Spouse of the Holy Spirit. Her nature as a woman was thus not outraged, but supernaturally fulfilled by her supernatural conception. Just as a marriage act, if it is a true marriage act, includes a free choice by the woman expressing her relationship with her husband, so Mary's fiat was a free act expressing her relationship with the Father of her divine Child, a relationship of obedience to the Father's will.

The Annunciation Compared and Contrasted with the Act of an Embryo Adopter

This act of Mary's has been compared to the act of a woman who, as a member of an adopting couple, admits an existing embryo into her womb. There is this similarity: in both cases, the person permitted to be in the womb already exists before the permission, and the act allowed by the woman is an act of a kind to impregnate her. However, Mary did not perform an act of admission, allowing an intromission of a kind to impregnate her. Her cooperation with the Spirit's impregnation of her was not the allowing of something into her. Jesus was made man in her womb by an action of the omnipresent God, who was already there inside her as He is inside all of us. Also, the father of the child, in Mary's case, was indeed his father and did generate him from her flesh, whereas the operation by which the woman who adopts an embryo is made pregnant is not an act of generation. The intromission admitted by the so-called adopting woman, the action which impregnates her, is not an expression of an intimate and permanent relationship between her and the person who does the intromitting. Even if the impregnator, the one inserting the embryo, happened to be her husband, the woman's letting him impregnate her in this way would not be unitive as a marriage act is unitive. This fact brings out the chilling impersonality of what she is allowing.

The word *impregnation* is nowadays used by scientists to mean the penetration and fertilization of the ovum by the sperm. However, the idea of a woman's being impregnated existed before people knew about these cells. Since people correctly consider normal pregnancy to have begun when the ovum has been fertilized, the distinction between impregnating a woman and fertilizing an ovum would be unimportant were it not for the fact of their having been separated by the technicians whose actions have given rise to the ethical question which is under discussion. The ovum has already been fertilized, but by having embryos put into her, the adoptive woman has also been impregnated. The fact of the earlier impregnation does not mean that the woman is not impregnated or that the intromission of the embryos is not an intromission of impregnating kind. It is precisely that, since to be made pregnant is to be made to have an infant in one's abdomen outside the digestive tract.

Why Just Adoption?

It is strange that people present this particular kind of embryo rescue, that is, the kind referred to as adoption, as the acceptable one, the one that should be allowed. If there were a baby abandoned and lying in the gutter, it would not be reasonable for a passing bachelor to say, "I should not save this baby. My menage is an unsuitable one in which to raise a child or even welcome it." Nor would it be reasonable to say about an adopting couple, "The couple that wishes to adopt this baby is acting from selfish motives. They just can't have children of their own, so they want to adopt. Since this is what moves them, they should not be allowed to adopt this needy child." If heterologous embryo transfer is allowable, then any woman physically suitable for it has good reason to volunteer for it, in that the abandoned embryos need to be rescued if they are to enjoy a normal human life, just as in extreme situations anyone who can foster a child may have good reason to do so. But is heterologous embryo transfer allowable? Some might say that, in the case of what is called embryo adoption, embryo transfer is not heterologous, since the woman is an adoptive parent, having agreed with her husband to adopt a particular child as their own, a child who now needs the medical assistance of transfer to her womb. But it remains the case that the child is not flesh of their flesh, and this is why I call the transfer heterologous, even if, by some legal action, they are calling the embryo their own.

Part 2: Objections to Embryo Adoption

Embryo adoption is presented as being an expression of a loving relation between the couple that is doing it. This presentation is designed to escape the sense that this intromission, which is of a kind to impregnate a woman, is in some way a violation, that it in some way exploits and abuses her. But this remains the case when a woman adopts an embryo, though the exploitation is self-exploitation and the abuse is self-abuse. Wrap it up as a loving act in which the woman and her husband lovingly agree, and the whole thing can be seen as virtuous. But what is happening here is like what happens when a man masturbates, causing himself to do what the husband does in the marriage act but without a wife and, therefore, without generation. The woman admitting an intromission of impregnating kind is doing what a wife does in the marriage act but without a husband or male seed and, therefore, without openness to generation. In both cases—in the case of solitary vice and in the case of a woman's allowing an impregnating intromission of an embryo—there is a defective marriage act. (The word *defective* here is a privative qualification: a defective marriage act is not a marriage act, as a dead man is not a man and a forged banknote is not a banknote.)

Inevitably, where the link between natural generation and pregnancy is let slip by our teachers, the embryos in the world's freezers become a resource for the use of Catholics who cannot conceive. Presenting the obtaining of children in this way as a loving act of the married couple is a cosmetic operation.

Objection to Embryo Adoption

My objection to embryo adoption or rescue is that it involves the woman in performing an act of admission whereby she allows an intromission of impregnating kind, in this way imitating the female marriage act in respect of a function which, in the context of a true marriage act, is a unitive function. This objection is much misunderstood. An example of such misunderstanding is shown by Christopher Tollefsen when he accuses me of saying that making a woman pregnant by intromitting an embryo is making procreation occur through her.[1] I have never said this. He does not mention

---

1. Christopher Tollefsen, "Divine, Human, and Embryo Adoption: Some Criticisms of *Dignitas Personae*," *National Catholic Bioethics Quarterly* 10.1 (Spring 2010): 75–85, esp. 76, doi: 10.5840/ncbq201010173.

what I objected to, which is the woman's act of admission, the female act of admitting an impregnating intromission. Because the intromission is of a kind to impregnate the woman, her act shares a certain description with the feminine marriage act. That her act allows an intromission which is not in fact of a kind to generate a human being is one of the things which makes it unlike a marriage act and, therefore, defective.

The Nature of the Female Marriage Act Contrasted with the Male Act

In the marriage act, two human actions take place: the masculine act, which essentially includes ejaculation and other motions of the flesh, and which is an act of intromission, and the feminine act, which is an act of admission allowing the intromission. The feminine act is most enjoyed (and, I suppose, more likely to be effective) if it includes its own proper motions of the flesh. However, a true marriage act can take place without these happening. Whatever the will of the man may be, if he does not ejaculate, the marriage act has not taken place. Except in the case of contraceptive intercourse, if he does purposely ejaculate in his wife's vagina and the woman freely admits this intromission, the marriage act does take place, whether the woman has concomitant motions of the flesh or not.

It is possible for a man to perform something which is like the marriage act but is not a marriage act: an act of rape, an act which is in some way deliberately rendered unfit for generation, or an act of solitary vice. These acts are contrary to the virtue which is proper to human sexuality. It is also possible for a woman to perform an act which is like a female marriage act but is not fit for generation, there being no male counterpart to the act taking place. Also, just as the female marriage act itself does not have to include the appropriate motions of the flesh, so an act can be unacceptably like the female marriage act without including these motions. The act of admission whereby a woman allows an impregnating intromission which is not of the generative kind is such an act, whether or not she feels sexual feelings about it.

It follows from the differences between the male and female marriage acts that the virtue having to do with reproductive behaviour is different in the two sexes. Male reproductive acts necessarily include motions of the flesh—erection and ejaculation. Female ones do not—not necessarily. Because men are like this, moral theology has treated the virtue of chastity as a part of temperance—as a virtue having to do with fleshly pleasure. The male perspective sees all sex as being like the masculine act, as involving enjoyable motions of the flesh. However, chastity does not have to do only with pleasure but with the fact that this species of fleshly pleasure is what leads to the generation of new human life, and the enjoyment of such pleasure is properly placed in the context of marriage, which is for the generation and rearing of children.

Reproductive Integrity, the Greater Part of Chastity

There is more than temperance involved in chastity: there is this greater thing, which I have called reproductive integrity, which has to do with the part played by intention in each of the two human acts by which a couple cooperates in a true marriage act. Part of the intention of a woman in the marriage act is that she intentionally admits an intromission which is of a kind to impregnate her. The fact that she is doing this is unitively significant. She is laying herself open to an action of a kind to cause her to bear her husband's child within her—thus, of a kind not only to generate but to achieve the bodily self-giving involved in pregnancy. Even if generation is impossible, it is a part of the significance of the act that she is admitting into her something which is of a kind to make her pregnant. Therefore, to admit an intromission of impregnating kind is to imitate the marriage act in respect of a unitively significant function.

I maintain that this is what it is to abuse human sexuality: to imitate the marriage act in respect of unitively significant function. When people use contraceptives, for instance, they are not performing marriage acts. They are imitating the marriage act in respect of its unitively significant function, in that the fleshly union itself, without having generative significance, imitates the unitively significant copulation of a true marriage act. To separate the unitive and the procreative in the case of contraception or, say, sodomy is not to do something having the unitive meaning of a marriage act but without the procreative meaning. It is to do something which has neither meaning but imitates the marriage act in respect of the unitively significant function of copulation. When people commit in vitro fertilization, they imitate the unitively significant function of uniting human flesh to flesh so as to bring about a new human being. When people commit acts of simple fornication, they imitate the marriage act so closely that this is counted among the least of mortal sins against chastity.

When a woman who adopts an embryo admits an intromission which is of a kind to impregnate her, she does not do anything which has either unitive or procreative significance but does something which does imitate the marriage act in respect of admitting an intromission of impregnating kind. I do not think that any people who have publicly criticized my argument about this have seriously addressed my actual words. They speak of my objecting to the intromitting behaviour involved but fail to acknowledge the specifically feminine part of the act that I say the woman performs: an act of *admission* whereby she allows an intromission of an impregnating kind. Privately, one well-known philosopher has objected to this description as implying that there is something sexual about the woman's act. He objected to the argument on the ground that there is nothing sexual about what is done in embryo transfer.

Feminine Aspect of Reproductive Integrity

The sexes are two: male and female. What distinguishes the sexes is that for a woman to perform a marriage act is for her to act in a way which is apt to make her pregnant. This fact is part of what gives specifically feminine unitive significance to the female marriage act. So, using the word *sex* in its proper and original meaning, it is not true that the woman's act, whereby she allows herself to be made pregnant with some embryo, does not have to do with sex. It does, in that it is specifically female. Part of specific femininity is that it is possible, even if unpleasant, to perform a marriage act without its proper physiological accompaniments. Thus, if such accompaniments are unsought by or absent from the act of a woman who admits an impregnating intromission, this does not make this act unsexual.

How a Woman Should Get Pregnant

The Virgin's fiat was an actualization of her specifically feminine nature. However, she was not attacking her own reproductive integrity, because she was giving to the Father of her Child the central act owed to him in virtue of their relationship, that is, an act of obedience that was not unquestioning, but unconditional. This was not an imitation of the female marriage act. Rather, marriage is itself an image of the relation of the Virgin, of the Church, and of the human soul to our Master, who is God. A woman should not become pregnant except through an act on her part which is the central expression of her preexisting, profound, and permanent relation to the begetter of the child within her, a relation exclusive of sexual relations with anyone else. Such was the relation expressed by Mary's fiat, something much more profound and permanent than a marriage act.

Should we say that the woman who, with her husband, agrees to adopt embryos is also fulfilling her specifically feminine nature? She has a natural desire to bear a child, and the transfer of the embryos to the womb fulfils this desire in some way, particularly if the embryos thrive. However, the desire to bear a child is properly expressed in the marriage act, where it is a desire to bear the husband's child. The couple who adopt an embryo are missing both the husband's part in the marriage act and the generation of the child. That event which took place at the Annunciation did not lack the engendering male act, but this occurred in a way which was more real, more loving, and more personal. More real, as God is more real than we are, and as his action was immediately generative; more loving, as God's love for Mary exceeded all merely human love; and more personal, as God loved the person Mary was at the deepest level.

Replies to Defences of Embryo Adoption

An excuse offered for embryo transfer is that, by agreeing to do this, the woman is providing that which the embryos need and to which they have a right. How can it be shown that, failing the mother's womb, the embryos have a right to the womb of some other woman? They cannot have a right to a non-maternal womb if a virtue proper to a woman is undermined by the nonmarital act of admission whereby an adopting woman allows an intromission of impregnating kind—that is, if such an act is contrary to the specifically feminine aspect of the virtue of reproductive integrity.

This virtue shows itself in the reaction of disgust which virtuous matrons and other women have at the suggestion of embryo rescue, because it *feels* wrong. But as with other manifestations of connatural knowledge, the women who feel this disgust are not necessarily able to say why they find the suggestion repulsive. The capacity for such feeling is a part of one's sexuality. A faithful wife who is propositioned by a would-be adulterer may have a similar feeling: a shuddering repulsion.

The Sisters of Life, whose vocation is to live and pray for the sake of those whose lives are threatened by the various evil things done by the medical profession (and for the sake of the mothers of these) do not rescue embryos by using their own wombs to accommodate them. When I asked their superior, some years ago, whether she would do such a thing, she said no, it felt like a violation, but she could not say why. Here is an example of the connatural knowledge of which I have spoken, and it was as well that the good sister had this, as in her position, she could have corrupted many of her community had she not had this knowledge. It may be replied that this would not be embryo adoption, as the sisters are not married and could not welcome an embryo into a family. So an adopting couple would offer a better context for the gestation of an embryo than a religious community devoted to life who could hand the babies over to childless people? Or maybe the community could form a new kind of family, where God is seen as the father and all the mothers identify with the Blessed Virgin? But they do not do this. The fact that human wickedness has produced freezers full of human beings who can continue to normal life only if women biologically not their mothers admit them into their genital tracts does not mean that women should do this.

Ecclesiastical authority has been invoked supposedly to show that impregnation of women with embryos is permissible, since it does not harm them and since Magisterial documents have pronounced that it is permissible to conduct therapeutic procedures which do not harm the embryo.[2] So should these pronouncements be taken to mean that anything done with an embryo which does not harm it is allowable? This *anything* would include nonvoluntary impregnation of women whose babies could be surrendered at birth. To reject this, while invoking ecclesiastical authority for embryo adoption, would be to treat the argument from authority like a bus which you can get off at any stop you like before the terminus. With any such rule, there is a tacitly understood provision "or others." A child who is told that he can do what he likes with an object provided he does not damage it, cannot use this permission to defend hitting someone with it. Similarly, you should not do anything to any embryo which harms anyone other than the embryo. It is the harm to the woman's reproductive integrity which is the basis of my attack on embryo adoption.

---

2. Elizabeth Bothamley Rex, "The Magisterial Liceity of Embryo Transfer: A Response to Charles Robertson," *National Catholic Bioethics Quarterly* 15.4 (Winter 2015): 712, doi: 10.5840/ncbq201515471. Her argument from authority leads to the conclusion that anything may be allowed with an embryo which does not harm it, though she does offer further defense of embryo adoption.

PART 2: OBJECTIONS TO EMBRYO ADOPTION

What do I mean by reproductive integrity? It is the virtue having to do with reproductive behavior. In a woman, it entails a kind of self-protectiveness more than it does in a man, and a sense of disgust and a sense that one's body is not to be violated are part of this self-protectiveness. A nonmarital act whereby one admits an intromission of impregnating kind is a gross outrage to this sense and is liable to damage if not to destroy it. In a man, the virtue of reproductive integrity has more to do with his genital activity, though this is also important in a woman. But an assault on reproductive integrity is not necessarily a piece of genital activity. It may consist in allowing something to be done to one's body. The virtue entails not dividing the different parts of human reproduction: the unitive and the procreative.

It is unitive in the context of a real marriage act that the woman lays herself open to an intromission which is of a kind to impregnate her. What is done by an embryo-adopting woman imitates the marriage act in this respect. Her act is, therefore, a defective version of the marriage act. A human act which is sufficiently like the marriage act to be a defective version of it is defective as a human act and, therefore, intrinsically evil.

Conclusion

Moral theologians have mostly been men, so there is a tradition of thinking about sexual morality from a masculine perspective. What is in question here requires that specifically feminine actions should be thought about. The woman does, in the marriage act, admit an intromission of impregnating kind, and it is an important part of the unitive significance of her marriage act that she does this. The main contention of those who want embryos rescued or adopted is that women may allow something to be done to impregnate them outside the marrige act. It is vital to consider whether such allowance is consistent with specifically feminine virtue. Normally, the act by which women allow themselves to be made pregnant is the central expression of a preexisting, profound, and permanent relationship with the father of the child being begotten, a relationship exclusive of sexual intercourse with anyone else. Such was the act by which Mary allowed the conception of our Saviour. Any act admitting impregnation without expressing such a relationship is contrary to that part of the virtue of chastity which I have called reproductive integrity.

8

Arguments against Embryo Adoption from the Perspective of Theology of the Body

Kent Lasnoski

For the sake of brevity and clarity, this chapter employs the disputatio format of the Scholastics, first presenting the objections to my position, then a reason to reconsider (*sed contra*), followed by a succinct argument for my position, and finally, a specific response to each objection not already refuted in the central argument. Elsewhere I have argued in favor of embryo adoption, though here I argue against its liceity.[1]

Question:
Is Embryo Adoption Morally Licit from
the Perspective of Theology of the Body?

Article 1. Whether Embryo Adoption Is a Matter of Sexual Ethics Relevant to Theology of the Body

Objection 1. It seems that embryo adoption is *not* a matter of sexual ethics relevant to Theology of the Body. Procreation properly speaking refers to the generation of a new person through the combination of gametes. Procreation is completed upon the spermatozoon's impregnating the ovum.

---

1. Kent Lasnoski, "Setting the Captives Free: Precedent for Embryo Adoption in Scripture and the Catholic Tradition," *Josephinum Journal of Moral Theology* 20.1 (2013): 88–112.

Part 2: Objections to Embryo Adoption

Gestation properly speaking refers to internal nutrition and shelter. Embryo adoption, which is a matter of gestating and eventually raising a child as a couple's own, is more analogous to postnatal adoption of a genetic stranger than it is to heterologous insemination. The principles of sexual ethics as expressed in Theology of the Body and elsewhere (e.g., a spouses may become pregnant only through a gift of self with her spouse and through the conjugal act) do not apply to this situation.

Objection 2. Further, embryo adoption is an application of the works of mercy as described in Matthew 25 and the Gospel declaration of Jesus in Luke 4 rather than an attempt to procreate apart from the conjugal act. The principles of sexual ethics as expressed in Theology of the Body and elsewhere in Catholic magisterial teaching, therefore, do not apply.

Objection 3. Further, the magisterial teachings of both Pope St. John Paul II and the Congregation for the Doctrine of the Faith demand that the human rights of the embryo be recognized and that the embryo be treated with available therapeutic means.[2] Embryo adoption is a simple fulfilment of the duty made explicit in the Church's instruction *Donum vitae*, namely, that the embryo "must also be defended in its integrity, tended and cared for, to the extent possible, in the same way as any other human being as far as medical assistance concerned."[3] This duty is to provide therapeutic actions toward the embryo. Since embryo transfer is principally a therapeutic action for the embryo, it is to be considered not under the rubric of sexual ethics but rather under medical ethics.

Objection 4. Further, embryo adoption is pursued as an expression of the preferential option for the poor rather than as an expression of one's desire to procreate apart from conjugal intimacy. This principle governs Catholic social teaching rather than sexual ethics. Therefore, the sexual ethic of Theology of the Body is irrelevant to embryo adoption.

---

2. See John Paul II, Address to Participants in the Symposium on "*Evangelium Vitae* and Law" and the Eleventh International Colloquium on Canon Law (May 24, 1996).
3. Congregation for the Doctrine of the Faith, *Donum vitae* (February 22, 1987), I.1.

Sed contra, *Dignitas personae* states, "It has also been proposed, solely in order to allow human beings to be born who are otherwise condemned to destruction, that there could be a form of 'prenatal adoption.' This proposal, praiseworthy with regard to the intention of respecting and defending human life, presents however various problems not dissimilar to those mentioned above."[4] These problems relate to surrogate motherhood and infertility, both of which are considered in terms of sexual ethics.

Respondeo, Sexual ethics concerns any use of the procreative faculty, which includes any actions that introduce the ontological change of "becoming a mother," that is, the real relations of *mother* and *offspring* as those relations pertain to both the woman and the child. Sexual ethics also extends to the full function of the sexual organs, even beyond procreation per se to the nurture of gestation itself. Finally, in the thought of John Paul II's Theology of the Body, the conjugal act must speak the language of the body, that is, its spousal meaning, its being ordered toward indissoluble exclusive union with the other and the consequences that follow from that union, namely, procreation, gestation, and postnatal education. Since gestation and postnatal education are anticipated by the conjugal act, they are understood under the rubric of sexual ethics.

***Adversus* 1.** Understood in its limited, essential sense, procreation is complete at conception; however, procreation refers more broadly to the entire process of generating, gestating (nurturing), and even educating—each of which is relevant to the theological approach of Theology of the Body.

***Adversus* 2.** The assertion is true: a person holds the fulfillment of a work of mercy as the remote end, that is, the intention, of the embryo transfer. This intention is pure and good. Nonetheless, this pure intention does not rectify the disordered object. The object of the act is to become pregnant by means of an embryo transfer. The object is a synthesis of the immediate means, which is the technical procedure of the embryo transfer, and the most proximate end, which is the resulting pregnancy. Impregnating acts are assessed under the rubric of sexual ethics, for example, those principles expounded by John Paul II's Theology of the Body. An impregnating act

---

4. Congregation for the Doctrine of the Faith, *Dignitas personae* (September 8, 2008), n. 19.

apart from the gift of conjugal love in the consummation of a marriage is intrinsically evil, on account of its violating the exclusivity of the gift of self in marriage.

One might object, saying that the object is more accurately described as the synthesis of embryo transfer (immediate means) and the gift of self as shelter and food (most proximate end). On this account, the pregnancy could still be the intention (a more remote end) but is in fact an anticipated and hoped for consequence rather than the object of the act itself. Such an analysis is compelling, because the embryo rescuer would still feel as though she had completed the action even if she never becomes pregnant. She will have made herself available for the child's basic human goods, despite the fact that the child did not flourish. Since the action itself terminates in the mind of the agent apart from pregnancy itself, the object is truly the work of mercy rather than the pregnancy. Even if this second analysis is more accurate, the action still falls under the criteria of sexual ethics, since it instrumentalizes the procreative organs as a means and because it holds the pregnancy as an intention.

***Adversus* 3.** The embryo is in fact the subject of rights, and embryo transfer is a therapeutic action for the embryo. Nonetheless, the act is *also* an intervention upon the woman related to her procreative faculties. The action, therefore, is subject to the criteria of sexual ethics, for example, those expressed in John Paul II's Theology of the Body.

***Adversus* 4.** Embryo adoption expresses preferential option for the poor precisely by engaging the procreative faculties; therefore, it must satisfy the criteria for morally praiseworthy use of those faculties, even if the action is not driven by any sexual motivation.

Article 2. Whether Embryo Adoption Is an Authentic Gift of Self and Reception of the Other in Accord with John Paul II's Hermeneutic of the Gift

Objection 1. It seems that embryo adoption is an authentic gift of self and is, therefore, licit. Quoting the Second Vatican Council, *Gaudium et spes*, John Paul II writes in *Man and Woman He Created Them*, "Man, willed in this way [for his own sake] by the Creator from the 'beginning,' can only find himself through a disinterested gift of self."[5] A person makes himself a gift when he, without expectation of repayment and for the benefit of the other, puts himself at the disposal or service of the other. One must intend himself positively to become somehow a good for the other. Such an action is self-donative, moreover, when it is not motivated by, or seeking for oneself, any end other than one's own intrinsic, internal good, that is, one's own becoming a free, loving subject. In other words, in making a gift of self, the agent wants for himself or herself only to become fully a man or a woman according to Christ's revelation of humanity's true nature and fulfilment. By saying the gift must be disinterested, John Paul II emphasizes the purity of motive, the absence of seeking extrinsic benefit for oneself. A couple seeking embryo adoption for the sake of rescuing a frozen person and raising the child as their own make a free, loving, disinterested gift of self. Therefore, embryo adoption is morally licit.

Objection 2. It seems that embryo adoption is the kind of self-gift by which a woman fulfills her precisely feminine vocation as described in the thought of John Paul II's Theology of the Body and *Mulieris dignitatem*: "The mystery of femininity is manifested and revealed completely by means of motherhood, as the text says: 'she conceived and bore ...' The woman stands before the man as a mother, the subject of the new human life that is conceived and develops in her, and from her is born into the world."[6] Christopher Oleson explicates the passage well: "This conceiving, developing, and bearing into the world is a unique manifestation and revelation of motherhood because of the special openness to the new person that the Holy Father says specifically characterizes the woman's part in parenting. It is in this openness, in conceiving and giving birth to a child, [that] the

---

5. John Paul II, *Man and Woman He Created Them: A Theology of the Body*, trans. Michael Waldstein (Boston: Pauline Books and Media, 2006), 15:3. For the hermeneutic of gift, see 13:2 and 16:1.

6. John Paul II, *Original Unity of Man and Woman* (Boston: St. Paul Editions, 1981), 155.

woman discovers herself through a sincere gift of self."[7] John Paul II goes on to say that "motherhood is *linked to the personal structure of the woman and to the personal dimension of the gift.*"[8] Embryo adoption establishes motherhood and is, therefore, a fulfilment of the woman's self-realization according to the hermeneutic of the gift.

Objection 3. It seems that embryo adoption is an authentic reception of the other for his own sake. John Paul II writes, "We can say that inner innocence (that is, the rightness of intention) in the exchange of the gift consists in a reciprocal 'acceptance' of the other in such a way that it corresponds to the very essence of the gift; in this way, the mutual gift creates the communion of persons. It is a question, therefore, of 'welcoming' the other human being and of 'accepting' him."[9] Couples performing embryo adoption welcome and accept the child with this rightness of intention, regardless of defect, race, gender, or genetic likeness to themselves. Their intention is perhaps purer than that of a couple who desires a child from conjugal intimacy to fulfill their own hopes of self-preservation or natural perfection and happiness. Embryo adoption is, therefore, morally licit.

Objection 4. It seems that embryo adoption fits the hermeneutic of the gift and is, thus, morally licit, because the couple adopting an embryo must see the frozen child and their own bodies with a redeemed vision likened unto that of original innocence. John Paul II argues that all the world, and especially the body of man and woman, constitutes a "primordial *sacrament* … understood as a *sign that* efficaciously *transmits in the visible world the invisible mystery hidden in God from eternity.* And this is the mystery of Truth and Love, the mystery of divine life, in which man really participates."[10] The couple sees in their own bodies a sign of God's loving providence for the frozen child and sees the child as a sign of God's goodness

---

7. Christopher Oleson, "The Nuptial Womb: On the Moral Significance of Being 'with Child,'" in *Human Embryo Adoption: Biotechnology, Marriage, and the Right to Life*, ed. Thomas V. Berg and Edward J. Furton (Philadelphia: National Catholic Bioethics Center, 2006), 184, citing John Paul II, *Mulieris dignitatem* (August 15, 1999), nn. 18, 30, 31, internal quotation marks omitted.
8. John Paul II, *Mulieris dignitatem*, n. 18, emphasis original.
9. John Paul II, *Man and Woman He Created Them*, 17:3.
10. John Paul II, *Man and Woman He Created Them*, 19:4, emphasis original.

that must be defended and brought to flourishing for its own sake. Out of this sacramental vision comes their motivation to perform embryo transfer. Their action, then, is an expression of the redeemed vision John Paul II invites couples to discover through the sacrament of marriage. Therefore, embryo adoption is morally licit.

Sed contra, John Paul II writes, "The mutual gift creates the communion of persons," which "is a question, therefore, of 'welcoming' the other human being and of 'accepting' him or her precisely because in this mutual relationship, about which Genesis 2:23–25 speaks, *the man and the woman become a gift, each one for the other, through the whole truth and evidence of their own body in its masculinity and femininity.*"[11]

Respondeo, The attempt to use the hermeneutic of the gift in the context of embryo adoption is well-intentioned but fundamentally misplaced. An action's being a gift of self is not a sufficient account of its moral plenitude. Man does find himself in free, loving gift of self, but certain gifts of self are limited to the conjugal covenant (namely, those of the procreative kind), and certain gifts of the self are limited to persons outside the conjugal covenant (e.g., the radical availability of a consecrated person). The self-gift and reception of the other spoken of in Theology of the Body are those that reveal, enact, and speak the language of the body's spousal meaning. These are limited to marriage *and* require the action of *both* spouses together rather than the action of merely one.[12] The logic of authentic, disinterested self-gift applied by John Paul II sits squarely in the context of the marital covenant. Discussion of self-gift through Theology of the Body, therefore, is relevant principally to the spouses' gift of self to each other and their reception of each other directly and, more precisely, sexually.

The fundamental acceptance John Paul II refers to is the man's reception of the woman as gift. The fundamental gift he refers to is not only the gift of creation but most precisely the woman's giving of herself (and

---

11. John Paul II, *Man and Woman He Created Them*, 17.3, emphasis added.
12. See John Paul II, *Man and Woman He Created Them*, 20:4. "Together they thus become one single subject, as it were, of that act and that experience, although they remain two really distinct subjects in this unity."

her simultaneously being given by God) to the man.[13] In this disinterested, reciprocal giving and receiving, the receiving itself becomes a giving, and the union of the body that flows from it sets the conditions for yet another gift—that of God's creating a person within the one originally given. Therefore, an attempt to apply the language of self-gift directly to an embryo transfer is misplaced. Gift of self relates to the ethics of childbearing in Theology of the Body only insofar as that childbearing is a fruit of the body's speaking its spousal meaning in the conjugal act.

Furthermore, John Paul II asserts that the conjugal act must always retain both its unitive and its procreative meanings.[14] This insistence is another way of saying that the only proper object of the sexual act is to consummate one's marriage, accepting the full possibilities of what might follow from that communion of persons. The sexual faculties, therefore, may never be properly used if they are instrumentalized toward *any* particular end, whether procreation or union alone. They may be used to consummate a marriage, an act which carries a procreative and unitive meaning.[15] Procreation itself is a potency and potential consequence of the act's internal structure. It is not an end toward which the act is directed as a means. Since embryo adoption would instrumentalize the procreative faculties (albeit toward a good end of gestating and raising a discarded child), such an action is not equal to the dignity of the procreative faculty, which is properly a power for consummating a marriage.

***Adversus* 1.** I concede that embryo adoption would constitute an authentic, disinterested gift of self; it is, nonetheless, an illicit gift of self on the

---

13. John Paul II, *Man and Woman He Created Them*, 17:4–7.
14. John Paul II, *Man and Woman He Created Them*, 118:6. He writes, relying on Pope St. Paul VI's *Humanae vitae* n. 12, "Since 'the conjugal act'—at one and the same time—'deeply unites husband and wife' and together 'makes them able to generate new lives,' and since the one as well as the other thing comes about 'by its innermost structure,' it follows that the human person 'must' (this is the necessity proper to reason, logical necessity) read, *at one and the same time*, the '*two meanings* of the conjugal act' and also the '*inseparable connection* between the two meanings of the conjugal act'" (emphasis original).
15. The language of *meaning* was developed by Herbert Doms and Dietrich von Hildebrand, validated by the Second Vatican Council, and relied on most especially in *Humanae vitae*.

woman's part. John Paul II writes that procreation is a matter of mutual self-gift and knowledge: "Procreation brings it about that 'the man and the woman (his wife)' *know each other reciprocally in the 'third,' originated by both*."[16] With embryo adoption, procreation (understood broadly) does not result from a mutual knowledge of the other through reciprocal gift, nor does it result in a third person originated by both and through whom the spouses may know each other. John Paul II refers here to the fact that the child is, in some way, a continuation of both parents, and they come to know themselves and each other through that person. This situation does not obtain in the case of embryo adoption, and the action, therefore, does not fit the hermeneutic of the gift in John Paul II's Theology of the Body.

***Adversus* 2.** John Paul II argues that maternity does actualize and reveal the gift of self particular to a woman, but revelation and actualization come about *always and only* through the woman's conjugal communion with her husband. That is, she discovers and becomes fully woman when she becomes one flesh with her spouse. The knowledge man and woman have of each other in begetting includes also the consummation of marriage, the specific *consummatum*; in this way, one obtains the grasp of the objectivity of the body, hidden in the somatic powers of man and woman, and, at the same time, the grasp of the objectivity of man, who is this body. Through the body, the human person is husband or wife; at the same time, in this particular act of knowledge mediated by personal masculinity and femininity, one seems to reach also the discovery of the pure subjectivity of the gift: that is, mutual self-realization in that gift: "Procreation brings it about that 'the man and the woman (his wife)' *know each other reciprocally in the 'third,' originated by both*."

In becoming mother to a third who is not generated by the reciprocal knowledge of each other in the communion of the spouses, a woman does not in fact live out her particularly feminine self-gift and realization.

***Adversus* 3.** The child may be accepted with pure intention for his own sake and is truly not commodified, yet the acceptance does not demonstrate the logos of Theology of the Body. The child must be accepted for his own sake *as a fruit of a reciprocal self-gift between the spouses in the conjugal act*.

---

16. John Paul II, *Man and Woman He Created Them*, 21:4, emphasis original.

Part 2: Objections to Embryo Adoption

As John Paul II writes in *Gratissimam sane*, the child is the instantiation of the common good of the marriage, namely, the incarnation of the spouses' indissoluble union of nature strengthened by grace.[17] The frozen embryo cannot be accepted as the fruit of reciprocal self-gift of the adopting spouses, regardless of how ardent their desire to save the child may be. The procreative faculties cannot be engaged except to invite God's gift of life through the spouses' gift to each other. Therefore, embryo adoption cannot be justified by recourse to the logos of Theology of the Body.

***Adversus* 4.** While the couple does have a redeemed sacramental vision of the child as a window into the goodness of God's life-giving love, the child is not a visible sign of the spousal meaning of their own bodies or of God's spousal love for the Church in Christ. In procreation, if the child is to be revelatory in the way imagined by Theology of the Body, the child must be the result of the spouses' own reciprocal, disinterested gift of their masculinity and femininity *to each other*. The child conceived in vitro still reveals the goodness of God and the spousal meaning of his own body, but precisely on account of the spousal meaning of his *own* body, the child demands being accepted *as the fruit of a conjugal gift* and desired for his own sake.

The impossibility of saving the child is a rebuke presented to the world exactly on account of the human body's spousal meaning. If a woman receives in her womb any life except that created in the reciprocal self-gift of conjugal intimacy, she inevitably and necessarily countermands the integrity of her body's spousal meaning. On these grounds, one can say even the genetic mother of the child conceived in vitro would witness against the spousal meaning of her body by taking that same child into her womb through embryo transfer. Again, the absurdity of being unable to save the child constitutes a condemnation of us who have created a world with such situations.

---

17. See John Paul II, *Gratissimam sane* (February 2, 1994), n. 11. "In the newborn child is realized the common good of the family. Just as the common good of spouses is fulfilled in conjugal love, ever ready to give and receive new life, so too the common good of the family is fulfilled through that same spousal love, as embodied in the newborn child. Part of the genealogy of the person is the genealogy of the family, preserved for posterity by the annotations in the Church's baptismal registers, even though these are merely the social consequence of the fact that 'a man has been born into the world' (Jn 16:21)."

9

Some Moral Contraindications to Human Embryo Adoption

Rev. Tadeusz Pacholczyk

My aim in this paper is to present the reasons why I believe embryo adoption is illicit and unlikely ever to be sanctioned by the Catholic Church. In addition, I will briefly consider the related question of the fate of the many cryopreserved embryos currently in storage.[1] We are facing a tragic situation. With more than a million human beings having been cryopreserved and suspended in the surreal wasteland of industrialized frozen orphanages, there is a strong desire to address a situation that is radically unjust. The large number of supernumerary embryos on ice creates significant pressure to discern the moral lines, especially as the numbers in the United States continue to increase each year. That sense of urgency itself, however, can end up being misdirected if it is not checked and regulated. The crux of the urgency is not, What should we be doing with all the frozen embryos? but rather, Why are we allowing the grave injustice of producing and freezing

---

1. This chapter is based on the following works: John Haas and Tadeusz Pacholczyk, "Moral Contraindications to the Adoption of Abandoned, Frozen Human Embryos," *Linacre Quarterly* 90.2 (May 2023): 139–144, doi: 10.1177/00243639231165252; Tadeusz Pacholczyk, "Some Moral Contraindications to Embryo Adoption," in *Human Embryo Adoption: Biotechnology, Marriage, and the Right to Life*, ed. Thomas V. Berg and Edward J. Furton (Philadelphia: National Catholic Bioethics Center, 2006), 37–53; and Tadeusz Pacholczyk, "Frozen Embryo Adoptions Are Morally Objectionable," in *The Catholic Citizen: Debating the Issues of Justice*, ed. Kenneth D. Whitehead (South Bend, IN: St. Augustine Press, 2004), 84–101.

human beings to continue unabated in the first place?[2] I would suggest that it is more important to focus our sense of urgency on shutting down the assembly line production of human beings that is occurring in every major metropolitan area in the United States, rather than on trying to legitimize embryo rescue.

Each of these ensnared human embryos is a being with full dignity and human rights. If we can agree that there is no licit way to resolve this injustice, we will also recognize how these kinds of acts result in permanent negative consequences. Of course, we would like to be able to avoid any such permanent negative consequences, so advocates of embryo adoption attempt to offer a so-called rescue solution for those who were unjustly created via in vitro fertilization (IVF). But certain kinds of actions, like IVF, are so disordered at the core of the choice being made that they result in a situation where many of the consequences not only are extremely serious but are, morally speaking, likely to be incapable of being reversed. Gravely immoral acts tend to play out that way. To consider a particular example, once an act of adultery has been committed, followed by divorce and destruction of a particular family, the complex web of delicate interpersonal relationships cannot be restored to their former innocent state. Or once an act of abortion has been chosen and completed, the life that was ended cannot be brought back. I believe that engendering frozen embryos through IVF results in similar irreversible damage and that the moral impropriety of embryo rescue is a manifestation of the core grave moral disorder that is operative in these situations.

The key questions under consideration revolve around the final step of the IVF process, which involves embryo implantation attempts: (1) whether transferring one or several of those embryos into the mother's own uterus raises fundamental moral concerns, and (2) whether transferring one or several of them into the womb of another woman, either before or after cryopreservation, raises fundamental moral concerns. Here I will focus primarily on heterologous embryo transfer (transfer to the womb of a woman who is not the genetic mother), as my intention is to morally

---

2. Tadeusz Pacholczyk, "Germany and Italy Have Done It—Shouldn't We?," *Making Sense of Bioethics* 42 (December 2008): 1–2.

evaluate embryo adoption. However, because the moral questions surrounding homologous embryo transfer (husband and wife using their own embryos rather than the embryos of others) are relevant as well, they will also be addressed in context.

Arriving at moral conclusions when facing circumstances involving cryopreserved embryos can be challenging. As we seek to evaluate these matters, I think it is helpful to begin by considering the odd character of encountering human embryos outside the body, that is, extracorporeal embryos. Today we find ourselves in the strikingly unnatural situation of routinely handling human embryos in sterile laboratory settings, far removed from a woman's womb. It is not uncommon to come across a scanning electron micrograph of an early human embryo sitting on the point of a needle. Fifty years ago, such a photo would have been unthinkable. When we see pictures of an eight-cell human embryo sitting on the point of a sewing needle or of a slightly older human embryo of a few hundred cells at the blastocyst stage, only five or six days old, it is apparent that, in some important moral sense, we are not meant to see human embryos in this manner.

Our actions of visualizing them, whether through microscopy or other means, should help trigger the awareness that we are now operating in an inappropriate context, one that potentially involves enormous boundary transgressions and grave ethical violations. By splaying out these very young human bodies, so far removed from the nurturing, sheltered protection of the maternal body, and transposing them into a commercial or research setting, we open the door to their being manhandled, manipulated, flash frozen and exploited in countless unjust ways. The problem is an enormous one today, as the infertility industry in the United States and abroad expands its lucrative business model, largely devoid of any meaningful ethical oversight. We cannot avoid confronting the radically abnormal circumstances in which the human embryo has become inextricably lodged because of the IVF process.

Eric Cohen, who often writes about issues of technology and society, offers some trenchant observations about the peculiarity of extracorporeal embryonic life: "How are we to reason rightly about the human embryo, especially the early stage embryo outside the human body so severed as it is from its natural human contacts?" He then cites an article published by Yuval Levin in the first issue of the *New Atlantis*:

Part 2: Objections to Embryo Adoption

We look at this creature, which has been manufactured, molded, examined, and up to a certain point developed under the lights of the laboratory. It is growing but can only grow so far without further biotechnical intervention. It is living but only because the scientists have created it artificially. It is human to the extent that our humanity is in our genes and our potential. It is useful as a resource for medical research, but would develop into a mature human adult if implanted into the body of a woman and permitted to grow. What in the world are we supposed to do with this thing? How is ethics supposed to serve us in this circumstance?[3]

Having crossed the Rubicon, we suddenly find ourselves in an unfamiliar, even surreal setting. In considering the embryo in this new and entirely unnatural venue, we face a vexing challenge when it comes to resolving ethical questions pertaining to embryo adoption. Cohen continues, "With IVF, we created human embryos outside the body—by uniting sperm and egg in the laboratory—bringing the very earliest stages of embryological development to new light. The significance of doing so is something we have barely begun to fathom; it is a boundary we crossed with little forethought and little reflection; and it may turn out to be a profound turning point in the history of human life and human culture. All the absurdity, all our dilemmas stem from this new reality."[4] Hence, we find ourselves grappling with completely novel questions, like the permissibility of embryo adoption, arising directly out of monumental boundary transgressions. By dissociating the gametic generative powers of man and woman from the setting of marital intimacy and transposing them into the setting of the laboratory or clinic, we have entered highly unfamiliar terrain.

I will argue herein that embryo implantation *as a form of pregnancy initiation* constitutes an intrinsic evil because of the instrumentalization and misuse of the goods of marriage when a woman is made pregnant using an IVF-derived embryo, apart from a unifying marital act with her husband. As an exceptionless norm, this means that under no circumstances would

---

3. Yuval Levin, "The Paradox of Conservative Bioethics: Taboos, Democracy, and the Politics of Biology," *New Atlantis* 1 (Spring 2003), cited in Eric Cohen, "Of Embryos and Empire: What the Embryo Debate Can Teach Us about American Civilization," *New Atlantis* 2 (Summer 2003): 12.
4. Cohen, "Embryos and Empire," 11.

embryo implantation, as a way of initiating pregnancy, ever be morally permissible, regardless of motivating factors or good intentions.

A brief personal story may help launch a discussion of both the natural law aspects and the marital aspects of this important moral question. Years ago, I was talking with a Catholic friend, a thoughtful and reflective scientist and father of six. Not being a bioethicist himself, he inquired rather out of the blue, "What about the morality of embryo adoption?" In reply, I asked him to ponder the possibility on a more personal level by asking him directly about his wife: "Well, how would you feel if Janet were implanted with somebody else's embryo?" After hesitating for a moment to ponder the question, he offered an insightful reply: "Well, she should get pregnant only through me." He seemed intuitively to grasp the importance of the marital covenant that bound him and his wife together, and the exclusivity implied within that covenant, hinting at a root problem with engaging or calling forth her gestative powers in a manner apart from marital acts with him.

His answer struck me as touching on something vitally important, if not key, to the discussion. On some level, there appears to be a violation of the root exclusivity that stands at the core of marriage—and a violation of the meaning of fatherhood and motherhood—in the proposal to sanction embryo adoption. His response spoke to the need to safeguard marital exclusivity in all its depth and implied that embryo adoption involves a failure to respect the spousal orientation of human procreative-generative gifts, including gestation and the state of pregnancy itself, all of which are so intrinsically a part of the marital state.

Along this same line of analysis, Brian Caulfield refers to a forceful comment from a Catholic woman to the effect that, although she was unpersuaded by the arguments against embryo adoption, "she did admit that opening her womb to a life produced by strangers was not what she had in mind when she took her marriage vows."[5] Her comment echoes the same basic concern in this debate, namely, that, on some level, a violation of marriage and of motherhood necessarily transpires in the decision to pursue heterologous embryo transfer. I am convinced that these kinds of primary intuitions about violations of marriage and parenthood merit further

---

5. Brian Caulfield, "Where Do Frozen Embryos Belong?," *Human Life Review* 27.3 (Summer 2001): 11.

scrutiny to help unveil and explicate the fundamental moral objectionability of human embryo adoption.

I have previously argued that the notion of procreation, understood in a full sense, involves a broad reality that should acknowledge the full generative powers of the woman, including gestation. This refers to *begetting or procreating children* in the inclusive sense of the entire act of marital self-giving, with its corresponding pregnancy and gestation, leading up to and culminating in childbirth. This refers to something that extends well beyond the physical act of intercourse of husband and wife, well beyond the mere generation of an embryonic human.

This view has been misunderstood by some as suggesting that procreation is somehow incomplete until gestation has concluded or birth occurs. My suggestion that the procreative unity or generative continuum is important to the moral analysis should not be confused with a position suggesting that the coming into being of an embryo, that is, the creation of new life, is not a discrete or punctual occurrence. As Rev. Thomas Williams correctly notes, "Since being and nonbeing are mutually exclusive, procreation is necessarily and essentially punctual."[6]

I am arguing that, while we recognize that the nature of embryo creation is punctual, it should not be misconstrued in a way that would allow us to completely reduce the complex and nuanced reality of human procreation to the mere joining of a sperm to an egg or the combining of pronuclei or some other related punctual notion, because to do so fails to acknowledge the broader reality (moral and otherwise) of the human procreative continuum and the singular interconnectedness of maternal and fetal life as constituted by pregnancy and gestation in all its fulness and glory.

Hence, we might say that a proper understanding of the term *procreation* must extend beyond the biological events of fertilization and take into consideration the entire process of *pro*-creation, or that which is done *on behalf of* the creation of a new child through conjugal acts of self-giving love. In other words, a more expansive grasp of the process of procreation, which properly construes implantation and gestation, is required if we are going to properly appreciate its broader meaning and richness.

---

6. Thomas D. Williams, "Heterologous Embryo Transfer and the Meaning of 'Becoming a Mother,'" in Berg and Furton, *Human Embryo Adoption*, 243.

Some authors claim that embryo adoption has practically nothing to do with procreation. They argue that the embryo in the deep freeze represents a post-procreative reality and that the procreative step occurred when sperm and egg were joined together in the clinic. But to declare that the procreative act is de facto completed in vitro is not correct. IVF may be a *creative* act, in the sense of creating something new, but it is not genuinely *procreative*, because procreation, in the full and proper sense, always and uniquely derives from conjugal acts. In the final analysis, when speaking of IVF, one is referring to an *alternative* to the procreative act. When referencing the case of fertilization in vitro, one might say that the procreative act itself has not actually been initiated, since a substitution for that act has instead taken place—one capable of engendering life in a technical sense that is far removed from the procreative order. I would argue that embryo adoption likewise involves an alternative kind of action from procreation, as the powers of the human procreative order are partially engaged to achieve the pregnant state apart from the concrete acts of marital intimacy which need to serve as the necessary precondition to, and setting for, that state.

Procreation, in this broad context, includes the inscribed intentionality of the conjugal act up to its implied finality at birth and encompasses all the stages of pregnancy. The gestational aspect of pregnancy should not be misconstrued as a kind of superaddition to procreation, an incidental form of nurturing or fostering which happens as a post-procreative reality; it is, rather, an integral and deeply expressive manifestation of human procreation-begetting itself. This understanding of procreation as a broad process that includes gestation-pregnancy does not imply in any way that women who miscarry do not procreate. If a woman conceives but only goes partway through the pregnancy before the child dies of natural causes, she undoubtedly participated in the beautiful procreation of a new life that regrettably failed to achieve its natural finality by coming to term in the birth of her child. Prior to the miscarriage, the couple certainly achieved another important finality, namely, that of engendering a new human being, a child of their own, deserving of full respect, esteem, and love during all stages of his or her life.

As a corollary, I would offer the simple observation that the separation of child from mother at birth constitutes a significant point of inflection. The procreative-gestative course has ended, and through the process of parturition, the infant is born and the mother is no longer pregnant. *Birth constitutes a significant boundary where procreation-gestation transitions into a new reality. In other words, birth is a threshold where something comes to an end and something else begins, as the biological unity of mother and child is severed and a new developmental stage ensues.*

Some have asserted that no Church document supports the notion of birth as a significant boundary in the work of procreation. Whether we can find any particular Church document that supports such a claim is not essential to the question of whether reason itself can discern a significant threshold in the birth of a child at the conclusion of gestation. In fact, reason identifies a profound threshold there, with the newborn now manifesting a radical degree of independence because of his or her bodily separation from the former state of internal intimacy and intertwining with maternal support systems, even as new external supports for the life and integrity of the child become possible, such as breast feeding. The generative continuum implied by the internal character of maternal-fetal gestation transitions to an external developmental continuum for the newly born individual.

In terms of magisterial documents, some hints of guiding principles for addressing the moral issues involved in embryo adoption may be discernible in *Gaudium et spes*, the Second Vatican Council's *Pastoral Constitution on the Church in the Modern World*. In paragraph 51, when discussing objective criteria governing decisions about married love and the transmission of life, reference is made to "criteria that respect the total meaning of mutual self-giving and human procreation."[7] While this passage from *Gaudium et spes* was clearly not written with the question of embryo adoption in mind, it seems to suggest a general insight pertaining to marital love and life: those actions which are compatible with married love and responsible procreation will integrally respect the "total meaning of mutual self-giving," while actions that invoke or impinge upon married love and the transmission of life, but that prescind from or otherwise attempt to circumvent the total meaning of mutual self-giving inscribed within the conjugal act, are likely to be morally suspect.

---

7. Vatican Council II, *Gaudium et spes* (December 7, 1965), n. 51, cited in *Catechism of the Catholic Church*, 2nd ed. (Washington, DC: US Conference of Catholic Bishops / Libreria Editrice Vaticana, 2018 update), n. 2368. The Vatican's official English translation references "objective standards" that "preserve the full sense of mutual self-giving and human procreation."

In the case of a wife, she is capacitated to conceive and give birth to a child—capacitated to enter into the pregnant state—through conjugal acts with her husband. In his apostolic letter *Mulieris dignitatem*, Pope St. John Paul II noted how pregnancy is properly linked to the marital union and to the mutual self-giving of spouses: "In this openness, in conceiving and giving birth to a child, the woman 'discovers herself through a sincere gift of self.' The gift of interior readiness to accept the child and bring it into the world is linked to the marriage union, which ... should constitute a special moment in the mutual self-giving both by the woman and the man."[8] Hence, there is a special kind of receptivity and self-giving implied in a woman's fertility and in her nurturing capacity through pregnancy, and that special feminine receptivity, I would argue, ends up being reoriented and disturbed at a fundamental level through an act of embryo adoption. In other words, embryo adoption violates the language of a woman's body, because the very mode of self-giving written into her body becomes subverted as she dissociates gestation-pregnancy from marital self-giving and unity.

Let me offer a parallel example to shed light on the kind of interconnectedness of meaning I am seeking to capture in this discussion. I have always been troubled, along with many others who reflect on the importance of understanding human origins correctly, by the tendency of some to propose that once sperm and egg have joined and a human embryo has been engendered in the fallopian tube, a woman remains nonpregnant until such a point as that embryo attaches itself to the maternal body in one way or the other, whether implanting in the uterus or ectopically elsewhere. This claim is a fallacy, given that the mother is *with child* even prior to any implantation event, and she is relationally in a new space, because she no longer subsists alone in the particular quadrangle of space and time delineated by her postcoital bodily reality. She is now intimately sharing that space with another being who is as human as she is, albeit in a far more vulnerable and dependent posture. This willingness to constrict the notion of pregnancy around the implantation event, as we are aware from discussions surrounding the morning-after pill, is even used to foster faulty moral analyses and draw incorrect moral lines by suggesting that actions directed against the unimplanted embryo are contraceptive rather than abortive in essence.

Returning to embryo adoption, I am convinced that constricting the notion of procreation-generation to a kind of punctual joining of sperm

---

8. John Paul II, *Mulieris dignitatem* (August 15, 1988), n. 18.

and egg may likewise be used to justify moral mistakes. By failing to grasp the procreative unity of human engendering, and the singularly unified reality of the generative continuum, we risk fragmenting the clear inner signification of the coming together of man and woman, in their highly particularized reproductive structures, and their bodily and spiritual complementarity, which enables them to bring forth and care for children. By reducing the command to "be fruitful and multiply" to a kind of one-and-done view, followed by a series of substitutable and putatively nonessential steps that may be performed on embryos once they have arrived on the scene, we have already stepped away from the proper perspective and context. This disintegrative tendency, clearly motivated by the very best of intentions when it comes to a desire to rescue embryos, draws us away from discerning the inherent and required interconnectedness of conception and gestation and from properly embracing the telos of the procreative unity and the generative continuum inscribed into sexuality at its most core and foundational level.

As an initial consideration, I would suggest that the proper mode for a woman to open her womb to new life always occurs indirectly, that is to say, through the mediation of her husband. The wife does not open her womb directly to life but opens her body up to her husband, and through this uniquely marital action, her womb is fittingly unsealed and rendered receptive to life. Implicit in the proposal of those who favor embryo adoption is the idea that a woman has the right to offer her body, or more specifically, her womb, to gestate an embryo. Yet I would argue that a woman does not possess this putative right to turn over her gestative powers to an extrinsic embryo in this manner, since those powers do not in fact belong to her alone, or even to her and her husband alone, but to their marital union, the essential properties of which stand outside the determination of the participants. Looked at from a theological perspective, married life in its procreative and gestative potential involves three persons: husband, wife, and God, and the structures that God has inscribed into the bodies of the man and the woman and into their shared communion must objectively inform the analysis of the morality of embryo adoption. Invoking these essential powers of the woman's body, including the state of becoming pregnant, is an action inherently and necessarily interwoven into the broader meaning and context of the marital act.

Sometimes it is noted that if a woman is free to offer a kidney to save the life of another, should she not likewise be able to offer her uterus in a type of donation to save the life of another? The answer is that these two actions are not directly comparable, because uteri have an orientation toward individuals of the next generation and, in this way, are distinct in character from organs, likes hearts and livers, that have an orientation toward individuals of the present generation and their organismic continuity and homeostasis. This orientation of the reproductive organs toward the next generation implies that their functions are discernibly tied in with the above-mentioned shared communion of spouses.

To put it another way, we ought to be able to recognize, in the human engendering of offspring, a generative and procreative continuum: a conjugal act occurs, maybe a few days later fertilization will follow as the embryo arises, and six days later implantation occurs, so that nine months later one anticipates the birth of the child. The gestational reality of pregnancy is quintessentially nested within this generative continuum.

I posit that the extrinsic implantation of a human embryo as a means of initiating a pregnancy cuts across the grain of the generative order by treating the state of being gravid as if it were a separable entity able to be extricated from the unified reality of spousal procreative intimacy, and that such a proposal is, at its core, unacceptable, even for praiseworthy motives and ends, such as attempting to rescue or save embryos from the unjust imprisonment of cryopreservation. The desired outcome or end state is certainly good, that is, the offering of life and growth to young humans trapped in liquid nitrogen, but the means chosen to realize those good ends appear to involve grave violations of marriage and parenthood and are, therefore, intrinsically problematic. As Charles Robertson has summed it up, "The opponents of embryo rescue, on the other hand, see pregnancy as having specifically marital significance. They see pregnancy as belonging essentially to the procreative dimension of human sexuality and so rightfully willed only as the consequence of a marriage act."[9]

We may also approach the matter from a slightly different angle, noting that the implantation of extrinsic embryos into a woman's uterus stands outside the order of reason, because it engages a technical process, in substitution for the proper mode of invoking a woman's generative faculty,

---

9. Charles D. Robertson, "Generation, Gestation, and Birth: An Important Element in the Embryo Adoption Debate," *Linacre Quarterly* 85.1 (February 2018): 37, doi: 10.1177/0024363918756388.

through the expertise of the technician who is tasked to perform the physical action of inserting the embryo inside the woman. To suggest that this task of insertion could be adjusted so that the husband performed it in the place of the hired technician would not constitute any kind of authentic workaround to the fundamental ethical concern. The role of a husband is not to impregnate his wife in ways apart from personal acts of one-flesh union and marital intercourse. To sum up, then, the broad ethical concerns: a woman ought not freely direct, hand over, or share the potency of her gestative faculty with anyone apart from her spouse, so as to respect the exclusive and covenantal importance of the one-flesh communion with her husband and his generative faculty.

The invoking of the gestative faculty of a human being who is female, in order to be morally acceptable, will necessarily entail or presuppose vaginal intercourse between her and the male who is her spouse. In opting to receive an embryo into her body through embryo transfer, the woman chooses and intends to become pregnant apart from marital intimacy, and such a decision, I am convinced, stands as a root misappropriation of her generative faculty by fundamentally, albeit subtly, deflecting the telos of her uterine gestative capabilities. Rather than engaging her generative faculty in a manner compatible with its proper object, which would be vaginal intercourse with the male human being who is her husband, she turns to a third-party clinician who then acts upon her in a transitive way, invoking and activating elements of her generative capacity with his technical arts and causing a state of pregnancy within her. The clinician does not act in generative bodily communion with her as her husband would. This profound and radical difference, I believe, is of essential ethical significance.

Even husband and wife together are unable, morally speaking, to make decisions that invoke their procreative-gestative powers in ways that are dissociated from their intrinsic designs. For example, a husband and wife may not choose to introduce the sperm of the husband derived from masturbation into the wife's uterus using a catheter or cannula, even if they mutually agree that they would willingly raise any child conceived in this fashion.[10] The conception of a child, in this case, would not result from the

---

10. Congregation for the Doctrine of the Faith (CDF), *Donum vitae* (February 22, 1987), II.B.6.

marital act. Simply deciding together, in this delicate arena, is insufficient to overcome the inherently problematic character of the procedure, even though the child would be conceived in vivo and the gametes would be derived from the parents themselves. Mutually agreeing to the implantation of an extrinsic embryo could arguably represent a parallel situation. Even their shared decision and intention to do so, I would suggest, is unable to overcome or supplant the inherently problematic character of the procedure.

In a sense, then, a woman cannot consent to pregnancy directly. The state of being pregnant is not within her purview to directly consent to. Her consent is always indirect, because pregnancy is the seamless continuation of fertilization, to which she also consents indirectly whenever she consents to intimate sexual relations with her spouse. The previous choice or decision on the part of the woman in the form of consensual sexual relations should always include the implied consent to become pregnant, so that pregnancy becomes ultimately an expression not only of her own fruitfulness but also of the unity with, and fruitfulness of, her husband.

When we consider the procreative powers of a man or of a woman, we must be precise about what it is that we are referencing. The procreative powers of the man include his male ejaculatory powers, which may be invoked only by his wife through marital acts, precisely because, in complement to her, they are ordered and oriented toward opening her womb to new life. Any other modality of invoking these powers of his, for example, masturbation to enable artificial insemination, will be illicit.[11] When we speak about the procreative powers of the woman, these include her ability to receive the seed, the ejaculatory gift of her spouse, exclusively through a marital act and in a way that is open to the reception of new life through conception and the resultant pregnancy. Her fruitfulness, her ability to become pregnant, is accessed or realized only through this initiating procreative moment of bodily sharing with her spouse.

For a woman to misappropriate her generative faculty through embryo adoption is to violate the meaning of her motherhood as well as the

---

11. CDF, *Donum vitae*, introduction, 5: "Human procreation requires on the part of the spouses responsible collaboration with the fruitful love of God; the gift of human life must be actualized in marriage through the specific and exclusive acts of husband and wife, in accordance with the laws inscribed in their persons and in their union."

Part 2: Objections to Embryo Adoption

fatherhood of her husband, constituting an act contrary to human reason. Our human generative potential is properly aligned with the order of reason only when a woman's gestative potential is uniquely initiated by a marital act with her husband, thereby respecting and safeguarding the human generative continuum in its essential integrity.

If we argue that human embryo transfer involves an intrinsically disordered kind of an action, does this suggest a somewhat inferior or defective status for the extracorporeally produced embryo, as some have suggested this analysis would imply?[12] It does not imply an inferior status based on the essence of the embryo, but it implies a diminished status in the sense that a grave injustice has been carried out against him or her by the initial action of creating him or her extracorporeally, creating a subclass—those humans who we treat by a clearly different metric in our willingness to freeze them and trap them in a static state. Humans are not the kind of creatures who ever ought to be created in glassware and frozen away, and any time we act unjustly toward them by treating them as unequal to ourselves in this manner, we express our willingness to diminish them and lessen their status, and such injustices need to be categorically resisted. The moral impossibility of transferring such extracorporeally produced embryos into women's uteri itself suggests that, were we to go ahead and perform such transfers, we would be carrying out an additional injustice toward those embryos and diminishing them further, as counterintuitive as that might seem on first consideration.

How could it be the case that one shows greater respect for the extracorporeally produced embryo by not transferring him or her into a woman's uterus than by carrying out such a transfer? I would suggest one objectively manifests greater respect for the extracorporeally produced human embryo by declining to engage in steps, procedures, or processes that constitute objectifying interventions, and any time we pull the embryo further away from the unique procreative continuum or procreative unity that he or she is properly entitled to, we extend such objectifying tendencies and fail to respect the human embryo's properly deserved state and status. In other

---

12. Edward J. Furton, "Embryo Adoption Reconsidered," in "Responses to *Dignitas Personae*: Part II of II," special issue, *National Catholic Bioethics Quarterly* 10.2 (Summer 2010): 337, doi: 10.5840/ncbq201010256.

words, we commit further wrongs against both mother and extracorporeal child (and against her husband) by insisting that the objective order of the woman's maternal generative powers and sexuality be contravened by initiating pregnancy through an ab extra implantation action.

Some have suggested that viewing the procreation of new life as having a broader intrinsic meaning than merely the act of fertilization implies that children conceived in vitro would be in some sense "partially procreated children," which they claim represents an "absurd situation."[13] Yet we must acknowledge that creating life outside its proper context does in fact result in an absurd situation whereby, for example, that new life ends up not in the nurturing body of his or her mother but in the deep freeze at the clinic; this in fact constitutes an absurd situation of the highest order and further implies a profound failure to achieve completion or realization of one's destiny—a kind of partial thrust or launch toward the fulness of human maturation, followed by a lockup. It would not be unreasonable to conclude that the absence of gestation, that is, the cryogenic imprisonment of the embryo, constitutes a kind of voided procreation whereby the full reproductive meaning of conception, gestation, and birth are profoundly torqued away from their intrinsic meaning, order, and realization.

Sometimes the argument is advanced that pregnancy is really a sophisticated form of nurturing rather than a part of procreation. If we may nurture a child who is not our own through breastfeeding, should we not be able to nurture an embryo that is not our own through pregnancy? But pregnancy and breastfeeding are two very different kinds of nurturing. Pregnancy signals and embodies a unique and exclusive relational bond between mother and child and is linked, in a discernible way, to the exclusive character of sexual self-giving between a man and a woman. Nursing a baby does not signal or embody that same unique relational exclusivity, since the procreative threshold of birth has now been crossed, and the baby's being out and away from his mother signals a new stage of availability for other relational encounters, including the encounter with other women who may serve as wet nurses. Drawing an analogy between the offering of one's uterus for embryo adoption to wet-nursing or other nurturing after birth "ultimately fails to recognize the radical interiority of 'two persons in one' that is

---

13. Williams, "Heterologous Embryo Transfer," 243.

Part 2: Objections to Embryo Adoption

integral to pregnancy, a seamless continuation of fertilization, in which the child 'feeds on and inside the mother's very substance.'"[14] So pregnancy is procreative and exclusive in its essential nature, while breastfeeding is not. In other words, pregnancy bespeaks the exclusive, relational language of human sexuality in a fundamentally different way than nursing does.

It may also be worthwhile to inquire whether there might be, on some occasions, a disordered dynamic that is operative in the scenario of embryo adoption. Is not there an important sense in which we are attempting to secure a child through embryo adoption as an end or a goal? The basic structure of marital sexuality embodies a very different end or goal. What one is willing or choosing to do, on a deeper level, nested within the marital bond, is not to seek a child as an end but rather to give oneself in totality to one's spouse in an act of complete openness, surrender, and donation of body and spirit. The inner meaning and language of human procreation is essentially one of total self-giving and only derivatively one of seeking or pursuing a baby. In other words, as the Congregation for the Doctrine of the Faith's 1987 document, *Donum vitae*, puts it, the spouses are meant to "cooperate as servants and not as masters in the work of the Creator."[15] Manually implanting embryos into uteri seems to invoke the manipulative dynamic of masters rather than servants within the delicate procreative arena of marriage, not unlike the dynamic which created the embryos in the first place through IVF. Serious concerns are thus raised by a procedure like embryo adoption that profoundly redirects, if not restructures, the sacred inner order of human procreation.

Pope Pius XII notes the intrinsic connection between conjugal love and procreation when he condemns the pursuit of either of these two realities in isolation from the other: "Never is it permissible to separate these different aspects so as to exclude positively either the aim of procreation or the conjugal relation."[16] Recognizing that the Holy Father was not addressing

---

14. Thomas K. Nelson, email to author, December 7, 2005.
15. CDF, *Donum vitae*, II.B.4.C.
16. Pius XII, Address to the Second World Congress on Fertility and Sterility, May 19, 1956, *Acta Apostolicae Sedis* 48 (1956): 470, quote translated in Donald P. Asci, *The Conjugal Act as Personal Act: A Study of the Catholic Concept of the Conjugal Act in the Light of Christian Anthropology* (San Francisco: Ignatius Press, 2002), 60.

embryo adoption in promulgating his insight, his words speak, nevertheless, to the problem of obviating the conjugal relation while pursuing a procreative aim or outcome. This pursuit of a procreative aim or outcome in strict separation from its required conjugal relation, as occurs in embryo adoption, does indeed seem to be incompatible with the inner order of marriage.

The restructuring of the inner order of human procreation that occurs during embryo adoption also has the effect of causing a profound rupture or fissure in parenthood. This fissure is introduced into both motherhood and fatherhood by virtue of the fact that embryo adoption fails fully to respect the exclusive nature of the couple's marital covenant and the exclusive reality implied by their conjugal union. A passage from *Donum vitae* stresses the profound exclusivity of parenthood in marriage: "The bond existing between husband and wife accords the spouses, in an objective and inalienable manner, the exclusive right to become father and mother solely through each other."[17] In other words, it is only in and through marriage, and specifically through the inherent unity of the marital act, that a man and a woman are capacitated to engender a child through each other.

The procreative expression on the part of the husband in marriage is much more limited than that available to his wife. This becomes especially manifest when considering embryo adoption, where a profound fissure is introduced into the proper order of fatherhood. In the general scheme of marriage under normal circumstances, the procreative expression afforded the man is uniquely manifested in and through the conjugal act, since this is the principal manner in which he becomes a full participant and partner in the pregnancy and gestation of his child. In the case of embryo implantation, however, the man's inner bodily connection to the gestating child through the conjugal act is systematically precluded. Under normal circumstances in married life, prior to the birth of a newborn, the father is incidental to practically everything except the conjugal act itself, while his wife does all the heavy lifting of undergoing significant bodily changes and carrying the pregnancy. In the case of embryo adoption, meanwhile, the man becomes entirely incidental to the whole nine-month-long prenatal enterprise. His one, all-important link to his child, the causal link through spousal bodily union, has now been severed. In this foundational sense, both fatherhood

---

17. CDF, *Donum vitae*, II.A.2.

Part 2: Objections to Embryo Adoption

and being a husband are fundamentally violated by the decision to adopt and implant a frozen embryo into his wife's uterus.

One may ask, If traditional postnatal adoption of an infant does not raise any moral problems, then what is the key difference with embryo adoption that renders it morally problematic? In postnatal adoption, of course, a pregnancy is not involved. By embracing an infant or child born of a different biological mother, one is *becoming an adoptive mother or father*, which is distinct from *becoming a mother or father* in the categorical sense. One is not violating any of the goods of procreation by adopting an already born child, because nobody needs to become pregnant and no uterine gestational steps are required for such an adoption to occur. No one is required to invoke their own procreative powers or transgress the exclusive marital meaning of their own bodies. In such an adoption, questions of respecting the generative continuum and the use of procreative faculties do not enter into the mix in any essential way. That is to say, there is no violation of the procreative goods entrusted to us by God. Hence, no intrinsic moral objection is discernible in the act of traditional adoption of a birthed child.

In embryo adoption, on the other hand, the woman pursues the role of gestational mother without having conceived that embryo through conjugal union with her husband. This is in actuality the essence of surrogacy, understood broadly, which violates the goods of motherhood and the goods of procreation by implanting an embryo generated extracorporeally into one's uterus. Embryo adoption thus raises the problem of a woman's misuse of her procreative powers as she pursues a kind of surrogacy or partial motherhood. Surrogacy, in the final analysis, is most essentially described by the decision of a woman to receive an embryo into her uterus in a way other than as a consequence of conjugal relations with her husband or with another man.

Surrogacy is sometimes argued to be intrinsically wrong because it can involve payment: a woman consents to gestate an embryo for a fee, and this kind of payment would comprise the essential evil of surrogacy. It has also been suggested that the idea of gestating an embryo on behalf of another person rather than for oneself constitutes the illicitness of surrogacy. In other words, it is the decision to gestate an embryo that one does not intend to raise as one's own child that would be morally problematic. Still others have suggested that the evil of surrogacy lies fundamentally in gestating any non-genetically related embryo, while gestating an embryo that is genetically related (e.g., derived from IVF) would not constitute surrogacy and might be licit. I would suggest, however, that surrogacy, in its morally problematic dimension, can be most amply categorized and analyzed as the choice to receive an embryo ab extra into one's uterus as a means of initiating pregnancy, that is, an embryo which is not the direct fruit of a particular act of sexual self-giving between a man and a woman. This seems to represent surrogacy at its most fundamental level.

In other words, a surrogate mother becomes such through an improper agent or means, through the persons or techniques involved in reproductive technology. One should not attempt to become a mother in such a semi- or pseudo-procreative manner; one should not make use of this special part of marital exclusivity outside its proper and reserved context. Surrogacy fails to respect the integrity of marriage by commandeering the privileged realities of conception and gestation that are uniquely ordered to arise from those exclusive acts of freely chosen conjugal self-giving between husband and wife.

The ramifications of this line of reasoning can be illuminated by considering a hypothetical scenario where a husband and wife decide to advert to IVF in the face of apparent infertility. Suppose they show up at an infertility clinic one day to donate their gametes, their egg and sperm cells. The technicians join their gametes together and place them in growth medium in a petri dish. The couple returns home to allow the resultant embryos to grow for a few days. The wife then comes back to the clinic to have some of the embryos implanted. In the meantime, however, she has been thinking about what she and her husband did earlier, leading her to the point of regretting ever having generated the embryos in the first place. What should she do now? Should she allow the technician to implant the embryos into her? I believe that the morally proper step for her would be a rather radical one: to leave the clinic without implanting the embryos, even though they are in fact her own children. By this bold step, she would put the brakes on an intrinsically disordered chain of events that she and her husband had initiated and step away from a second evil act, namely, the act of becoming a surrogate mother to the couple's own embryos generated earlier at the clinic.

Overall, then, I would argue that a double violation is discernible whenever one becomes pregnant through IVF, even if it involves homologous IVF. The first violation flows from allowing one's gametes to be used generatively outside the body and apart from the conjugal act. The second transgression occurs at the point of embryo transfer by attempting to become a gestational mother without being properly capacitated for that role in mutually consenting and unifying sexual relations with her spouse.

Part 2: Objections to Embryo Adoption

I would conclude that both heterologous and homologous embryo transfer constitute intrinsic evils and cannot, therefore, ever be licitly chosen.

The designs over motherhood and fatherhood as given to us by God always imply an act of total, mutual, and exclusive self-giving between spouses. This is inscribed within the structure of the conjugal act, which is that special and unique human act that affords the necessary precondition to capacitate a woman and a man to each become parents through the other. Any attempt to become parents by invoking the procreative-gestative powers of their bodies outside the specific setting of committed marital intimacy represents a violation of their gift of mutually committed sexuality and a violation of its intrinsic order and meaning as established by God in the beginning. Because embryo adoption would always involve the husband and wife in a transgression of this nature, I conclude that it cannot be morally licit.

At this point, it is worth reiterating the broader perspective, namely, how human persons, being made in the image and likeness of God, are crafted for profound and fruitful interpersonal communion in a manner that elevates and changes the meaning of our human sexuality from being simply biological to unitive. Human sexuality cannot be exclusively framed in reproductive terms nor completely paralleled to that of animals, so while it will be allowable to use, for example, artificial insemination with livestock and pets, with humans it will not. The relational meaning and the dimension of interpersonal communion inscribed in our sexuality have powerful and important moral implications in humans and extend the umbrella of our sexuality into a different sphere.

Careful reflection is needed to grasp these unitive, personal dimensions of sexuality and to avoid improperly reducing them to raw bodily or instinctual occurrences. Perhaps *Donum vitae* puts it most clearly: "God, who is love and life, has inscribed in man and woman the vocation to share in a special way in his mystery of personal communion and in his work as Creator and Father. For this reason marriage possesses specific goods and values in its union and in procreation which cannot be likened to those existing in lower forms of life. Such values and meanings are of the personal order and determine from the moral point of view the meaning and limits of artificial interventions on procreation and on the origin of human life."[18]

---

18. CDF, *Donum vitae*, introduction, 3.

It should also be noted that there are substantive counterarguments in the practical realm to embryo adoption. First, it is noteworthy that the action of thawing out embryos is not a risk-free undertaking, and there remain, even with improvements in freezing and thawing technologies, significant dangers in terms of embryonic demise during the process. During thawing only 65–70 percent of embryos survive, and many are damaged by the process, with only about 30–35 percent surviving with all cells being viable.[19] Hence, the intentional decision to subject humans stored in the deep freeze to defrosting appears to constitute a disproportionate bodily risk for them.

Second, there is the serious concern that standardizing the practice of adopting human embryos would encourage the production of more embryos in the future, because those very clinics where IVF is being done, and where new embryos are being created, will be able to say, Now we don't have to be too concerned about producing as many extra embryos as we wish, because there will always be some couples willing to adopt any that are left over. This offers the clinics something of an excuse to continue their current immoral practices, if not to expand them. In other words, embryo adoption threatens to involve those who are adopting the embryos in a type of complicity with evil. From a business point of view, one could extend this scenario a step further: clinics might be tempted to set up a two-tiered marketing strategy to assist infertile customers. One tier would involve offering standard IVF technologies. The second tier would involve a potentially more economical alternative: for those who did not feel the strong need for a child of their own flesh and blood, they could be offered the opportunity to adopt a premade embryo from another couple. Maintaining a stockpile of sufficiently diverse human embryos to allow for the choosing of desired characteristics could further improve the customer experience and the lucrativeness of the business model.

I have attempted to offer arguments identifying the intrinsic evil of human embryo adoption as an instrumentalization and misuse of goods proper to marriage and procreation. These goods, and the goods of parenthood itself, are intended to be accessed uniquely and exclusively through the conjugal acts of husband and wife with each other.

---

19. Peter A. Clark, "Cryopreserved Embryos: A Catholic Alternative to Embryonic Stem Cell Research and Adoption," in *Embryonic Stem Cells: Basic Biology to Bioengineering*, ed. Michael S. Kallos (London: IntechOpen, 2011), 36.

Part 2: Objections to Embryo Adoption

Christopher Reilly has argued against my position by noting, "Some Catholic thinkers claim that saving the life of a cryopreserved (frozen) human embryo through adoption is an immoral act, maybe even 'inherently evil.' What they are proposing, however, is a hopelessly unreasonable conflict among the goods of life, mercy, and marriage that elevates juridical logic over central Christian teachings."[20] Rather than juridical logic, I would suggest that my view represents ethical logic. His claim is further flawed, because identifying those actions that ought never to be chosen by Christians is a helpful and eminently reasonable activity, precisely because it allows us not only to recognize and protect the truth but also to become conformed to the inner logic of moral order that permeates all authentically Christian teaching. The assiduous defense of that inner logic, and the consequent conforming of one's life and choices, offers the essential path to authentic human liberation, while safeguarding the great goods of life, mercy, and marriage.

In another place, Reilly mentions "the call to mercy and sacrifice for the sake of the other. Consider that very few moralists would argue that it is fundamentally unacceptable for a person to put their very life in danger to save the life of someone else. If risking one's life can be acceptable to save another, why should we consider it a sin for a mother to offer her womb to save an embryonic person?"[21] One of the flaws in this argument revolves around the claim that one is saving a life in embryo adoption, since the embryo is not imminently facing death and actually remains quite alive while in the deep freeze—living, in fact, for potentially a very long time in that state, even for much longer than the lifespan of a typical human adult.

An important point must be borne in mind with respect to these conclusions. The immorality of embryo adoption says nothing about the blessing that any child born by this technology represents. Children who come into the world are always a gift and a blessing, no matter how they arrive, whether by IVF, by embryo adoption, or even by cloning. The child is always an innocent bystander in the deployment of these technologies,

---

20. Christopher M. Reilly, "Rescuing the Good Samaritan in Embryo Adoption and Beyond," *National Catholic Bioethics Quarterly* 20.3 (Autumn 2020): 487–488, doi: 10.5840/ncbq202020345.
21. Christopher M. Reilly, "Embryo Adoption: A Radically Counter-Cultural Act of Mercy," *Dignitas* 27.1–4 (Spring–Winter 2020): 30.

and absolutely no fault or blame of any sort can be imputed to the child. All responsibility is properly attributable only to the parents and other parties involved in forming a deliberative decision to exploit these technologies.

A deeper difficulty relating to the choice to use these technologies lies in our misunderstanding of God's laws and mercy. I have had the opportunity to meet children who have been born by various reproductive technologies, including artificial insemination and IVF, and most recently, I met a beautiful little girl born from embryo adoption. What is most difficult for many people to begin to fathom is how one could affirm that it would be a better state of affairs if that beautiful, joyful child had never been born; that is to say, we seem to have to conclude that if we affirm that the parents should have chosen to follow the moral path and never done IVF or artificial insemination or embryo adoption (if it is correct that embryo adoption is immoral), then we also would have to affirm that this wonderful child should never have become a part of our lives.

First, God can and does bring good out of our mistakes, even if this never justifies our sins or errors. While a child born out of rape or adultery is still an infinitely valuable human person made in the image of God, this cannot ever be used to justify rape or adultery. The proper response here does seem to lie in the hidden and mysterious affirmation that a better state of affairs will ultimately prevail whenever we choose to pursue the right and the good rather than to violate the moral law and pursue our own will. Although certain goods that we might be attracted to initially will not be ours if we decline to violate the moral law, other goods of a different and more profound kind will in fact accrue to us whenever we resolve to embrace the liberating fulness of moral truth. We sometimes suppose that we have a grasp on what constitutes the best state of affairs for ourselves when it comes to moral decision-making, even though our vantage point is so drastically curtailed when compared with God's. It is further curtailed by being tilted toward ego and our own desires and willfulness through the harsh and unrelenting reality of original sin within us. While it is the better part of wisdom to submit ourselves to the One who has a broader and more complete plan for all things, including a plan for the suffering and trials we may experience such as infertility, each of us has, nevertheless, succumbed at times to the temptation to appropriate the decision about good and evil to ourselves and our desires.

What, then, is to be done with the multitude of embryos that remain held in cryostasis in fertility clinics and laboratories throughout the world?

Part 2: Objections to Embryo Adoption

What other options might exist for the disposition of frozen human embryos? A simple answer to this question seems elusive. As a well-known passage from *Donum vitae* described the matter, "In consequence of the fact that they have been produced *in vitro*, those embryos which are not transferred into the body of the mother and are called 'spare' are exposed to an absurd fate, with no possibility of their being offered safe means of survival which can be licitly pursued."[22] Notwithstanding the contextual particulars of this passage—that it was not written to directly address the question of embryo adoption—it is, nevertheless, clear that extracorporeal human embryos raise profound difficulties in terms of deciding their fate.

One solution that has been proposed is to allow the liquid nitrogen that is sustaining the frozen embryos to evaporate, so they would end up thawing and dying a natural death. The argument is sometimes offered that the liquid nitrogen may be analogous to the instrumentation and tubes which are sometimes used in medical settings at the end of a person's life. In a traditional moral analysis, these means of support can become disproportionate, or extraordinary, when death is imminent. In the case of the embryo, it is argued that death is very imminent if the liquid nitrogen is removed; in other words, the liquid nitrogen may be serving as a disproportionate means of life support that would not be morally obligatory. Hence, one might be able to stop replenishing the liquid nitrogen, so that the levels would gradually decrease through the natural process of evaporation. Finally, the embryos would warm up to room temperature, thaw out, and expire.

This analogy between liquid nitrogen and extraordinary means of support, however, does not seem to be compelling, because the early embryos are actually destined, in the right environment, not for immediate death but for growth and development into adults. The proper environment simply happens to be unavailable to them. Moreover, the claim that liquid nitrogen is disproportionate seems dubious. As I have pointed out elsewhere,

> In fact, however, the decision to continue cryopreserving an embryo in liquid nitrogen is not likely an instance of using extraordinary means, since the burden and costs associated with taking care of embryonic children in this way are actually minimal. When we have children, we have a duty to clothe, feed, care for, and educate them, all of which costs plenty of money. When our children are frozen, we don't need to clothe, feed, or educate

---

22. CDF, *Donum vitae*, I.5.

them; our care for them can only be expressed by paying the bill each month to replenish the liquid nitrogen in their storage tanks. This way of caring for our children is obviously unusual, but it does not seem morally extraordinary in terms of achieving the desired end of safeguarding their physical integrity.[23]

Hence, the analogy with extraordinary means is arguably an untenable one. Moreover, to call their death natural when we choose not to replenish an easily available, low-burden means may instead be a euphemistic description of what could more properly be characterized as neglect of our offspring.

Perhaps the closest we can come to finding a morally acceptable path would be to maintain those embryos that currently exist in the frozen state, while ensuring that no further embryos are produced and stored in this way in the future. With the passage of time, the currently frozen embryos should become less and less viable and eventually decay of their own accord, without our directly participating in their death. One could even make use of nonhuman primate embryos to experimentally determine how rapidly primate embryos tend to decay in frozen storage. Perhaps after a few hundred or a few thousand years, all the embryos would be unable to be thawed, since their lives would have ended spontaneously during their time in their frozen orphanages. This, at least, would not involve us in the direct moral agency of actively terminating their lives by withdrawing what is keeping them alive, namely, the liquid nitrogen, and might be somewhat analogous to a natural process of aging. It also leaves open the opportunity for rescue if another means, such as an artificial uterus or incubator, becomes available in the future, though such a development would likely raise further moral questions and complications.

All of these difficult considerations remind us how the initial decision to violate the moral law through IVF invariably has grievous repercussions that lead us into the kinds of quandaries considered here, where there is no easy way out. One might say that the relational rupture caused by IVF is so severe that it cannot be reversed. The birth of a baby is a kind of relational rupture that cannot be physically reversed. Similarly, the generation of extracorporeal embryos through IVF results in a relational rupture that does not seem to be resolvable by man through his own efforts. As emphasized earlier, certain evil choices have permanent consequences that cannot

---

23. Tadeusz Pacholczyk, "What Should We Do with the Frozen Embryos?," Making Sense of Bioethics 48 (June 2009): 1.

be undone. The frozen embryos stand as a sad and enduring testimony to the prior disordered decisions that have been made and are continuing to be made within our society. They represent something of a permanent scar marring the face of our times, inviting us to deeper and more circumspect moral reflection and resolve.

10

The Next Steps If Embryo Adoption Is Illicit

Irene Alexander

The authors of the preceding chapters of this volume have provided a compelling account of why embryo adoption is illicit. More precisely, it is the act of artificially impregnating a woman, which is contrary to the natural moral order, and not the praiseworthy intention to save a human life, which defines the moral character of the practice and renders it an illicit one. One inevitably reaches this conclusion after reexamining the underlying rationale in *Dignitatis personae* and *Donum vitae* on other artificial reproductive technologies, such as in vitro fertilization (IVF), artificial insemination, surrogacy, and the transfer of embryos for infertile couples (an embryo adoption of some kind), all of which were condemned in these two documents as either formally illicit or not ethically acceptable.

When moral theologians listen with care and renewed attention to the underlying rationale in these documents, a single common thread emerges: the reality of what I call conjugal agency, namely, that licit actions in reproductive bioethics must respect the role of the spouses in being agent-causes of procreation and pregnancy and that this agency must be exercised through conjugal union. The determining criteria for what constitutes a licit

---

An earlier version of this chapter was published as "Frozen Embryos, Unwanted Pregnancies, and Artificial Wombs: Which Options Are Morally Licit?," *Nova et Vetera* 19.4 (Fall 2021): 1111–1145, doi: 10.1353/nov.2021.0064. Reprinted with permission of the publisher.

clinical procedure versus an illicit one emerges very clearly in these documents once theologians grasp this logic at its root. When this logic is then applied to the question of embryo adoption, it becomes clear that it is illicit for an agent other than the husband to impregnate his wife, and in addition, it is illicit for such impregnation to take place outside conjugal union. For this reason, I concluded that both heterologous and homologous embryo transfer are intrinsically immoral.[1]

This article is intended to address the next question that naturally arises from my conclusion: What, then, are the licit moral options? This question is certainly not merely a theoretical one but, in many cases, a pressing and immediate concern for couples who have used IVF in the creation of their family and now repent of their mistake but have frozen embryos remaining. What options can licitly be pursued if it is true that embryo adoption is illicit and contrary to the unity of marriage? Is leaving these embryos frozen morally acceptable? Is allowing them to thaw and die considered murder? Does it go against the teaching in *Donum vitae*, which states, "It is therefore not in conformity with the moral law deliberately to expose to death human embryos obtained 'in vitro.'"[2]

I will address in detail the remaining moral options for the situation of frozen embryos: (1) leaving them in their frozen state and (2) thawing them and allowing them to die naturally.[3]

---

1. Irene Alexander, "Is Artificial Impregnation Opposed to the Unity of Marriage? A New Look at Embryo Adoption," *Nova et Vetera* 16.1 (Winter 2018): 47–80, doi: 10.1353/nov.2018.0003. Here I was careful to demonstrate that the Congregation for the Doctrine of the Faith has not formally declared embryo adoption to be illicit but seems to intuit a problematic connection between this practice and the already-condemned practices. I demonstrated with clarity what exactly that problematic connection is and responded to criticisms of this view by other scholars.
2. Congregation for the Doctrine of the Faith (CDF), *Donum vitae* (February 22, 1987), I.5.
3. Another question is whether artificial wombs could be a licit way of saving the lives of these frozen embryos. This technology is already on the horizon, with the successful artificial gestation of premature lambs, so it is probably only a matter of time before it will be available for humans too. However, this possibility requires its own discussion, which is outside the scope of this chapter.

The Future of Frozen Embryos

I believe that there are fundamentally two reasons why proponents of embryo adoption are so vocal and insistent in their opinion that the practice is licit, despite not providing strong and compelling arguments to support their view.[4] The first and main reason is that the alternatives do not look very good. The cry that embryo adoption must be licit and is the only moral option seems to stem from an urgency that rightly recognizes the poverty of the alternatives. Yet beginning by looking at all of the alternatives and then deciding on which one seems to provide the most therapeutic outcome is a problematic way of navigating difficult issues in moral theology. It is characteristic of a more consequentialist approach, which examines the outcomes as determinative of which actions are licit. Pope St. John Paul II is very critical of this way of reasoning in *Veritatis splendor*. To be clear, my remark is not to suggest that well-meaning Catholic ethicists are

---

4. See Alexander, "Is Artificial Impregnation Opposed to the Unity of Marriage?," 74–80. See also Melissa Moschella, "Gestation Does Not Necessarily Imply Parenthood: Implications for the Morality of Embryo Adoption and Embryo Rescue," *American Catholic Philosophical Quarterly* 92.1 (Winter 2018): 21–48, doi: 10.5840/acpq20171130137. Moschella, in my opinion, successfully demonstrates that genetic, rather than gestational, parenthood makes a more significant moral claim. Yet for those who oppose embryo adoption, the key issue is not who the true mother is (genetic, gestational, or adoptive) but whether the *act of artificial impregnation* is itself morally licit. Moschella does not address the heart of the issue at all. To a difficult objection raised by Nicholas Tonti-Filippini that "in HET [heterologous embryo transfer] a woman becomes a mother through 'an event from which her husband is, in effect, excluded,'" she replies that this concern is "based on the assumptions that (1) gestation creates a special biological relationship in a way that wet nursing or other post-natal caregiving does not ... and (2) that gestation in and of itself makes a woman a mother in the focal sense," which she has taken the time to disprove (44). Yet the objection to HET is not at all about the specific communion between mother and child but about whether an agent other than her spouse should make her pregnant in the first place. Does this role not belong specifically to the husband? Should a technician be the one who says to the woman through the act of HET, "I am the one making you pregnant, not your own spouse?" Moschella does not sufficiently address the problem that embryo adoption by nature is contrary to the unity of marriage, a violation of the union between spouses, not the union between mother and child.

functioning through a consequentialist mode of reasoning; I do not deny that they intend to defend moral absolutes. But on this particular issue, I do believe that the poverty of the alternatives fuels a more particular urgency to promote embryo adoption over a more careful consideration of how the biotechnology ruptures the integrity of the natural law.

The second reason why proponents of embryo adoption insist on its liceity and do not immediately see its problems concerns a deeper, in-house issue among scholars in moral theology regarding how to specify moral objects in the Catholic tradition. The novel theory initiated by Germain Grisez and his colleagues considers a good moral act to be one in which the moral agent does not intentionally desire to damage any of the basic human goods. While it is clear that, in choosing abortion, a woman intentionally destroys human life, how could something as good-hearted as adopting an orphaned embryo into one's own body be, in any way, an act that is intentionally opposed to a basic human good? Even if it is opposed to marital unity, in that a pregnancy comes about outside conjugal union, there is no deliberate intention within the acting subject to harm the marital good.[5]

The key issue here, however, is that Grisez's method of specifying moral actions, which forms the basis for what is called new natural law theory, is his own novel yet influential theory; it is distinct from the old natural law theory, which takes into account the nature of the action in its causal aspects and does not rely solely on the agent's intention toward or against a basic human good as an adequate moral description of the human act.[6] Even Janet Smith, in her commentary on Grisez's action theory, states very explicitly, "Grisez denies that reason must conform itself to nature. ... Their analysis, especially in its terminology, in many ways resembles traditional

---

5. E. Christian Brugger, "In Defense of Transferring Heterologous Embryos," *National Catholic Bioethics Quarterly* 5.1 (Spring 2005): 95–112, doi: 10.5840/ncbq20055170.
6. Christopher Tollefsen, "Is a Purely First Person Account of Human Action Defensible?," *Ethical Theory and Moral Practice* 9.4 (August 2006): 441–460. For a defense of the moral meaning of nature in the old natural law theory as distinct from the new natural law theory, see Edward Feser, "In Defense of the Perverted Faculty Argument," in *Neo-Scholastic Essays* (South Bend, IN: St. Augustine Press, 2015), 378–415.

modes of analysis; these resemblances can mislead the reader into thinking that their analysis is more aligned within the tradition than, in fact, it is."[7]

The embryo adoption issue has brought to the forefront of contemporary bioethical thinking an underlying philosophical divide that Catholic bioethicists cannot ignore: the new natural law analysis of the moral object eschews the underlying philosophy of nature as integral to defining what a moral act is.[8] The new approach eclipses something far more fundamental from the very beginning, and exploring this issue far exceeds the limits of this chapter. However, I mention it because what follows is my contention that sound moral thinking, especially in bioethics, requires the ethicist to consider the nature of the action chosen in specifying the moral object. This is distinct from a purely first-person perspective, where a moral object is determined by reference to a strict view of the agent's intention—that is, what he understands himself to be doing through his own interior choice—which he then projects onto a morally neutral external act. My arguments will proceed by taking seriously the philosophy of nature more aligned with the tradition, as distinct from the novel theory of intentionality toward basic human goods.[9]

---

7. Janet Smith, *"Humanae Vitae": A Generation Later* (Washington, DC: Catholic University of America Press, 1991), 353.
8. For my critique of the new natural law position on describing moral objects, see Irene Alexander, "Redefining Direct and Indirect Abortions through 'the Perspective of the Acting Person': A Misreading of *Veritatis Splendor*," *Linacre Quarterly* 86.1 (February 2019): 28–46, doi: 10.1177/0024363919838852.
9. For more on this debate, see John Finnis, Germain Grisez, and Joseph Boyle, "'Direct' and 'Indirect': A Reply to Critics of Our Action Theory," *Thomist* 65.1 (January 2001): 1–44, doi: 10.1353/tho.2001.0014; Christopher Tollefsen, "Response to Robert Koons and Matthew O'Brien's 'Objects of Intention: a Hylomorphic Critique of the New Natural Law Theory,'" *American Catholic Philosophical Quarterly* 87.4 (Fall 2013): 751–778, doi: 10.5840/acpq201387455; Steven A. Long, "A Brief Disquisition regarding the Nature of the Object of the Moral Act according to St. Thomas Aquinas," *Thomist* 67.1 (January 2003): 45–71, doi: 10.1353/tho.2003.0037; and Steven J. Jensen, "Causal Constraints on Intention: A Critique of Tollefsen on the Phoenix Case," *National Catholic Bioethics Quarterly* 14.2 (Summer 2014): 273–293, doi: 10.5840/ncbq201414230.

PART 2: OBJECTIONS TO EMBRYO ADOPTION

Leaving Embryos in Cryopreservation

Rev. Tadeusz Pacholczyk suggests that leaving the frozen embryos in cryopreservation is the only currently available ethical choice, aside from the future possibility of artificial wombs:

> The simple answer is that ethically there is very little we can do with our frozen embryos except to keep them frozen for the foreseeable future. No other obvious moral options seem to exist. ... Parents have an obligation to care for their children in this way until some other option becomes available in the future (maybe a sophisticated "embryo incubator" or "artificial womb" of some kind), or until there is a reasonable certainty that they have died on their own from decay or "freezer burn." ... Perhaps after a few hundred years, all the stored embryos would have died on their own, and they could finally be thawed and given a decent burial.[10]

Pacholczyk is not alone in this judgment. Catholic bioethicist Rev. Nicanor Austriaco, OP, holds a similar position. He suggests that "adoptive parents, instead of implanting their adopted embryo into his adopted mother's womb, could pay to maintain the cryopreservation necessary for the survival of their child until incubators capable of bringing him to term are invented."[11]

Before one can carefully evaluate these arguments, it is important to appreciate the rationale for the condemnation of cryopreservation that the Congregation for the Doctrine of the Faith (CDF) gives in *Donum vitae*: "*The freezing of embryos,* even when carried out in order to preserve the life of an embryo—cryopreservation—*constitutes an offense against the respect due to human beings* by exposing them to grave risks of death or harm to their physical integrity and depriving them, at least temporarily, of maternal shelter and gestation, thus placing them in a situation in which further offenses and manipulation are possible." Furthermore, like IVF, cryopreservation "establishes the domination of technology over the origin and destiny

---

10. Tadeusz Pacholczyk, "What Should We Do with the Frozen Embryos?," Making Sense of Bioethics 48 (June 2009): 1, 2.
11. Nicanor Pier Girorgio Austriaco, *Biomedicine and Beatitude: An Introduction to Catholic Bioethics* (Washington, DC: Catholic University of America, 2011), 109.

of the human person. Such a relationship of domination is itself contrary to the dignity and equality that must be common to parents and children."[12]

A conceived embryo ought to come into being beneath the heart of his mother. Her pregnancy is the reception of her spouse's conjugal gift. Conversely, through IVF and subsequent cryopreservation, clinicians and consenting parties use technology to act in a way contrary to the order of nature. Cryopreservation not only participates in an offense against marital unity but, even more damaging, rips the human person away from his or her natural maternal home by actively disrupting the normal process of gestation.

It is worth sitting for a few minutes with this image of freezing a human being. Would parents ever put their young children in their own freezer at home? Doing so would be a grave crime, because it would indeed "expose them to the serious risk of death or physical harm," just as cryopreservation does. The CDF also notes that "a high percentage [of embryos do] not survive the process of freezing and thawing."[13] Yet despite the destruction of a high percentage of embryos in the process, the purpose of cryopreservation is precisely to keep them alive for further use or, at least, until further decisions can be made about their fate.

Finally, cryopreservation does further damage to the embryonic children by exposing them to destructive manipulation and experimentation as victims of great moral evil—not unlike the Nazis' imprisonment of human persons and their highly unethical experiments on them. Embryonic children are prisoners of war—the culture war—over the personal meaning of human sexuality and the dignity of the human person.

The Object of Cryopreservation Violates the Order of Nature

One of the strongest condemnations of cryopreservation of human persons in *Dignitatis personae* is on the following grounds: it is fundamentally "incompatible with the respect owed to human embryos."[14] While most Catholic bioethicists see the reasons that I have articulated above as the grounds for condemning the process of freezing embryos to begin with,

---

12. CDF, *Donum vitae*, I.6; II.B.5, emphasis original.
13. CDF, *Dignitas personae* (September 8, 2008), n. 18.
14. CDF, *Dignitas personae*, n. 18.

Part 2: Objections to Embryo Adoption

few have reflected sufficiently on the unique abomination cryopreservation is according to the natural law. Unlike almost *any* other kind of technology, the process of deep-freezing living embryos causes them to be utterly suspended in their development. For example, an embryo frozen for five years and later implanted in a woman and birthed is actually a five-year-old while simultaneously a newborn—odd as that sounds. That is why I am convinced that ethicists must look closer at what cryopreservation does to the human person in relation to the inclinations of the natural law.

According to the order of nature, the soul, as the form of the body, is constantly striving for self-preservation with a view to exercising the person's higher powers—the flourishing in human excellence. The good of the body, such as health, is ordained to the good of the soul. St. Thomas Aquinas describes the natural law not as moral rules nor even as human goods necessarily, but as natural inclinations of the human person toward various ends. The Thomistic tradition recognizes that the moral law follows the order of nature. The natural world is not merely physical but follows an order that is morally determinative. Aquinas describes it this way: the human person shares the inclination to self-preservation in common with all living things; he also possesses the inclination to procreation and education common with animals; as a rational creature, he possesses the inclinations to know the truth, especially the truth about God, and to live in society.[15] While he shares common inclinations with other lower creatures (plants and animals), he carries them out in a fundamentally human and personal way.

If we look closely at the philosophy of nature here in Aquinas's description of the natural law in terms of its inclinations, we can see much more clearly the evil of cryopreservation. Bioethicist Nicholas Tonti-Filippini describes the process of freezing a human person as follows: "Parts of the embryo are separated by the chemical solution and, in that state, the parts of the whole do not relate to one another in any physiological sense except perhaps by being related spatially. The separating effect of the chemical solution and the effect of super-freezing means that the embryo is not integrated

---

15. Thomas Aquinas, *Summa theologiae*, trans. Fathers of the English Dominican Province (New York: Benzinger Bros., 1911–1925), I-II.94.2 corpus: "According to the order of natural inclinations, is the order of the precepts of the natural law."

or dynamic in the way in which we normally consider to be essential to being a living organism."[16] Therefore, because cryopreservation inhibits the embryo's growth and development as a living organism, it is not only the initial freezing but the actual current state of the embryo which gives great cause for alarm.

I believe that when we hold a magnifying glass up to the current state of the frozen embryos, it becomes clear that they suffer a profound moral evil of an intrinsic kind. Cryopreservation not only exposes the embryos to various physical harms (frost bite, death) or leaves them exposed to potential experimentation. Even if these were not real risks, the use of a technology that causes suspended animation of a human person is an evil contrary to nature. This type of technology actively prevents the exercise of the human person's natural inclinations toward the hierarchy of goods. There is no way in which a technology that has this effect on a human person can be compatible with the natural law and the good of the human person. It is for this reason, most of all, that cryopreservation is fundamentally "incompatible with the respect owed to human embryos."

In order to see this reality more clearly, it may be helpful to illustrate the contrast with an adult patient on a ventilator. The ventilated patient needs assistance in breathing. The air pushed into the body of the patient assists the patient's own natural inclination toward self-preservation; it does not actively hinder the inclination. But the continued cryopreservation of frozen embryos actively inhibits the human being's inclinations to self-preservation and growth. It contains the ungodly power of suspending the human person in development and, therefore, in time. If ethicists look only at the consequence of these two different technologies—both keep persons alive—they will misdiagnose the precise reason why cryopreservation is a moral evil. Ethicists must always keep in mind that the right use of technology assists the human person in restoring the order of nature, whereas the "domination of technology" takes place when that order is disregarded or destroyed by the technology.[17]

---

16. Nicholas Tonti-Filippini, "The Embryo Rescue Debate: Impregnating Women, Ectogenesis, and Restoration from Suspended Animation," *National Catholic Bioethics Quarterly* 3.1 (Spring 2003): 134, doi: 10.5840/ncbq20033181.
17. CDF, *Dignitas personae*, n. 17. See also n. 12, citing CDF, *Donum vitae*, introduction, 3: "Techniques which assist procreation 'are not to be rejected on the

Part 2: Objections to Embryo Adoption

To clarify again by contrast, the imprisonment of an innocent adult is a grave crime. He or she is unjustly denied certain basic freedoms. But the suspension and paralysis of a human being so that he or she can no longer function in a dynamic human way according to the inclinations of his or her being is significantly worse—indeed, it is unimaginable. It is in itself contrary to the order of nature and, therefore, intrinsically evil. Regardless of what this conclusion might imply, it is imperative that ethicists come to terms with the reality of cryopreservation vis-á-vis the natural law. One cannot properly grieve the embryos' situation without adequately reflecting on the full depth of their depravity. Not only was freezing the embryos immoral to begin with, but their continued existence in a trapped state of being is incompatible with the natural law.

I will provide one final clarification. A paralyzed or even unconscious patient still exercises the inclinations of the natural law toward self-preservation, toward development, both physically and spiritually, even if there is a form of physical impairment. A frozen embryo is not merely physically and temporally paralyzed. The inclinations or natural strivings of the human person are actively hindered until they totally cease. That is why these embryos do not age while frozen. Nor do they need nourishment to survive. The nutritive faculty has been completely suspended. A patient experiencing paralysis endures physical but not moral evil. By contrast, a frozen embryo suspended in his being is *currently* experiencing a moral evil unlike anything that man has created in the history of civilization. No human invention or technology has ever halted the human person's natural dynamic striving as cryopreservation has. Injuring a human being is not the same as entirely halting his or her dynamic human activity.

Toni-Filippini makes a similar argument:

> Keeping a human embryo in an induced state of arrested development indefinitely does offend against the good of life. It is a quasi-living existence, lacking the characteristics such as biological activity, growth, development, and maturing that are usually associated with life. The living dynamism of the cryopreserved, anhydrous embryo is on hold.

---

grounds that they are artificial. As such, they bear witness to the possibilities of the art of medicine. But they must be given a moral evaluation in reference to the dignity of the human person.'"

> It is difficult to describe what exactly the frozen-anhydrous state is. It is not like a general anesthesia, because even in general anesthesia the body continues to function. Further, the anesthesia is only properly willed in order to block pain experience and to immobilize so that surgery can be completed without muscle reflexes causing movement. Similarly, it is not like hypothermia caused accidentally through prolonged immersion in cold water or exposure to other cold environments, or the induced hypothermia sometimes used for long and complex surgery on highly vasculated areas or areas of metabolic significance in which a slowed-down metabolism would help. In each of those cases, while functions are slowed down and some are suppressed, some dynamic living activity continues. But in a frozen-anhydrous state all activity ceases.[18]

While Toni-Filippini does not explicitly use the language of "an intrinsic moral evil," it seems that he would agree with me in the use of this term to condemn a technology that causes suspended animation of a living human person.

For this reason, then, I disagree with Pacholczyk, who calls the continued cryopreservation care for the human embryo and, more specifically, ordinary care rather than extraordinary care. He, therefore, encourages parents of these children to continue to pay to keep them cryopreserved:

> Some have suggested that a morally acceptable solution to the frozen embryo problem might come through applying the principle that "extraordinary" means do not have to be undertaken to prolong human life. They argue that to sustain an embryo's life in a cryogenic state is to use extraordinary means and this is not required.
>
> In fact, however, the decision to continue cryopreserving an embryo in liquid nitrogen is not likely an instance of using extraordinary means, since the burden and costs associated with taking care of embryonic children in this way are actually

---

18. Tonti-Filippini, "Embryo Rescue Debate," 134. For this same reason, even the cryopreservation of an adult would be morally evil, and this may be a moral issue in the not-so-distant future. From the outside, one might argue that it is just putting someone to sleep with the intent of rehydrating him or her in fifty or one hundred years. But in reality, the person is not sleeping, which is, in fact, a biologically active process.

minimal. When we have children, we have a duty to clothe, feed, care for, and educate them, all of which costs plenty of money. When our children are frozen, we don't need to clothe, feed, or educate them; our care for them can only be expressed by paying the bill each month to replenish the liquid nitrogen in their storage tanks. This way of caring for our children is obviously unusual, but it does not seem morally extraordinary in terms of achieving the desired end of safeguarding their physical integrity.[19]

My reply to this argument is that the distinction between extraordinary and ordinary care does not even apply in this case, because the current state of suspended animation is an intrinsic evil. It is not care for the human person at all, either ordinary or extraordinary, because care always assists and does not hinder the natural inclinations of the human being. Cryopreservation does not "safeguard their physical integrity" but profoundly disrupts it, even if it continues their existence. The chemical solution disrupts the organism's physical integrity so that the parts of the embryo no longer communicate with one another as one integrative whole. That is precisely why the embryos do not age while frozen.

Both those who argue that embryos can remain frozen because the care is ordinary and those who argue that they can be removed because the care is extraordinary are missing the essential point that this distinction concerns care or assistance for the human person, not imprisonment of a human organism's dynamic animation. This aspect is what most Catholic bioethicists are missing when analyzing the issue. Care fosters the natural human inclinations toward life and health, with the body itself actively participating in its own reintegration; care does not chemically separate the communication of the parts of the body and so entirely halt the animation of the human person. For example, artificial nutrition and hydration aid the human person toward homeostasis, with the human body itself being the agent of its own recovery by taking in nutrition toward growth and healing. Suspended animation disrupts and halts the agency of the organism. That is why the embryos do not need nutrition to survive—odd as that is.

---

19. Pacholczyk, "What Should We Do with the Frozen Embryos?," 2.

Similarly, even extraordinary ventilation assists the human person's own living and dynamic striving for self-preservation by providing air and assisting in circulation. A frozen embryo is not breathing, nor does he or she have active circulation. Suspended animation does not assist but actively hinders the dynamism of the living human person in an utterly unique and abominable fashion.

The conclusion from this analysis, then, is that there is, in fact, a moral imperative to remove the frozen embryos from an intrinsically evil state immediately. Every moment of their being frozen is a new moment of grave moral evil. The embryos should be immediately thawed. This process involves rehydrating them and returning them to a warm and temporarily stable environment where they can resume their dynamic human activity.[20] The object of the moral act in this case is restoration from an intrinsically evil state of suspended existence into a restored state of dynamic human existence. Unfortunately, there are no morally licit ways of returning the rehydrated embryo to the womb of a woman. Within a few days, the recultivated embryo will die from a lack of stable environment. How, one might ask, can this action be morally licit, if one knows ahead of time that the embryos will die?

Thaw the Embryos and Allow Them to Die Naturally

The decision to thaw the embryos, although one foresees ahead of time that they will not long survive, is actually very similar to the situation of an ectopic pregnancy. Frozen embryos are actually "ec-topic" or "out of place." Ethicists should begin to use the language of *ectopic embryos*, since it is technically precise and because it is easier to see the ethical similarity with ectopic pregnancies. The frozen ectopic embryo is in a place where he cannot thrive, much like an embryo which implants in the fallopian tube of a woman. One is morally obligated to take action to save the mother's

---

20. In normal conjugal conception, the female body anticipates receiving a new embryo during the menstrual cycle by increasing her temperature shortly after ovulation. Her body releases progesterone (pro-gestation) to receive and nurture this new being. From the first moment of their conception, babies are meant to be received in a *warm* and nurturing environment. The female body anticipates and prepares for this reception.

life, even though one knows ahead of time that the young embryo will not survive, and the procedure is justified under the principle of double effect.[21]

The same logic applies to ectopic frozen embryos. The act itself is good, namely, a process of thawing and rehydrating that restores the embryo to a state of dynamic human existence. The good effect, returning the embryo to a dynamic state, is intended, and the undesirable one, the embryo's death, is unintended and caused indirectly. Importantly, the embryo's death is a true secondary effect of an act that achieves the good effect, not the means of achieving it. The process of thawing and rehydrating removes a tiny human being from one place where morally he ought not to be *and ought not to remain* to another, authentically restorative place. That he also will not long survive and will die from the lack of a stable environment are foreseen but unintended secondary effects of this process. Furthermore, thawing and rehydrating do not involve any direct damage to the embryo, which would hasten his death and constitute a direct abortion. The technician is not lacerating or chemically burning the young life or directly expelling the child from an otherwise hospitable womb.

Finally, there is real proportionality between the good and bad effects, because the embryo is continually subjected to a profound intrinsic moral evil. Consider an innocent person kidnapped and taken to a private cell where he is repeatedly tortured, albeit deliberately kept alive because he may at some point be useful. Is it morally right to allow this person to be subject to continued torture? No, of course not! One ought to immediately free him, even if one knows ahead of time that, as a result of his capture and profound abuse, he will not long survive. Likewise, cryopreservation is abusive. It does not merely keep the embryo alive; it traps him in a way absolutely contrary to his nature as a human being—in a way totally impossible and unheard of in the entire history of the world until the last few decades. The injustice to the embryo did not happen only once in his or her initial freezing. Every day of existing as a frozen human person with the natural inclination to develop, while being simultaneously hindered in that development, is a new day of

---

21. See Irene Alexander, "The Error of Intentionalism," *National Catholic Bioethics Quarterly* 17.3 (Autumn 2017): 399–408, doi: 10.5840/ncbq201717341. That is to say, certain procedures are justified. I have defended why salpingectomy is the only licit procedure and why salpingostomy and the use of methotrexate are direct abortions and unjustifiable rather than indirect abortions.

profound and inconceivable injustice. That is, freeing someone from a state that is incompatible with the natural law is proportionate to allowing him to die naturally. Consequently, there is a grave moral reason to take action.

Both the intention and the specific act of releasing the embryo from his state of imprisoned animation are morally laudable, even if, as a secondary effect, the embryo will not long survive. In the end, it is a tragedy much like the loss of life in an ectopic pregnancy, but the moral act of thawing and restoring the embryo is licit and justifiable.

The real moral tragedy, however, is that, unlike a surprise ectopic pregnancy, technicians knew ahead of time what the process of IVF would cause. It is not merely a medical abnormality. The technicians and couples deliberately chose to separate procreation from the conjugal act, with all of its accompanying lethal effects. There is moral injustice not in the act of thawing and restoring a human child from suspended animation to living dynamic activity, albeit for a brief time, but in deliberately choosing the procedures in the first place which left him to this tragic fate.

I would like to consider an important objection to my argument. In *Donum vitae*, the CDF states that "it is therefore not in conformity with the moral law deliberately to expose to death human embryos obtained 'in vitro.'" Have I not argued in favor of the very thing *Donum vitae* calls unlawful? No, not at all. The context of this passage is addressing the specific question "How is one to evaluate morally the use for research purposes of embryos obtained by fertilization 'in vitro'?" The CDF here condemns the voluntary destruction of embryos used in experimental research, even with the noble intention of contributing to new medical discoveries. In fact, it condemns all "methods of observation or experimentation which damage or impose grave and disproportionate risks upon embryos obtained *in vitro*."[22] The sentence I quoted above is the response to a scientist who might ask, Given that we already have these IVF embryos, shouldn't we at least use them for scientific research, since they will likely die anyway? What difference does it make if they die through our experiments? At least they may give us useful knowledge for treating other ailments.

Note how different that issue is from the situation of embryos already frozen. I have argued that properly respecting their dignity as persons

---

22. CDF, *Donum vitae*, I.5.

requires their immediate removal from suspended animation to a restored and dynamic state of human existence. Furthermore, while the secondary effect of this act will be that the embryos will not long survive, the technician does not immediately cause the death of the embryo as the scientist would in the case above. The moral difference is as clear as the difference between an indirect abortion and a direct abortion. The latter immediately causes the death of the embryo, whereas the former does not.[23]

To those who remain unconvinced by my argument because, in the end, no life is saved, unlike a typical ectopic pregnancy, which at least saves the mother, I would call attention to the true purpose of the moral life and its foundation, as wonderfully put by John Haas, then-president of the National Catholic Bioethics Center, in the inaugural issue of the center's quarterly journal: "Catholic bioethics, and any bioethics that would be compatible with it, must recognize that the human person has a destiny which transcends physical existence. Death is the lot of every human being. But every human being has a destiny, an ultimate fulfillment, beyond death. …The only thing which would ultimately and in the final analysis do violence to the human person would be actions that placed one's ultimate destiny in jeopardy."[24]

Haas aptly reminds ethicists that moral evil is worse—indeed, profoundly worse—than physical evil, which includes even death itself. That is why I am arguing that the embryos should be thawed immediately. Many moral theologians have made errors in judgment by subscribing to the idea that one must save a life at all costs. The Catholic tradition has never held this position, nor could it, if we know philosophically that the good of life is not on par with other human goods but is a necessary prerequisite for flourishing in human excellence. The good of the body is ordained to the good of the soul. John Paul II found it necessary to reiterate this point by quoting the Latin poet Juvenal in his encyclical *Veritatis splendor*: "Consider it the greatest of crimes to prefer survival to honour and, out of love of physical

---

23. See Alexander, "Redefining Direct and Indirect Abortions," 28–46. There has been significant confusion over what ought to be a clear teaching on direct and indirect abortion.
24. John Haas, "Bioethics in the New Millennium," *National Catholic Bioethics Quarterly* 1.1 (Spring 2001): 18–19, doi: 10.5840/ncbq20011170.

life, to lose the very reason for living."²⁵ It is more human and, therefore, more important to refrain from grave moral evil, even if it means accepting that not every human life can be saved.

Haas rightly claims that the root reason for this conclusion is that the moral life finds its foundation in the eternal law of God and the hierarchy of the created ends of the human person: "There are theologians today who teach that sinful actions are only those which 'harm' the person. However, the Catholic Tradition has understood sin as a departure from the Eternal Law, which is the Mind of God ordering all things toward their created ends, as the ultimate harm to the human person. But one needs a long view to see this and a confidence that the created order reflects an intelligible and loving design."²⁶

While Haas probably wrote these words in reference to dissenting theologians who described themselves as proportionalists, his point remains perpetually valid. Whether one intends to harm is not the sole criterion for moral judgment in the Catholic tradition, nor is looking merely at outcomes. The eternal law is the key foundation for the moral life; that is why John Paul II returned to this theme in great depth in *Veritatis splendor* when he found so many errors in moral reasoning from academic theologians.

Given the moral imperative to free the ectopic frozen embryos from their absurd state of suspended animation immediately, the only moral choice is to thaw and rehydrate them and to anticipate and mourn their death. This option is the only one that Catholic bioethicists should recommend as an ethical solution.

On a pastoral note, Catholics in this position should seek to baptize their ectopic frozen children with a view to their eternal destiny as beloved sons and daughters in Christ.²⁷ While parents of these children will

---

25. John Paul II, *Veritatis splendor* (August 6, 1993), n. 94, citing Juvenal, *Satires* VIII.
26. John Haas, "Bioethics in the New Millennium," 19.
27. The Baptism of frozen embryos presents certain clinical and canonical challenges. The process itself cannot be the direct cause of the child's death, so clinicians must take every precaution before proceeding. Two issues arise here. First, an embryo in such a nascent state may not be able to tolerate an immersion Baptism, and hence, the preferred method in this case may be what the Church also approves of for infant Baptisms: pouring water three times over

necessarily mourn the loss of the human good of life with their children, they can still exercise their own parenthood by offering them the supreme gift of sacramental grace. By baptizing their children, they can fulfill the hopes and aspirations of every parent of faith: to ensure that their children reach heaven, where they may again be reunited with them—for parents of frozen embryos, to lock eyes with their children for the first time. For those embryos that have been completely abandoned by their parents, I advise that, after the act of rehydration, either a health care worker or a volunteer should tenderly hold these tiny babies and love them in their final moments on this earth, just as parents would with their own dying child.[28] I further recommend that a specific ministry like Rachel's Vineyard be created for IVF parents to repent and grieve this profound human loss and to reclaim their parenthood of these children as a means to their own spiritual healing.

The "special word" of John Paul II in *Evangelium vitae* to "women who have had an abortion" will ring true for them as well: "You will come to understand that nothing is definitively lost and you will also be able to ask forgiveness from your child, who is now living in the Lord. With the friendly and expert help and advice of other people, and as a result of your own painful experience, you can be among the most eloquent defenders of everyone's right to life."[29] Upon receiving true forgiveness, they may also

---

the head. Yet (and here is the second issue) an embryo does not yet have a fully formed head. Even if a tiny pipette could be created for the purpose of Baptism, the canonical issue that needs to be resolved is whether Rome would consider such an action to be a valid Baptism. Perhaps the real potency in the living human embryo toward the formation of a head would suffice for the matter of the sacramental act, and a very small stream of water could be poured over the rehydrated embryo. I defer to the Catholic Church in Rome to advise and govern how these types of Baptisms could potentially take place. I am grateful to Rich Vigh for dialoging with me on this important aspect of the issue.

28. Obviously, this kind of action would need to be accomplished without risking vital harm to the embryo. It could be accomplished by holding a petri dish containing the embryo.
29. John Paul II, *Evangelium vitae* (March 25, 1995), n. 99, in *L'Osservatore Romano* (English ed.) April 5, 1995. Cf. John Paul II, *Evangelium vitae* (March 25, 1995), *Acta Apostolicae Sedis* 87 (1995): 515–516, n. 99.

wish to consider sharing their IVF experience with others and so fight for the dignity of life, marriage, and family.

Fidelity to Truth Requires Courage and Hope

To conclude my remarks about the future of frozen embryos, the only ethical option is to thaw the embryos and allow them to die naturally. The reason for this conclusion follows from the facts that I have now made very clear: continuing to keep them in cryopreservation is intrinsically evil. The only option that is not morally evil at all, but is in fact a laudable act, is to rehydrate and return the embryos to their dynamic human activity, though one knows in advance that they will not long survive. All other options violate the integrity of God's loving design and disrespect his law.

I would like to acknowledge openly that I sincerely empathize with those who find my conclusion difficult to accept. It is a heartbreaking issue and one that I have personally shed tears over as I examined it from all sides. At the same time, the mere fact that a conclusion is difficult does not mean that it is wrong. It means that fidelity to the truth calls for great courage and especially hope—that we can trust in the promises of God—that despite our cruel human folly and the tragedies we create here on earth through our sin, one day "He will wipe away every tear from their eyes, and death shall be no more, neither shall there be mourning, nor crying, nor pain anymore, for the former things have passed away" (Rev. 21:4).

Part 3:
Defenses of Embryo Adoption

11

The Procreative Dimension of Marital Union and Embryo Transfer

Christopher Tollefsen

Common to Catholic proponents and opponents of heterologous embryo transfer, whether as part of an attempt at in vitro fertilization by an infertile couple or as part of embryo rescue or adoption by persons not responsible for the embryo's existence, are a set of norms concerning marital intercourse and procreation articulated by the Catholic Church. The following are of special importance:

> The spouses' union achieves the twofold end of marriage: the good of the spouses themselves and the transmission of life. These two meanings or values of marriage cannot be separated without altering the couple's spiritual life and compromising the goods of marriage and the future of the family. The conjugal love of man and woman thus stands under the twofold obligation of fidelity and fecundity.[1]

> The bond existing between husband and wife accords the spouses, in an objective and inalienable manner, the exclusive right to become father and mother solely through each other.[2]

---

1. *Catechism of the Catholic Church*, 2nd ed. (Washington, DC: US Conference of Catholic Bishops / Libreria Editrice Vaticana, 2018 update), n. 2363.
2. Congregation for the Doctrine of the Faith (CDF), *Donum vitae* (February 22, 1987), II.A.2.

Part 3: Defenses of Embryo Adoption

> Surrogate motherhood represents an objective failure to meet the obligations of maternal love, of conjugal fidelity and of responsible motherhood.[3]

The first passage refers to what are often identified as the unitive and procreative dimensions of marital love. As Pope Pius XII said, "Never is it permitted to separate these different aspects."[4] Spouses do, or attempt to, separate them by the use of contraception, which attempts to achieve union while denying the possibility of procreation. And they do, or attempt to, separate them in the use of various artificial reproductive technologies, which create children outside the exclusive domain of marital intercourse.

The norm of the second passage follows from that of the first: if spouses are never to attempt separation of the unitive and procreative dimensions of the marital act, then as a consequence, neither spouse may attempt to become a parent independent of the other. The obligations that each spouse has in this regard include obligations of fidelity to the other and so are correlated to rights on the other spouse's part: either spouse's right is violated if the other attempts to become a parent in any way without the first spouse's consent and cooperation in the ways appropriate to becoming a parent.

The norm of the third passage is a corollary to that of the second: In the typical situation, surrogacy is a sign that the norms of the first two passages have broken down. A child has been conceived *ex utero*. For whatever reason, the biological mother or intended social mother is unable or unwilling to carry the child to term, and so another party is introduced into the reproductive equation. For example, in addition to the intended social parents, to heterologous sperm and oocyte donors, and to the various in vitro fertilization technicians, now a surrogate is added to the mix to carry the child before giving him or her back to the intended parents. Such a situation is indeed a failure "of maternal love, of conjugal fidelity and of responsible motherhood."

---

3. CDF, *Donum vitae*, II.A.3.
4. Pius XII, Allocution to the members of the Second World Congress of Fertility and Sterility (May 19, 1956), cited in US Conference of Catholic Bishops, Natural Family Planning Program, "Unitive and Procreative Nature of Intercourse," accessed November 6, 2023, https://www.usccb.org/issues-and-action/marriage-and-family/natural-family-planning/catholic-teaching/upload/Unitive-and-Proc-Nature-of-Interc.pdf.

To reiterate, these norms are part of the common patrimony of Catholic ethicists, moral theologians, and the faithful. None wish to contravene them. Thus, all discussion of embryo transfer (ET) and of embryo adoption (EA) must find its way back to these norms, either to show that, as is manifestly the case with heterologous in vitro fertilization, these norms are violated by ET or EA, or to show that ET and EA are by their nature sufficiently different from heterologous in vitro fertilization that they are not condemned by Catholic ethical norms.

Embryo transfer is the act most centrally in question, for it is the act that is common to in vitro fertilization, whether heterologous or homologous, to EA, and to ET for purposes of rescuing an abandoned embryo. If ET is intrinsically impermissible, then not only will the creation in vitro of a human embryo be morally impermissible, but so will the transfer of that embryo into the womb of the couple who commissioned its creation and who are genetically its parents, parents who now perhaps regret the initially sinful act but wish to do right by the created embryos. Similarly, embryo rescue and embryo adoption will also fall, as both require ET for their success.

Accordingly, this essay focuses primarily on ET in the context of responding to a specific family of arguments against it, arguments that make the case that an act whereby a woman is made to be pregnant in any way other than as the fruit of sexual union is itself an act that, in some way, attempts to separate the unitive and procreative dimensions of marriage and the marriage act. Those who make this argument typically think that ET involves a violation of the norm of the second passage, by making a woman a mother through no act of her husband, and of the third, by making the woman a surrogate mother. Indeed, some thinkers believe all three norms are violated even in the case of homologous in vitro fertilization, such that the biological mother will be a surrogate carrier of her own child if she chooses to undertake ET.[5]

---

5. See, for example, Tadeusz Pacholczyk, "Some Moral Contraindications to Embryo Adoption," in *Human Embryo Adoption: Biotechnology, Marriage, and the Right to Life*, ed. Thomas V. Berg and Edward J. Furton (Philadelphia: National Catholic Bioethics Center, 2006), 51–52.

Part 3: Defenses of Embryo Adoption

Rev. Nicanor Austriaco has characterized this family of arguments as involving the idea of "extended inseparability."[6] That is, these arguments all begin with the accepted principle that the unitive and procreative dimensions of marriage may not be separated and then extend the norm beyond the point at which a new human individual comes into existence—the point of conception and generation—through the stages of gestation and typically up to birth; the extended period is certainly inclusive of the moment, whenever it might be, at which the woman becomes pregnant. *That moment, like the moment at which the individual comes into existence, is not to be separated from the act of conjugal intercourse.*

In this essay, I address three forms of this argument. The first, put forth by Mary Geach, I have addressed before and will discuss here most briefly.[7] The second approach to extended inseparability, represented here by Stephen Long and Charles Robertson, is intended to be Thomistic; Long and Robertson argue that the natural teleology of procreation extends to gestation.[8] The third approach, represented by Nicholas Tonti-Filippini, Christopher Oleson, and Catherine Althaus, is broadly personalistic in the manner of Pope St. John Paul II's work on the Theology of the Body.[9] These

---

6. Nicanor Pier Giorgio Austriaco, "Embryo Adoption and the Extended Inseparability Argument," *National Catholic Bioethics Quarterly* 21.1 (Spring 2021): 29–35, doi: 10.5840/ncbq20212114.
7. Mary Geach, "The Female Act of Allowing an Intromission of an Impregnating Kind," in Berg and Furton, *Human Embryo Adoption*, 251–271; for my response, see Christopher Tollefsen, "Could Human Embryo Transfer Be Intrinsically Immoral?," in *The Ethics of Embryo Adoption and the Catholic Tradition*, ed. Sarah-Vaughan Brakman and Darlene Fozard Weaver (New York: Springer, 2007), 85–102.
8. See Stephen A. Long, "An Argument for the Embryonic Intactness of Marriage," *Thomist* 70.2 (April 2006): 267–288, doi: 10.1353/tho.2006.0019; and Charles Robertson, "A Thomistic Analysis of Embryo Adoption," *National Catholic Bioethics Quarterly* 14.4 (Winter 2014): 673–695, doi: 10.5840/ncbq201414470.
9. See Nicholas Tonti-Filippini, "The Embryo Rescue Debate: Impregnating Women, Ectogenesis, and Restoration from Suspended Animation," in Berg and Furton, *Human Embryo Adoption*, 69–114; Christopher Oleson, "The Nuptial Womb: On the Moral Significance of Being 'with Child,'" in Berg and Furton, *Human Embryo Adoption*, 165–195; Catherine Althaus,

authors also argue for a teleological extension of generation to gestation, but they focus less on natural teleology and more on the experience and significance of gestational intimacy.

I will argue that each approach fails to show that ET is intrinsically impermissible, or *per se malum*. First, in response to Geach, I will reiterate my earlier argument that, even if one grants a teleological directedness of conception to pregnancy, this teleology has no bearing on the specific way in which one or another aspect of that process affects the unitive dimension of the marital act; the unitive dimension is affected *only* by its relationship to the possibility of conception.

Second, I will address a challenge to the Thomistic analysis: Is it really the case that the alleged natural teleology of procreation to gestation and birth is morally normative? Here we will see that a familiar dialectic about the normativity of the natural plays a role in delineating at least some of the main approaches to ET and EA. But I will argue that St. Thomas Aquinas is not to be taken as an automatic ally of the opponents of ET.

Third, I will argue, in response to the more personalist approach, that such teleologies and intimacies as are to be found in the extended dimensions of human procreation include not just gestation and birth but subsequent nurturing, rearing, and educating. Viewed through an adequately wide lens, there is simply no ground on which to distinguish sharply what happens on the far side of birth as constituting something different in kind from the gestational period leading up to birth. Thus, attempts to include only gestation as within the extended inseparability argument fail.

Sexual Union, Generation, and Impregnation

Geach deserves credit as one of the earliest and most forceful defenders of the extended inseparability view. Her argument begins from the claim, with which I agree, that marriage is a great and fundamental good, a good that is treated with appropriate respect only by those who do not in any way

---

"Human Embryo Transfer and the Theology of the Body," in Brakman and Weaver, *Ethics of Embryo Adoption*, 43–67; and Catherine Althaus, "Establishing the Moral Object of Heterologous and Homologous Embryo Transfer," in *Contemporary Controversies in Catholic Bioethics*, ed. Jason Eberl (New York: Springer, 2017), 169–187.

disintegrate the unity of the marital act, the "one-flesh union of spouses ... per se apt for generation." But "this disintegration occurs when a man or woman imitates the marriage act in respect of any function which is specific to the one-flesh union and which in the context of the marriage act contributes to the unitive significance of that act." Geach believes that such imitation is present in a woman's "act of admission whereby she allows a carnal intromission of impregnating kind." For *that* is precisely what is done by a woman accepting ET: there is a carnal intromission—the intromission of the embryo—of an impregnating kind but outside the context of the marital act. Thus, Geach characterizes ET as "indecent" and not to be done.[10]

In a previous response to Geach, which I still believe sound, I argued that the marital act is not an act of an impregnating kind, but rather of a generative kind, and that generating and gestating are two different kinds of act, only one of which—generation—is central to the possibility of one-flesh union between spouses. For it is the marital act's per se aptness for generation exclusively that is responsible for the couple's becoming one with respect to the reproductive function in sexual intercourse. Subsequent gestational success (and indeed, actual *generational* success) does not contribute to the *biological* union of the couple, which is necessary in order that their vow of comprehensive union be realized at the level of their biological existence.

This view does justice both to the Church's teaching on marital sexuality, which holds that only sexual acts per se apt for generation are appropriate for marital intercourse, and to Catholic teaching on the *punctuality* of generation. That is, human beings are substances, which at any moment do or do not exist, and their souls are a matter of special divine creation.[11] The coming into existence of a human person is, thus, not a process in any meaningful sense. Rather, there is a substantial change from gametes, which go out of existence, to a new individual human being. It is the per se aptness of the sexual act for the punctual and precise generation of a new human being that capacitates that sexual act for realizing the comprehensive

---

10. Geach, "Female Act of Allowing an Intromission," 251, 259, 261.
11. The language of *punctuality* is introduced in Thomas D. Williams, "Heterologous Embryo Transfer and the Meaning of 'Becoming a Mother,'" in Berg and Furton, *Human Embryo Adoption*, 229–249. Used of generation, this seems unquestionably true; as I will discuss below, it is less accurate as regards procreation.

union of the spouses in one flesh, and philosophical attempts to extend what is necessary for the spouses' *becoming one flesh* beyond that punctual moment threaten to be false to both the biology and the metaphysics of human reproduction.

In addition to this fundamental objection to Geach's view, I hold that we should say that no intromission by the male in sexual intercourse is of a kind to *impregnate*, even when there is actual generation. Rather, when the marital union bears fruit and results in the generation of a human embryo, the agent of impregnation is the embryo itself, whose existence as such is sufficient to make his or her mother pregnant. Thus, impregnation is not as such an act that imitates the marital act.

Natural Teleology and St. Thomas

In this section, I offer a brief account of Long's and Robertson's defenses of extended inseparability. They believe their positions to be fundamentally Thomistic in their attention to the natural teleologies of the reproductive organs.

Moral Normativity of Natural Teleology

Long is concerned to identify the "per se naturally normative teleological order from paradigmatic cases taken apart from what is technologically possible" to determine whether heterologous ET is morally permissible.[12] That is, what is normatively teleological must be discernable in nature prior to what technology makes possible. It is no argument for ET that it is technologically possible; rather, the prior natural order must first be identified.

Long has no doubts as to the "densely intelligible narrative" of the natural teleology: "It must be affirmed that the carrying of the child exists for the sake of the integral purpose of procreation, whose purpose is not alone the mere conception of the child but the delivery of a live rather than a dead child."[13] There is, thus, a natural ordering: sexual union, to generation, to gestation, to live parturition. This order might be violated in one of a number of ways. For example, to *interrupt* this process is to interfere wrongfully in the "normative teleological order." But Long also holds that

---

12. Long, "Embryonic Intactness of Marriage," 272.
13. Long, "Embryonic Intactness of Marriage," 272.

for a married woman to implant in her womb an embryonic human being who is not conceived in a specific conjugal act with her husband is for her to take that which belongs to the spousal couple as spousal couple and give it to another. But all that which integrally and essentially is naturally necessary to the procreative end is included in the spousal donation as belonging to the couple alone. It follows that a married woman who implants an embryonic human being in her womb who is not conceived in a specific conjugal act with her husband violates marital intimacy, which is a *per se malum*.[14]

Thus, no part of the teleological order may be appropriated outside the context in which it finds its natural place: "Just as one may not share venereal activity with one who is not one's spouse, because these venereal acts exist for the sake of, and are necessary to, the generation and transmission of new life (i.e., the integral procreative end, which is not generation alone) in marriage, so one may not rightfully choose to share childbearing with anyone save one's spouse, as it exists for the sake of the transmission of the life conceived with one's spouse."[15]

Right of Spouses to Become Parents Only through Each Other

Robertson, speaking of the inalienable right that spouses have to become mother and father only through each other, asks, "Does procreation here refer only to the way in which a person is conceived, or does it include the gestation and birthing of the child?"[16] Robertson notes correctly that the woman's generative power is dependent for its operation on the proper functioning of the reproductive system of the woman, and he notes further, again correctly, that the reproductive system includes the organ of gestation, the uterus. This is a matter of natural teleology but has the following consequence: "The intention to give birth to a child, whether that child is one's own or not, always entails the choice to make use of the generative faculty."[17]

Still, this fact does not give a norm for action just as such. On Robertson's account, it is necessary to learn what intentions are permissible in

---

14. Long, "Embryonic Intactness of Marriage," 274.
15. Long, "Embryonic Intactness of Marriage," 274.
16. Robertson, "Thomistic Analysis of Embryo Adoption," 675.
17. Robertson, "Thomistic Analysis of Embryo Adoption," 677.

relation to the use of a faculty by consulting our natural inclinations. Such inclinations will be perfected by being ordered to their natural ends and disordered if not so directed. Following Aquinas, Robertson holds there is a natural inclination for reproduction, and he holds further that this inclination is and should be ordered not to the good of the individual but to the good of the species: "Hence, the fundamental, primary end of the reproductive power is the mature offspring of the parents that is the same in kind as its parents."[18]

Robertson then considers Aquinas's treatment, in the *Summa contra Gentiles*, of sexual ethics in light of this primary end of the reproductive power; the use of the generative faculty must be suitably directed, and for the woman, this suitable direction is toward intercourse with a man. Robertson's rendering of Aquinas's argument for the claim that not just any man will do, but only the woman's husband, is worth quoting at length:

> Further considerations, however, indicate that the proper object of her activity should not be just any man, but her husband. Aquinas continues his analysis in book 3, chapter 122, of *Summa contra gentiles* by looking more carefully at what is required for the rearing of offspring. He notes first that while some animals that are sexually reproduced do not need the care of their parents, others do. Of the latter, some need the care of one parent, and others need the care of both. Further, some need a longer period of care, whereas others need a shorter period. ...
>
> Human beings, however, are animals whose offspring require a very long period of care, which is best given by both parents because of the need the child has not only of the physical supports for the perfection of his body, but also for the formation of his properly human faculties both by instruction and correction. Hence, it is natural to human beings to form male–female partnerships of long duration for the good of the offspring. This partnership is nothing other than the society of matrimony.[19]

From all this, Robertson concludes that for a wife to make use of any aspect of her generative faculty with a person other than her husband

---

18. Robertson, "Thomistic Analysis of Embryo Adoption," 679.
19. Robertson, "Thomistic Analysis of Embryo Adoption," 683–684.

by means of marital union is to violate the rights of the husband to exclusive use of her generative faculty. By allowing herself to become pregnant through embryo transfer, the woman does exactly that: make use of her generative faculty with, typically, someone other than her husband (the in vitro fertilization technician) and, even if the technician is her husband, by some manner other than sexual union with him. Ultimately, "to use the generative faculty in a disordered way is a refusal to render to God his due by subordinating ourselves to the order He has established in nature."[20]

Response to Arguments from Natural Teleology

Consider again Long's description of the natural ordering of sexual union, to generation, to gestation, to live parturition. Let us accept this as a genuinely natural teleology: sexual union and subsequent generation occur *in nature* ultimately for the sake of live birth, an end mediated by gestation, without which there will be no such birth. This ordering is thought to be normative in at least two ways: First, the process is not to be interrupted, as when gestation and live birth are prevented by abortion or when generation is prevented by contraception. Second, the prior stages of the order are not to be dirempted from the latter by accomplishing some later stage of the order without what naturally precedes. Thus, for example, neither generation nor gestation nor live birth is to be achieved in the absence of sexual union.

The most fundamental question to ask about this natural teleology is one that generates radically different answers from competing philosophical standpoints: How is it that this natural teleology as such is normative for human beings? Why, to put this question in another form, should it *matter* to me or anyone like me, in my practical deliberations, that this is *nature's* order? The question is pressing, because nature's order does not converge regularly with either my desires or what I can accomplish in some extranatural way: I might very much wish to have sexual intercourse without generation or achieve generation without sexual intercourse. Why should it matter to me that, in the order of nature, one is for the sake of the other?

I, along with colleagues in the so-called new natural law school of thought, hold that there is no good answer to this question that does

---

20. Robertson, "Thomistic Analysis of Embryo Adoption," 685.

not presuppose some already normative or axiological claim. Convincing answers to the challenge must identify aspects of the agent's good, known by practical reason without inference from a bare claim about what is natural, that are implicated in the relevant human acts and natural processes. To see this, we need look no further than Aquinas's treatment of the nature and ethic of marriage and marital sexuality, from which Robertson draws so extensively.[21]

It is true that Aquinas repeatedly notes analogies between the human situation and that of other animals, such as birds, as regards sexual intercourse, the generation of offspring, and their rearing. Some animals do not require the work of both mates in order for offspring to successfully grow to adulthood; some require conjoined work only for a limited period of time. Thus, different animals display different mating patterns. Humans, contrasted with many other animals, require much more from both parents, lest the "proper upbringing of offspring [be] hindered," in large part because "the offspring needs not only nourishment for its body but also instruction for its soul." Children are not initially ready for such instruction, and once they are, it takes considerable time. Nor does Aquinas think, not for entirely sound reasons, that the woman alone is sufficient for this task. Consequently, "it is natural in the human race that the man should have not a short-lived but a long lasting fellowship with a definite woman: this fellowship is called matrimony."[22]

Now it is true that Aquinas says here of marriage, so understood, that it is natural that it should be a long-lasting fellowship. But it is natural because it is necessary, and the necessity is a practical necessity for those considering the ordering of human life toward the human good. That good encompasses a social good, the continuation of the species, and also a personal good, for the father wishes to see his successor flourish. This, too, Aquinas describes as natural. But *natural* here should be understood to mean "what is required by reason" rather than the other way round, and the entire discussion of marriage and sexual ethics in book III of *Summa contra Gentiles* begins, in chapter 121, with an assertion that the divine law directs these matters *in*

---

21. See, in particular, Thomas Aquinas, *Summa contra Gentiles*, trans. Laurence Shapcote (Green Bay: Aquinas Institute, 2018), III.121–125.
22. Aquinas, *Summa contra Gentiles* III.122.

accordance with reason. Aquinas should thus be read, in directing our attention to "natural facts and teleologies," not as identifying those teleologies as normative *per se*, but rather as *salient* in light of reason's direction to our good, prominently, the good of propagation of the species but also the good of having children of one's own.[23]

Moreover, Aquinas's discussion of the normative nature of marriage is deeply suffused with normative claims that simply have no natural teleological analogues but are framed in terms of the goods of friendship, equality, and fidelity between the spouses. Aquinas argues in *Summa contra Gentiles* III.123 that marriage should be permanent and that husbands should not be permitted to put away their wives both on grounds of fairness to the wife and because of the way in which friendship and equality would not be fostered between spouses were it known that the union could end. Similarly, chapter 124 argues against all forms of polygamy, and central to Aquinas's argument are the conditions necessary for the equality of marital friendship, for which relationships with multiple partners are unsuited. Here again, a claim about the human good—in this case, the good of marital friendship and *fides*—is what drives the argument, not a claim about natural teleology as such.

We should adopt a similar standpoint in our moral reflection on ET. The goods at stake are those identified by both proponents and opponents of the practice: marriage, paternity and maternity, solidarity with the vulnerable, a well-ordered society. There are also important facts about human beings that are relevant, such as the necessity that a child in the womb be given adequate nutrition and prenatal care if the pregnancy is to be healthy. But the norms for engaging with these goods in marriage or in the fertility lab, and for reckoning with the relevant facts and natural teleologies, are inferred not from those teleologies but instead from the most general norm of morality, that all one's willing should be consistent with integral human fulfillment. Such willing is always fair, is never directed toward the intentional damage or destruction of a basic good, and pursues the realities

---

23. John Finnis, *Aquinas* (New York: Oxford University Press, 1998), 153n91. As Finnis notes in his treatment of Aquinas's sexual ethics, "Aquinas' moral arguments never runs from 'natural' to 'therefore reasonable and right,' but always from 'reasonable and right' to 'therefore natural.'"

of those goods and not their mere or sham appearances. The fundamental question is whether the effort to transfer an embryo into the womb of a woman not its biological mother for the purposes of either rescue or adoption is contrary to any of these norms.

Personalism

The previous discussion of natural teleology leads, I believe, directly into the next set of figures in the extended inseparability debate, those whose work is more obviously indebted to John Paul II's writings on marriage than is the work of the previously discussed authors. Central to the Pope's thought is the idea of marriage as a mutual self-gift, encompassing all levels of the human person.[24] That idea naturally lends itself to thinking of that marital gift and its fruition in a child in a very holistic manner in the context of pregnancy, as we will see. John Paul II also gave attention to the complementary notion of what we might call gestational intimacy, a form of intimacy between pregnant mother and child that is an extension in some ways of the marital intimacy of the spouses. I find the accounts of these more personalist authors rich and insightful; the questions I will pose do not call into question the insights, only their role in arguments against ET.

Unparalleled Intimacy between Mother and Child

Tonti-Filippini asks whether the capacity of a woman to receive a child in her womb is a part of her generative faculty, a question similar to that asked by the Thomists of the previous section and one which they, like the Thomists and myself, agree should be answered in the affirmative. But then Tonti-Filippini traces an analogy between marital intimacy and its fruit—the child who has come to be—and gestational intimacy between mother and child, an intimacy that he says "has no parallel." Yet at the same time that the bond between mother and child is "unique," it also is an extension of the spousal bond in such a way that the husband shares in that intimacy as an extension of his wife's comprehensive gift of her self and her body to him in marriage: "Although it is the woman who carries the pregnancy and thus is intimately

---

24. See John Paul II, *Familiaris consortio* (November 22, 1981); and John Paul II, *The Theology of the Body: Human Love in the Divine Plan* (Boston: Pauline Books and Media, 1997).

related to the child in a way in which her husband cannot be except through her, nevertheless the child is the fruit and thus the sign and symbol of the union between this man and this woman. Far from being excluded, the husband stands bound ever more strongly to his wife through the coming into being of *their* child, the living consequence of their love." But heterologous ET breaks this extended form of marital intimacy by bringing the child into the unique gestational relationship independent of the spouse's marital love. In Tonti-Filippini's words, "The pregnancy is in fact achieved *outside the marital relationship*."[25]

Relationship between Marital Self-Gift and Gestational Intimacy

Oleson likewise connects marital self-giving with gestational intimacy: "Accordingly, when the wife *becomes a woman with child* through a natural act of conjugal love, the intimate communion that she now lives with the child in her womb has been made possible by the father, who participates in it. He is intimately and uniquely bound up in his wife having become with child, and thus shares in this new communion of persons."[26]

Oleson gives special attention to the gestational intimacy of mother and child, citing John Paul II, who wrote, "On the human level, can there be any other 'communion' comparable to that between a mother and a child whom she has carried in her womb and then brought to birth?"[27] Like Tonti-Filippini, Oleson focuses on the way in which bearing a child brings about an ontological change in the mother, a change that he wishes to say is not "merely biological and psychological" but, again in light of John Paul II's *Letter to Families,* personal and vocational.[28]

Finally, Oleson, like Tonti-Filippini, sees heterologous ET as an intrusion into a sphere of intimacy that, while it is paradigmatically between mother and child, ought nevertheless to be an extension and fruit of marital self-giving and intimacy. What ought to be a way in which the woman experiences marital intimacy no longer can be, as the child is not the son or daughter of the mother's husband.

---

25. Tonti-Filippini, "Embryo Rescue Debate," 84, 85, emphasis original.
26. Oleson, "Nuptial Womb," 175, emphasis original.
27. John Paul II, *Letter to Families* (February 2, 1994), n. 7, cited in Oleson, "Nuptial Womb," 178.
28. Oleson, "Nuptial Womb," 179.

Inclusion of Both Procreation and Gestation in the Conjugal Act

Finally, Althaus also wishes to extend "procreation beyond conception to include gestational motherhood" and to highlight the "ontological change" that becoming a mother brings about.[29] Althaus draws our attention to recent and insightful work on the gestational motherhood of Mary by John Saward; the period of Mary's pregnancy is again one of special intimacy between Mary and her Son. It is also a time in which his redeeming and sanctifying work has begun, not just a preparatory period before the Nativity of Our Lord.

Althaus's specific argument depends upon her description of what she calls the "object of the moral act" of ET, namely, to "seek pregnancy outside the marital act." This indicates that she wishes not just to extend procreation beyond conception but also to claim "that the conjugal act extends beyond conception to include gestational motherhood."[30] In a very direct way, then, Althaus believes that heterologous ET is a violation of the first norm identified at the beginning of this essay, that the procreative and unitive aspects of the marital act are not to be separated.

Response to Arguments from Personalism

I begin my critical assessment of the personalist version of the argument for extended inseparability by addressing a confusion present in these writers about my view and views similar to mine. Oleson, writing before any published work of my own on this topic but in regard to the view that I and other new natural law thinkers such as Christian Brugger and William May hold, writes that, on our view,

> no good of marriage is at stake ... in transferring a "spare" embryo into another woman's womb, and thus there is no problem becoming pregnant with a child that is neither hers nor (if she is married) her husband's. Everything morally relevant to the goods of procreation and procreative unity within marriage pertains only to *the marriage act itself*, and thus is no longer a factor after the genetic conception of embryonic life has taken place. Accordingly, these moralists see pregnancy, which is to say, a

---

29. Althaus, "Establishing the Moral Object," 171, 179.
30. Althaus, "Establishing the Moral Object," 169, 171.

woman's being with child, as having only biological and perhaps psychological significance, but no moral significance relative to her maternal vocation within marriage.[31]

Althaus delivers a similar critique of my own work: "I dispute Tollefsen's shortchanging his use of the term 'generation' to mean some sort of biological or purely material account only. While this physical reductionism is certainly not his intent, to say that procreation stops at conception has profound ontological meaning and implications."[32] Here Althaus echoes criticism made by Michel Accad of Rev. Thomas Williams, who had written of procreation that it is "necessarily and essentially punctual."[33]

However, Althaus conflates two different claims in criticizing my work. I had claimed that it is the possibility of generation only—a possibility that, when realized, *is* indeed punctual—that makes possible the two-in-one-flesh union that realizes, at the physical level of the couple's personal reality, their comprehensive marital commitment. That is, for the couple's sexual activity to be marital in kind, they must perform a sexual act that is by its nature per se apt for generation only. Failure to do that—for example, were they to engage only in manual stimulation to climax—is insufficient to make them one flesh, but an act per se apt for generation is *sufficient* to make them one flesh.

Thus, consider three couples: one incapable of performing a sexual act per se apt for generation, perhaps because of impotence on the part of man; a second capable of such an act but incapable of generation itself, perhaps because of infertility on the part of the man; and a third incapable of gestation, such that each zygotic human being conceived in the mother was destined to perish before even his or her first mitotic division. Only one of these couples is incapable of achieving a one-flesh union, namely, the first. For the possibility of one-flesh union is dependent solely on the act's ordering to the possibility of generation as such. As I wrote in the essay

---

31. Oleson, "Nuptial Womb," 167, emphasis original.
32. Althaus, "Establishing the Moral Object," 176.
33. Michael Accad, "Heterologous Embryo Transfer: Magisterial Answers and Metaphysical Questions," *Linacre Quarterly* 81.1 (February 2014): 43, doi: 10.1179/2050854913Y.0000000016, discussing Williams, "Heterologous Embryo Transfer," 243.

that Althaus critiques, "An account of the biological *union* of two fish, two sharks, two dogs, or two platypuses, would be complete once it had specified how members of the species did whatever was necessary in order to bring new members of the species into being."[34]

But immediately after saying that, I went on to note that any account of *human reproduction* or, one might equally say, of *human procreation* that stopped there would be radically incomplete, and incomplete not merely biologically but precisely as regards the marital communion between spouses. A full story of human reproduction or procreation would need to address, inter alia, "how the newly existing being would itself receive nutrition, how it would grow, in what environment it would live, how it would be educated and socialized, and so on."[35] These, I claimed in 2007 and still hold, are all aspects of human procreation and, for that reason, aspects also of the martial communion of spouses, of what it means for spouses to act as one in the procreation and education of their children.

But none of these aspects of human procreation are "performed as one physical organism," even when both spouses contribute to the performance in a cooperative manner:

> The reproductive process of a species—and the marital communion of spouses—thus goes beyond generation as such, but no aspects of the process beyond the generation of a new being are *biological* functions performed by a male and female organism acting as one. So, for human beings, no other aspects of the reproductive process are essential to the unitive significance of the sexual act, when performed by a married couple. It is, for example, normatively part of human reproduction and hence marriage in the wide sense, that both husband and wife should together educate offspring; but this togetherness is neither a physical unity, nor a part of the reproductive function of the marriage act.[36]

---

34. Christopher Tollefsen, "Could Human Embryo Transfer Be Intrinsically Immoral?," in Brakman and Weaver, *Ethics of Embryo Adoption*, 93, emphasis original.
35. Tollefsen, "Could Human Embryo Transfer Be Intrinsically Immoral?," 93.
36. Tollefsen, "Could Human Embryo Transfer Be Intrinsically Immoral?," 93, emphasis in original.

Part 3: Defenses of Embryo Adoption

What about the pregnancy itself? Is that something of moral significance to the marital union? It seems to me the answer is obviously yes. For example, husbands must be invested in the pregnancies of their wives, typically by working to support the mother and child, by providing needed forms of care for the mother, and by preparing spiritually for the work of being a good father. Moreover, it seems correct to me that the insights of the personalist approach to pregnancy should be taken onboard here. There is a special form of intimacy between mother and unborn child that is *or can be* an expression and sign of the marital intimacy of the spouses and in which the husband may share, and spouses should work together to maintain that extended form of marital intimacy. But I wish to qualify this claim in three ways, the third of which will lead to my final critical point of this essay.

First, what is the significance of my italicized qualifier "is *or can be* an expression and sign of the marital intimacy"? Olseon quotes John Paul II issuing a caution for thinking about gestational intimacy. Motherhood, whether at conception, gestation, or parturition, should not be thought of in purely biophysical and psychological terms. Rather, "motherhood is linked to the personal structure of the woman and to the personal dimension of the gift."[37] That is to say, *motherhood* is, in this context, a deeply normative term, encompassing the moral responsibilities that a woman takes on in light of having generated new human life and in light of further gift-responsibilities undertaken in marriage. Thus, like Aquinas's remarks about natural teleologies, claims about biological or psychological intimacy in gestation should not be taken as claims about nature's having normative implications as such, but as claims about nature with salience for those whose practical deliberations are informed by concern for marital, parental, and societal goods.

So, for example, in thinking about Judith Jarvis Thomson's famous defense of abortion, an adequate response will not cite gestational intimacy as a fact of intrinsic normative valence, for it is not always a fact, and indeed, Thomson's argument has worked culturally to erode its facticity. Rather, an adequate response will show how the real biological, psychological, and spiritual possibility of gestational intimacy is an *opportunity* in relation to the goods of marriage and parenthood. This, it seems to me, is

---

37. John Paul II, *Mulieris dignitatem* (August 15, 1988), n. 18.

the appropriate lesson of John Paul II's linking of gestation to the "personal dimension of the gift."

My second qualifying claim is as follows: while the opportunities for gestational intimacy are real and can be of profound moral significance, it is also possible to overstate those opportunities, a tendency sometimes evident in the discussion of ET and EA. The personalists I have discussed, for example, are keen to claim that the intimacy of gestation is different in kind and quality from that of nursing (given the standard analogy of embryo rescue with wet-nursing), and the unique nature of gestational intimacy is invoked more than once.

Gestational intimacy certainly *is* unique, by definition: it is the form of intimacy available exclusively to expecting mothers. It might also seem that there is no closer *physical* bond possible between two human persons than that between mother and gestating child, and that this physical bond serves as an affordance for intimacy in more personal dimensions that *also* exceed what is available at other stages of parenting. But beyond the tautological claim, these assertions seem questionable to me.

Consider first the physical bond of twins gestating together in the womb. While different in kind, their physical closeness is, like the gestational closeness of mother and child, extraordinary and surely contributes to the closeness experienced by many twins throughout the rest of their lives. And then there is the physical closeness of some conjoined twins: neither Hensel twin can live without the other, and their entire lives are shaped by the constant sharing of limbs, organs, and sensations, such as touch. If there is a candidate for the most physically close that two human beings can be, this is surely it.

But is not the intimacy afforded by gestation qualitatively deeper and more satisfying than that subsequently available after birth? I think we should hesitate before saying yes. Consider some of the noteworthy opportunities that birth makes possible as regards intimacy between parent and child: face-to-face connection, human touch, auditory experience, olfactory experience (everyone who has held a newborn knows the smell), immediate knowledge of a child's distress or contentment (by contrast, a child in the womb can be in distress or even die without the mother's awareness), *shared* physical care for the child between parents, and initiation into the Christian sacrament of Baptism. These forms of intimacy are not guaranteed: parents too often renege on their responsibilities. But the same is true of the forms of intimacy made available by gestation: mothers and fathers, too, forsake these opportunities and remain or become strangers to their children in the womb.

This leads to my third qualifying claim: seeing what is available between parents and gestating children, and then between parents and newborns, and conceptualizing those opportunities from within the frame of spousal, maternal, and paternal self-gift should lead us to press further. For what I would call the procreative forms of parental intimacy made available at later stages of parenting are, likewise, full of moral and personal significance. Catholics speak of marriage as bringing a responsibility for the procreation and education of children, and some contributors to the debate over ET draw a sharp boundary between these. But they are, from a suitable vantage point, simply the same duties. The entire context of human procreation is one in which parents beget, rear, and raise children with a view to their being free and flourishing adult human beings: this responsibility encompasses generation, gestation, birth, rearing, educating, and all the subsequent forms of care that children need even well into adulthood. All are equally the responsibilities of parents committed to being cocreators with God of new human life destined for the kingdom of heaven; all are equally parts of *procreation* in a reasonably extended sense that should flow from the intimacy and self-giving nature of marital communion.

Pro-life defenders of the unborn are accustomed to pointing out the arbitrariness of assigning full moral status at any point after conception; that is the moment at which a substantial change brings about a new human being, and every other subsequent change is merely a change of status. The claim has import in this context as well. There is no point at which parents can say that they are done with the tasks of procreation, in this extended sense, and are now engaged merely in education. Everything from the moment of conception onward is an effort of parents to continue to cocreate, to actualize the potentialities of, or to assist in the self-actualization of the potentialities of the being who, in an important sense, will always remain *in via* while here on earth, who will always be on the way toward being fully himself or herself.

So what I take to be the key insight of the personalists is vindicated: the work of procreation *is* extended. But the attempt to identify nine months of that work as uniquely different in kind and quality from all that follows is, I think, a mistake. That, in conjunction with the argument against Geach and the challenges I have raised to neo-Thomist objectors, should incline us in the direction of arguments in favor of embryo rescue and embryo adoption.[38] Just as fostering, adopting, and sponsoring children at a distance are compatible with the goods of marriage and human life, so embryo rescue and embryo adoption are opportunities available to those willing to serve those two essential human goods.

The debate over embryo transfer and adoption is unusual in Catholic bioethics, because it is conducted between Catholic moralists and theologians who are equally committed to the Church's teaching on the dignity and integrity of marital sexuality. This teaching is rejected by many others, yet in both my view and those of my interlocutors, it is essential to human flourishing and central to the Church's evangelistic mission. As I have shown, proponents and opponents of ET can and do share many other commitments as well: to the natural teleologies of generation and gestation, to the importance of gestational intimacy, and to the ways in which everything that unfolds in a person's life from conception on should normatively be understood as an extension and fruit of spousal love. My hope is that, through continued discussion, we will eventually also come to agree that the practices of embryo transfer and adoption are fully compatible with our most central Catholic commitments, as I believe them to be.

---

38. For a particularly rich treatment of such arguments, see Sarah-Vaughan Brakman, "*Real* Mothers and Good Stewards: The Ethics of Embryo Adoption," in Brakman and Weaver, *Ethics of Embryo Adoption*, 119–138; and Sarah-Vaughan Brakman and Darlene Fozard Weaver, "Embryo Adoption before and after *Dignitas Personae*: Defending an Argument of Limited Permissibility," in Eberl, *Contemporary Controversies in Catholic Bioethics*, 147–167.

12

Protecting the Dignity of the Child

Understanding the Rationale for the Inseparability Norm in the Context of the Embryo Adoption Debate

Melissa Moschella

Donum vitae highlights two "fundamental values" that are relevant to moral judgments regarding reproductive technologies: "The life of the human being called into existence and the special nature of the transmission of human life in marriage."[1] This essay will argue that both philosophical analysis and a close reading of *Donum vitae* reveal that these two values should be understood as inextricably intertwined, and that the primary reason why it is intrinsically wrong to use reproductive technologies is that these methods of procreation fail to respect the dignity of the child. Note that I use the term *reproductive technologies* to refer to any method of procreating apart from sexual intercourse, the most typical examples of which are in vitro fertilization (IVF) and intrauterine insemination (IUI). The use of reproductive technologies inherently involves treating the child as a product of manufacture—a *thing* subordinate to and made for the purposes of its producers rather than a *person* equal in dignity to his parents and intrinsically valuable. Once the child exists, parents may (and often do) treat the child as equal in dignity. Thus, the claim is not that these parents are bad parents who fail to love and respect their (born) children—a claim that is obviously false, at least for the vast majority of parents who conceive through reproductive technologies. Rather, the claim is that, at least in the act of *making*

---

1. Congregation for the Doctrine of the Faith (CDF), *Donum vitae* (February 22, 1987), introduction, 4.

the child through technological means, the child is necessarily treated as a product. Thus, I will argue that the rationale for the norm forbidding the separation of procreation from marital union is that such separation necessarily involves a failure to respect the dignity and rights of the child.

The essay will then go on to argue that, by contrast with IVF or IUI, heterologous embryo transfer (HET), pursued as an aspect of embryo adoption, does not involve this failure to respect the child's dignity and rights. For embryo adoption, like infant adoption in many cases, responds to a situation in which a fundamental injustice has already been done to the child by bringing that child into the world apart from marital sexual intercourse.[2] (In the case of embryo adoption, the child is made in a lab; in infant adoption, the child is often the result of extramarital sex.) And embryo adoption, like infant adoption, involves no *additional* injustice to the child but, on the contrary, seeks insofar as possible to remedy the harms resulting from that injustice by incorporating the child into one's family and providing him with the unconditional parental love he needs in order to flourish. Because of the inextricable connection between the two values highlighted by *Donum vitae*—the value of nascent human life and the value of the transmission of life in and through marriage—the fact that embryo adoption (by contrast with procreation through reproductive technologies) fully respects the dignity and rights of the child is strong evidence that it also respects the inseparability of the procreative and unitive aspects of marriage.

Before proceeding to the substance of the argument, a note on terminology is in order: Although it is common in the literature on this topic to discuss the permissibility of HET, this essay generally refers to *embryo*

---

2. While my focus here is largely on the injustice to children of being produced through technical means rather than procreated through the marital act, it is worth noting that St. Thomas Aquinas articulates the wrongness of fornication as a failure to respect the good of the child that might result from the act. He argues that "every sin committed directly against human life is a mortal sin," and that "fornication implies an inordinateness that tends to injure the life of the offspring to be born of this union," for the good of the child requires that the child be conceived within marriage, where he will be able to receive the care of both parents. Thomas Aquinas, *Summa theologiae*, trans. Fathers of the English Dominican Province (1920; New Advent, 2017), II-II.154.2 corpus, https://www.newadvent.org/summa/3154.htm.

adoption rather than *HET*, because HET is insufficient as an act-description for the purposes of moral evaluation. HET describes a physical process, but the object of a human act (which defines the act morally) is not "a process or event of the merely physical order." Rather, the "object is the proximate end of a deliberate decision which determines the act of willing on the part of the acting person."[3] For example, "giving money to someone" describes a physical behavior that could be specified morally in a variety of ways (depending on the proximate end determining the agent's choice)—for example, it could be specified *as* bribery, *as* paying a debt, or *as* almsgiving. Similarly, HET could be chosen *as* a variety of morally distinct types of acts—for example, *as* infertility treatment, *as* embryo rescue, or *as* embryo adoption. My aim in this paper is to defend the moral permissibility of HET as embryo adoption (both in principle and in practice), although I believe that the argument could easily be extended to defend the permissibility of HET as embryo rescue as well.[4]

Understanding the Inseparability Norm

It is a basic norm of Catholic sexual ethics that one ought never to violate the "inseparable connection ... between the unitive significance and the procreative significance which are both inherent to the marriage act."[5] We can call this the inseparability norm. *Donum vitae* invokes this norm

---

3. John Paul II, *Veritatis splendor* (August 6, 1993), n. 78.
4. Interestingly, while *Dignitas personae* mentions prenatal adoption, the description provided is actually a description of what the scholarly literature calls embryo rescue (attempting to gestate the child "solely in order to allow human beings to be born who are otherwise condemned to destruction"). CDF, *Dignitas personae* (September 8, 2008), n. 19. Thus, as Christopher Tollefsen has pointed out, the document fails to actually consider the possibility of embryo adoption as an act distinct in type from embryo rescue. Christopher Tollefsen, "Divine, Human, and Embryo Adoption," *National Catholic Bioethics Quarterly* 10.1 (Spring 2010): 75–85, doi: 10.5840/ncbq201010173. For a mapping of the various positions in the literature, see Melissa Moschella, "Gestation Does Not Necessarily Imply Parenthood: Implications for the Morality of Embryo Adoption and Embryo Rescue," *American Catholic Philosophical Quarterly* 92.1 (Winter 2018): 21–48, doi: 10.5840/acpq20171130137.
5. Paul VI, *Humanae vitae* (July 25, 1968), n. 12.

when it argues that the wrong of procreation apart from the conjugal act is analogous to the wrong of contraception, for both fail to respect the unity of the two aspects of the marital good.[6]

A brief account of the wrongness of contraception can, therefore, be helpful in understanding the inseparability norm before considering how it applies to reproductive technologies. When couples contracept (intentionally sterilizing their sexual acts), they violate the inseparability norm by attempting to enjoy the unitive aspect of the marital good while thwarting the procreative aspect. I say *attempting* to enjoy marital union because, in acting against the natural fruit of their marital union, contracepting spouses are indirectly acting against their union itself. Sherif Girgis explains the argument as follows:

> When spouses try to sterilize sex, they adopt a goal at odds with its marital quality. They choose to stunt what makes this act a candidate for bodily and therefore marital union: its link to a common bodily end, to the making of new life. And you can't both choose and fight that one thing. A couple may want to express affection and share pleasure—and there's nothing wrong with that! But they can't choose a sexual act to embody truly all-encompassing union if they're trying to stunt what makes this very act a bodily union, oriented to family life, in the first place. Even if their behavior looks the same, because they use a pill and not a barrier, they've crowded out the will to unite as one flesh, by willing to sterilize their act. They're fighting the total union that romantic love seeks in this act. They might have the right behavior for a marital act, but not the right will.[7]

Contraception, therefore, renders a sexual act nonmarital, and according to the natural law tradition (and to Catholic moral theology), only marital sex acts are morally permissible. The reason for this is that all nonmarital sex acts violate the good of marriage, which is the finality of the sexual act (the fulfillment of the person *qua* sexual).[8] For a sex act to be marital, two

---

6. CDF, *Donum vitae,* II.B.4a.
7. Sherif Girgis, "The Historic Christian Teaching against Contraception," *Public Discourse,* August 10, 2016, https://www.thepublicdiscourse.com/2016/08/17559/.
8. For a more detailed account of sexual ethics from a natural law perspective, and for additional references, see Melissa Moschella, "Sexual Ethics, Human

conditions must be met: (1) The act must truly unite the spouses as one flesh, joining the male and female halves of the reproductive system to form one organic unit cooperating for the joint biological end of reproduction (note that infertile couples can meet this condition, as it is biological coordination toward the joint biological end of reproduction, *not* the achievement of that end, that constitutes the one-flesh union). (2) The act must be done with the right intentions (i.e., to actualize and express one's marital union, understood as an all-encompassing, lifelong, and monogamous union with an inherent orientation to procreation and family life). The second condition requires that the couple be married—that is, have made the relevant marital commitments in the appropriate way. These marital commitments constitute a habitual intention that suffices for the second condition as long as it is maintained, but maintaining this habitual intention requires that no *contrary* intentions be present.[9] Such contrary intentions rendering one's sex acts nonmarital include the intention to thwart the procreative potential of one's union. Contraception is, therefore, wrong because it is an antiprocreative choice (intent) that is contrary to the intentions required for marital sex. Some scholars, following a long tradition of Church teaching, have also argued that contraception is wrong because it involves a contra-life choice, a choice directly against the basic human good of life.[10]

Having considered a brief explanation of the wrongness of contraception, we are now in a better position to return to *Donum vitae*'s claim that the wrong of reproductive technologies is analogous to the wrong of contraception. As with all analogies, there are both differences and similarities between the cases. The similarity is that both contraception and reproductive technologies violate the inseparability of the unitive and procreative

---

Nature, and the 'New' and 'Old' Natural Law Theories," *National Catholic Bioethics Quarterly* 19.2 (Summer 2019): 256–257, doi: 10.5840/ncbq 201919218. For a theological account, see John Paul II, *Familiaris consortio* (November 22, 1981).

9. John Finnis, "Marriage: A Basic and Exigent Good," *Monist* 91.3–4 (July–October 2008): 392–393.

10. Germain Grisez et al., "'Every Marital Act Ought to Be Open to New Life': Toward a Clearer Understanding," *Thomist* 52.3 (July 1988): 365–426. For an explanation and defense of this argument, see Melissa Moschella, "Sexual Ethics, Practical Reason, and the Magisterium: A Response to Irene Alexander," *National Catholic Bioethics Quarterly* 22.1 (Spring 2022): 99–127, doi: 10.5840/ncbq20222219.

PART 3: DEFENSES OF EMBRYO ADOPTION

aspects of marriage. The obvious difference is that, unlike contracepted sex acts, procreation through reproductive technologies need not involve any sex act at all and, therefore, cannot be contrary to the good of marriage in quite the same way or for quite the same reason as contraception.

This section argues that the reason that procreation should never be sought in isolation from the unitive aspect of marriage (actualized through marital sexual intercourse) is primarily that doing so always involves a failure to respect the dignity of the child. Thus, while contraception violates the marital good by *thwarting the procreative aspect of that good*, procreation through reproductive technologies violates the procreative aspect of the marital good by *seeking it in a way that is disordered*, because it is unjust to the future child. If one believes that the contra-life argument against contraception is sound (as I do), then that argument strengthens this interpretation of the analogy between the wrong of contraception and the wrong of procreation apart from the conjugal act. For both contraception and procreation through reproductive technologies fail to respect the good of life-in-transmission, though in different ways.

This point about the injustice to the child involved in procreation apart from the conjugal act is emphasized throughout *Donum vitae*, which states, "Only respect for the link between the [unitive and procreative] meanings of the conjugal act and respect for the unity of the human being make possible procreation in conformity with the dignity of the person." The document goes on to explain why this is the case, arguing that "in his unique and irrepeatable origin, the child must be respected and recognized as equal in dignity to those who give him life." The only way to do this, it is suggested, is for the child to "be accepted in his parents' act of union and love ... in the conjugal act wherein the spouses cooperate as servants not as masters in the work of the Creator who is Love." By contrast, conceiving a child "as the product of an intervention of medical or biological techniques" fails to respect the child's equal dignity by "reducing him to an object of scientific technology" and subjecting him "to conditions of technical efficiency which are to be evaluated according to standards of control and dominion."[11]

Donum vitae's argument hinges on the crucial difference between spouses' *accepting* a child as a gift that supervenes upon their "act of union and love"—an act in which they cooperate with the Creator as servants not masters—and spouses' choosing to *make* or *produce* a child in a lab (with the

---

11. CDF, *Donum vitae*, II.B.4c. See also CDF, *Dignitas personae*, n. 16.

help of technicians who act as their agents). In natural procreation, children are, as Oliver O'Donovan puts it, begotten not made.[12] In order to see the difference between *begetting* a child (accepting a child as a gift) and *making* a child, it is necessary to analyze how the object of the act differs in natural procreation by contrast with procreation through reproductive technologies. Although in common speech we might sometimes refer to procreation through sexual intercourse as "making a baby," this is an imprecise description of the object of the act. For in marital sexual intercourse, the object of the act is to seal, actualize, and express one's marital union (with procreation sought, if it is sought, as an aspect of the dual good of marriage, not in isolation from it).

Indeed, if marital union is not, at least implicitly, the object of the spouses' act of sexual intercourse, then their intercourse is not truly *marital*, even if those engaging in it are married.[13] Consider, for example, the historical case of King Henry VIII and his second wife Anne Boleyn.[14] While we cannot be sure of the king's precise intentions, his behavior—such as the fact that he fabricated treason charges against Anne and had her beheaded when she did not give him the son he desired—makes it plausible to claim that, at least in some cases, he engaged in sexual intercourse with Anne *merely* for the sake of producing an heir. Even if their marriage had been valid, such sex would not be truly marital and would fail to respect the dignity of both Anne (whose body was being used as a mere means to the production of a child) and any resulting child (who was, through natural means, being sought as a product to fulfill the king's desire for an heir).

In truly marital sexual intercourse, however, procreation is not the act's object but is rather a gift that supervenes on an act of marital union sought for the sake of the good of marriage itself. Procreation may be sought as an *aspect* of the good of marriage, but it is not just as such the object of marital sexual intercourse. Thus, if spouses engage in marital intercourse but do not

---

12. Oliver O'Donovan, *Begotten or Made?* (New York: Oxford University Press, 1984).
13. As noted above, spouses need not *explicitly* intend to actualize their marital union in order for their sexual intercourse to be marital. The commitments made in their marriage vows constitute a habitual intention that makes marital union the implicit object of their sexual intercourse unless any contrary intentions are present.
14. I am indebted to Robert George for this example.

Part 3: Defenses of Embryo Adoption

conceive a child as a result, they might be disappointed (if they were hoping to conceive), but their act would not be a *failure*, for it would still have achieved its object of expressing and actualizing their marital union. By contrast, in procreation through reproductive technologies, the object of one's act (or, more precisely, of the series of acts involved in the process) is literally and solely to make a baby, such that if a child is not conceived as a result, the act will indeed be a failure. In other words, the proximate end, which is the object of the agent's choice in reproductive technologies, is baby-making.

Baby-making (in the precise sense in which I am using the term) is intrinsically wrong, for it inherently treats persons as products made for one's purpose and at one's command, and the relationship of maker to product is inherently one of dominion over a being fundamentally inferior in dignity to oneself.[15] Indeed, the wrong of baby-making is analogous to the wrong of slavery, for both set up a relationship of domination, in which one human being is treated as fundamentally inferior in dignity to another, as existing for another's purposes. Even when such domination is relatively benign, as may have been the case with those who treated their slaves well, it is, nonetheless, inherently contrary to human dignity. It is revealing in this regard that much of the literature in defense of IVF and other reproductive technologies speaks of procreation as a right in a way that indirectly views children themselves as a right.[16] For in no other context—except slavery—

---

15. For further development of this point, see Christopher Tollefsen, "In Vitro Fertilization Should Not Be an Option for a Woman," in *Contemporary Debates in Bioethics*, ed. Arthur Caplan and Robert Arp (Hoboken, NJ: Wiley, 2014): 451–459; and Germain Grisez, *The Way of the Lord Jesus*, vol. 3, *Difficult Moral Questions* (Quincy, IL: Franciscan Press, 1997), q. 52. It is also worth noting here that Irene Alexander, whose view will be discussed below, clearly misunderstands Tollefsen's argument that when spouses procreate through marital intercourse, they do not *make* a child. She misinterprets this as a denial that the spouses are genuine causal agents of conception, thus completely missing his point, which is not about natural causality but about correctly identifying the object of the spouses' act. Irene Alexander, "Is Artificial Impregnation Opposed to the Unity of Marriage? A New Look at the Question of Embryo Adoption," *Nova et Vetera* 16.1 (Winter 2018): 68–69.
16. See, for example, Muireann Quigley, "A Right to Reproduce?," *Bioethics* 24.8 (October 2010): 403–411, doi: 10.1111/j.1467-8519.2008.00722.x.

have human beings considered themselves to have a *right* to another human being just as such.

It may sound implausible and harsh to claim that parents who procreate through IVF or other reproductive technologies adopt an attitude toward their children that is similar to the attitude of masters toward their slaves. For clearly there are many parents currently raising children whom they conceived through IVF who love and respect those children and do not view or treat them in ways that are even remotely similar to the ways masters viewed and treated their slaves. My claim here, however, is only that the act of baby-making itself inherently treats children as products made for one's own purposes and at one's command. This attitude of dominion is not necessarily malevolent, just as some slave owners may have treated their slaves well, even in some cases believing that their slaves were better off under their dominion than they would be if freed.[17] Further, there is nothing to prevent parents from changing their attitude to the child after he or she exists—indeed, such an attitude change seems likely at least after the child is born and her humanity becomes more obvious.

Nonetheless, the way parents typically treat the embryos they have produced through IVF, at least initially, *does* reflect an attitude of dominion over them that fails to respect their equal dignity. For IVF is typically done in a way that aims at the production of more embryos than can be inserted (at least initially) into the mother's uterus. The embryos produced are typically graded on the basis of embryologists' judgments of their quality, and the best embryo or embryos are selected to be transferred to the woman's uterus in the hopes of achieving a pregnancy (either immediately or after being cryopreserved for a short time to give the woman's body time to recover from the ovarian hyperstimulation and egg retrieval processes). The remaining high-quality embryos are typically maintained for an indefinite period

---

17. For evidence that many slaveholders believed sincerely (even if self-deceptively) that slavery was beneficial to the slaves, see Eugene Genovese and Elizabeth Fox-Genovese, *Fatal Self-Deception: Slaveholding Paternalism in the Old South* (New York: Cambridge University Press, 2011). To give just one example, the authors quote a letter from Methodist Bishop James Andrew to his wife expressing his judgment that it would be bad for the slaves if he freed them: "How could I free them? Where would they go, and how would they support themselves?" (4).

of time in a cryopreserved state, in case the couple would like to use one of them to attempt another pregnancy in the future, and those deemed to be of low quality are likely to be discarded or donated for research purposes. As *Donum vitae* emphasizes, all of this clearly reflects an attitude of dominion that treats the embryos as products rather than persons.[18] To bring this point home, just imagine how shocked we would be if parents treated infants in this way, intentionally creating more than they were willing or able to raise, selecting the best, discarding those of poor quality, and then cryopreserving the remainder in case they later decide that they want them.

I should emphasize here that I believe most infertile couples seeking to conceive through IVF are not aware of these ethical issues but rather are desperate for children and told by their doctors that IVF is the appropriate treatment for their infertility. Unfortunately, most are not aware of alternatives—like NaProTechnology (Natural Procreative Technology), which actually identifies and treats the underlying causes of infertility (rather than bypassing the problem as IVF does)—because standard medical training fails to educate doctors about this approach.[19] Further, during the IVF process, the objectifying treatment of the embryos is cloaked in clinical language that masks the injustices occurring, and parents often are not even aware that they could avoid some of these ethical problems by, for instance, insisting on creating only one or two embryos and committing to inserting both into the mother's uterus in the hopes of achieving a pregnancy. In one revealing podcast, a woman who conceived through IVF expresses deep regret and guilt over having produced many more embryos than she could ever possibly gestate and raise, and she criticizes the IVF clinic for failing to warn her about this possibility or give her the option to make fewer embryos. Despite this regret, however, she nonetheless unwittingly demonstrates the very attitude of dominion which I have argued is inherent in procreation through reproductive technologies. She demonstrates this attitude by refusing to

---

18. CDF, *Donum vitae*, II.B.4c.
19. St. Paul VI Institute, "NaProTechnology," accessed June 28, 2023, https://naprotechnology.com/. See also Katie Elrod and Paul Carpentier, "The Church's Best-Kept Secret: Church Teaching on Infertility Treatment," in *Women, Sex and the Church*, ed. Erika Bachiochi (Boston: Pauline Books and Media, 2010), 121–142; and John Steven Fisher, dir., *NAPRO: A Quiet Revolution*, YouTube, posted by Dominican Friars on December 9, 2016, https://www.youtube.com/watch?v=6JT-m4-iEWE.

consider placing the embryos for adoption, because—though she is not willing to raise any of the remaining embryos herself—she does not want someone else raising her children (an attitude which no one would consider morally acceptable if we were dealing with infants rather than embryos).[20]

Technically, it is possible for IVF to be done in such a way that only one or two embryos are made and all are transferred to the uterus, without grading or selection, thereby avoiding many of the injustices involved in standard IVF protocols. Even in such a case, however, the problematic attitude of dominion over the child, instrumentalizing the child as a mere means to the parents' fulfillment, is nonetheless present. For the parents must be acting for the sake of *some* benefit (otherwise their action would not be intelligible), and the benefit sought must be for themselves or some other existing person. They cannot be acting for the benefit of the child, because the child does not yet exist, and one cannot be benefitted unless one already exists. Thus, their act of making the child necessarily treats the child as a mere means to the benefit of themselves or others rather than as a person who must be respected as an end in himself. *Making* human beings is the prerogative of God alone, for only God—who lacks nothing and who, therefore, acts not to fulfill any lack in himself but out of a pure superabundance of goodness and generosity—can make human beings without undermining their dignity as ends in themselves.

Procreation as the fruit of marital sexual intercourse is the only way to bring a human being into the world that does not treat that person as a product made for one's purposes. For it is the only way to bring a person into the world in which procreation is not the immediate or sole object of one's act, but is rather sought as the fruit of an act of marital sexual intercourse that has a distinct intelligible purpose of its own—namely, actualizing one's marital union. Note, however, that even a married couple who procreate through sexual intercourse *could* seek a child in a way that treats the child as merely instrumental to their own ends—for example, merely for the sake of emotional gratification or (as in Henry VIII's case) to carry on the family line.[21] The difference between natural procreation and IVF, however, is that

---

20. Jennie (last name not given), "Embryos on Ice: Jennie's Story," interview by Kallie Fell, *Venus Rising*, podcast, season 4, episode 57, October 25, 2022, Center for Bioethics and Culture Network, https://cbc-network.org/2022/10/embryos-on-ice-jennies-story/.
21. Grisez, *Difficult Moral Questions*, q. 52.

Part 3: Defenses of Embryo Adoption

IVF *necessarily* involves this attitude of instrumentalization, whereas natural procreation does not.

This violation of the dignity of the child inherent in reproductive technologies is the fundamental reason why the use of these technologies is inherently immoral. Thus, in this context, the inseparability norm should be understood as serving and protecting the dignity of the child. In other words, these technologies violate the human good of marriage precisely because, in separating procreation from the unitive aspect of the marital good, they violate the requirements of procreation in conformity with the dignity of the child. Although much of the Catholic literature related to reproductive technologies and embryo adoption focuses on the proper use of the generative faculty or the biological finality of the sexual act, this is not the focus of *Donum vitae* or *Dignitas personae*.[22] Indeed, those documents do not even mention the term *generative faculty*, and while they do talk

---

22. See, for example, Charles Robertson, "A Thomistic Analysis of Embryo Adoption," *National Catholic Bioethics Quarterly* 14.4 (Winter 2014): 673–697, doi: 10.5840/ncbq201414470; and Nicanor Pier Giorgio Austriaco, "Embryo Adoption and the Extended Inseparability Argument," *National Catholic Bioethics Quarterly* 21.1 (Spring 2021): 29–35, doi: 10.5840/ncbq20212114. Rev. Nicanor Austriaco, for instance, argues that the principle of inseparability between the unitive and procreative aspects of the conjugal act should be extended to include pregnancy. He makes this argument based on the claim that "in the natural order, having sex leads to making a baby, which then leads to becoming pregnant" (34). He thus believes that because there is a teleological connection on the biological level among sex, procreation, and pregnancy, one ought never to seek one in isolation from the others. Alexander also makes an argument based on biological causality, claiming that we must discover the natural "order among causes that God has wisely inscribed in his Creation" and "then choose to act in accord with it" ("Is Artificial Impregnation Opposed to the Unity of Marriage?," 52). These arguments are, however, fundamentally flawed, for not all finalities in the natural (biological) order correspond directly to finalities in the moral order, as is obvious when we consider that there is no moral requirement to respect the biological finality of every one of our cells, organs, or organ systems. Rather, we recognize that the relevant human good—the finality of our cells, organs, and so on, in the *moral* order—is life and health, and thus that, while life and health must be respected, acting contrary to the finality of a particular cell, organ, and so on (by, say, taking diet pills that prevent one from digesting one's food) is not wrong, except insofar as it intentionally or unreasonably damages life or health.

about the inherent meanings of the conjugal act, they do not analyze the act in terms of its biological finality but rather in terms of its finality in the moral order—namely, the dual good (unitive and procreative) of marriage.[23] Thus, in explaining "why the act of conjugal love is considered in the teaching of the Church as the only setting worthy of human procreation," the reasons given are that procreation apart from the conjugal act "establishes the domination of technology over the origin and destiny of the human person" and that "such a relationship of domination is in itself contrary to the dignity and equality that must be common to parents and children." For only when procreation is the "fruit of a conjugal act" can the spouses "become 'cooperators with God for giving life to a new person'" rather than masters of a technical process aimed at making a child for their own purposes.[24] Likewise, in explaining why it is "ethically unacceptable to *dissociate procreation from the integrally personal context of the conjugal act,*" *Dignitas personae* says the following: "The blithe acceptance of the enormous number of abortions involved in the process of *in vitro* fertilization vividly illustrates how the replacement of the conjugal act by a technical procedure—in addition to being in contradiction with the respect that is due to procreation as something that cannot be reduced to mere reproduction—leads to a weakening of the respect owed to every human being." By contrast, "recognition of such respect is ... promoted by the intimacy of husband and wife nourished by married love."[25]

---

23. Crucial to this point is Aquinas's distinction among the natural, logical, moral, and technical orders, each of which relates to reason in a different way and is studied with different methods. Thomas Aquinas, *Commentary on the Nicomachean Ethics*, trans. C. I. Litzinger (Chicago: Regnery, 1964), I.1, https://isidore.co/aquinas/english/Ethics.htm. Tollefsen argues that each of the orders has its own normativity, and thus that while normativity in the natural order can be relevant to moral normativity (revealing possibilities and causal connections that practical reason can recognize as having ethical relevance), one cannot directly deduce moral normativity from natural normativity. Christopher Tollefsen, "Aquinas's Four Orders, Normativity, and Human Nature," *Journal of Value Inquiry* 52.3 (August 2018): 243, doi: 10.1007/s10790-018-9657-6. For a discussion of this point in relation to sexual ethics, see Moschella, "Sexual Ethics, Practical Reason, and the Magisterium," 99–127.
24. CDF, *Donum vitae*, II.B.5.
25. CDF, *Dignitas personae*, n.16, emphasis original.

Part 3: Defenses of Embryo Adoption

Application to Embryo Adoption

The previous section argued that the reason why it is wrong to seek the procreative aspect of the marital good apart from the unitive aspect is that doing so inherently violates the dignity of nascent human life. This section will show that embryo adoption, unlike procreation through reproductive technologies, does not violate the dignity of nascent human life, and that this in itself is strong evidence that it does not violate the norm prohibiting the separation of the unitive and procreative aspects of marriage.

First, embryo adoption, unlike procreation through reproductive technologies, does not involve making a child—for the child already exists—and thus does not inherently treat the child as a product or set the parents in a relationship of domination over the child. Further, because the child already exists, the adoptive parents need not treat the child as merely instrumental to their own ends, for they can act for the good of community with the child, a truly common good in which all share. Of course, it is possible for adoptive parents to adopt for purely selfish motivations, merely seeking to fulfill some lack in their lives or erroneously considering the adoption a treatment for infertility, but these problematic motivations are possible when adopting a child at any age, not specific to the case of embryo adoption.[26]

Second, none of the acts involved in embryo adoption necessarily treats the child as a product or involves any failure to respect the child's dignity. Indeed, the Snowflakes embryo adoption program run by Nightlight Christian Adoptions—which is the oldest embryo adoption program and the one with which I am most familiar—is explicit in its recognition of and commitment to the fundamental dignity of every human life, beginning at conception. For instance, the program's web page prominently cites Jeremiah 1:5, "Before I formed you in the womb I knew you, before you were born I set you apart," features a link to a video with the title "It is not potential life but it is life with potential," and states, "We believe life begins at conception."[27] This commitment to the dignity of nascent human life is also

---

26. For more on this point, and on the type of attitude that prospective adoptive parents should have, see Tollefsen, "Divine, Human, and Embryo Adoption," 75–85.
27. Nightlight Christian Adoptions, "Home Page," Snowflakes Embryo Adoption Program, accessed December 1, 2022, https://nightlight.org/snowflakes-embryo-adoption-donation/embryo-adoption/.

reflected in the program's structure, which involves all of the same steps and safeguards as postnatal adoption. Although not legally required (for the law unjustly treats human embryos as property, not as persons), the Snowflakes program requires that all prospective adoptive parents go through a rigorous home study process and complete extensive pre-adoption education, just as is typically required for postnatal adoptions.[28]

Then, just as in postnatal adoption, there is a process of matching prospective adoptive parents with parents placing their embryos for adoption, in which each set of parents views the other's profile and decides whether to accept the match. In this way, placing parents can be assured that their children will be raised by a loving family, the families can agree in advance about the level and type of communication that each desires or is open to, and the adoptive parents can decide if, for instance, they are comfortable with the number of embryos to be adopted or with the family's medical history (which might be predictive of health problems for the embryos).[29] Such factors are also involved in the matching process for postnatal adoption. Snowflakes forbids both genetic testing of the embryos for any reason and gender selection, even if the gender of the embryos happens to be known from prior testing done by the placing family.[30] Embryo adoption, therefore, actually allows for *less* selection than most postnatal adoption programs, which typically do allow for gender selection or for backing out of the adoption if it is discovered (before or at birth) that the baby has a significant health problem.

The Snowflakes program also tries to keep biological siblings together to the extent possible, asking prospective adoptive parents to adopt all of the remaining embryos in a particular sibling group. It is recognized, however, that unforeseen circumstances may lead to a situation in which it is

---

28. Nightlight Christian Adoptions, "Home Study," Snowflakes Embryo Adoption Program, accessed December 6, 2022, https://nightlight.org/snowflakes-embryo-adoption-donation/embryo-adoption/adopter-process/home-study/.
29. Nightlight Christian Adoptions, "Matching," Snowflakes Embryo Adoption Program, accessed December 5, 2022, https://nightlight.org/snowflakes-embryo-adoption-donation/embryo-adoption/adopter-process/matching/.
30. Chris and Kari S., "A Letter to You from a Snowflakes Adopting Family," Snowflakes Embryo Adoption Program, accessed June 28, 2023, https://nightlight.org/wp-content/uploads/01-AP-General-Information-Packet-7.18.2022.pdf; and Nightlight Christian Adoptions, "Matching."

impossible or imprudent for the adoptive family to attempt a pregnancy with all of the embryos, and in that case, the remaining embryos can be made available to be adopted by another couple.[31] This, too, is similar to postnatal adoption, in which agencies generally try to keep siblings together but will sometimes place them with different families when this is not feasible.

Finally, in line with currently accepted best practices for postnatal adoption and the best available research on what is best for adopted children, Snowflakes counsels adoptive parents to be open and honest with children about their adoption story from the very beginning and allows only open adoptions, in which there is at least some level of communication between the placing and adoptive parents, thus making it possible for the children to have some knowledge of their genetic parents and siblings.[32] While no adoption agency can guarantee that adoptive parents will have an appropriate attitude toward their adoptive children, the Snowflakes program is clearly structured to foster an attitude of respect for the equal dignity of the embryos being adopted and to prevent (as far as possible) couples from seeking to adopt embryos as a remedy for infertility. Indeed, standard adoption education for both embryo and postnatal adoption includes a lesson on the need to grieve the loss of genetic children and come to terms with one's infertility in order to be able to approach adoption with the right attitude (of generously welcoming a child in need of care into one's family rather than seeking to fill a void left by the absence of genetic children).[33]

Those who believe that embryo adoption is not morally permissible may agree that none of the above practices is problematic, for their concern generally focuses specifically on HET—that is, transferring an embryo not conceived with the egg and sperm of the woman and her spouse—done with the intent of achieving a pregnancy (defined narrowly

---

31. Nightlight Christian Adoptions, "Matching."
32. Nightlight Christian Adoptions, "Matching."
33. See, for example, the domestic infant adoption education package offered by Creating a Family, a highly respected nonprofit organization dedicated to adoption and foster care education. Creating a Family, "Domestic Infant Adoption (10 Hours)," accessed July 11, 2023, https://www.creatingafamilyed.org/bundles/domestic-infant-adoption-package. See also Nightlight Christian Adoptions, "Embryo Adoption Education Requirements," Snowflakes Embryo Adoption Program, July 2019, https://nightlight.org/wp-content/uploads/Embryo-Adoption-Education-Requirements-July-2019.pdf.

as successful implantation of the embryo in the uterine lining). While, as argued above, HET is a physical process that could be chosen under several act-descriptions (e.g., infertility treatment, embryo adoption, or embryo rescue) that specify it for purposes of moral evaluation, one can nonetheless consider whether anything about HET in itself (regardless of the act-description under which it is chosen) fails to respect the equal dignity of the child. Perhaps someone might argue that being gestated in the womb of a woman who is not one's genetic mother is inherently contrary to the dignity of the child. But I cannot see why this would be inherently contrary to the child's dignity any more than being nursed or raised by someone other than one's genetic mother. Perhaps, more plausibly, one might worry that HET is contrary to *Donum vitae*'s statement that "the child has the right to be conceived, carried in the womb, brought into the world and brought up within marriage."[34] Yet this statement obviously cannot mean that, when injustice or tragedy make this ideal impossible, we must leave the abandoned or orphaned children to die rather than allow them to be raised by someone other than their married biological parents. Such an interpretation certainly would prove too much, implying that postnatal adoption would also be impermissible. Rather, *Donum vitae* is here stating an ideal that is the norm for responsible procreation that fully respects the dignity and rights of the child, an ideal in which there is no rupture between genetic, gestational, and social parenthood.

While *Donum vitae* is clear that the ideal is for there to be no rupture between genetic, gestational, and social parenthood, the Church is also clear in praising adoption (when done with the right intentions).[35] Thus, when

---

34. CDF, *Donum vitae*, II.A.1.
35. John Grabowski and Christopher Gross argue that, from a Catholic theological perspective, "the relationships that are formed through adoption are equal to or transcend biological ties, because … adoption itself is a form of covenant. Adoption, as a covenant, contains a declaration of fidelity that is as important as blood or biological relation." John S. Grabowski and Christopher Gross, "*Dignitas Personae* and the Adoption of Frozen Embryos: A New Chill Factor?," *National Catholic Bioethics Quarterly* 10.2 (Summer 2010): 307–328, doi: 10.5840/ncbq201010255. Grabowski and Gross ultimately conclude that embryo adoption, though permissible in principle, is morally problematic, because it involves material cooperation with the IVF industry and risks causing scandal. Sarah-Vaughan Brakman and Darlene Fozard Weaver convincingly respond to these concerns, arguing, for instance, that there is no evidence that

Part 3: Defenses of Embryo Adoption

a rupture between the various aspects of parenthood has already occurred because of injustice or tragedy—as when a child is conceived out of wedlock to parents not capable of raising her—it is obviously not wrong for another couple to step in and adopt the child. This is not the ideal, but it is the best that can be done for a child conceived in such nonideal circumstances. The same is true with embryo adoption; an injustice was done to the embryos by conceiving them apart from the marital act, and a further injustice was done by creating extra embryos and cryopreserving them. But the adoptive couple does not cooperate with those injustices in any way. Rather, the adoptive couple steps in to provide the best care possible for these children in nonideal circumstances, welcoming them unconditionally into a stable, loving family.

Indeed, from the perspective of the child, being adopted at the embryonic stage involves less psychological rupture than being adopted after birth, just as being adopted soon after birth involves less rupture than being adopted at an older age. For just as a child adopted at age five suffers a greater psychological rupture than an infant, because he has formed stronger psychological bonds with his biological parents, so, too, does an infant suffer a greater psychological rupture than an embryo, for the infant has already formed psychological bonds with his mother in the womb, but the embryo has not.

---

the possibility of embryo adoption makes couples more likely to pursue IVF or to create excess embryos, and also that failure to adopt embryos would likely cause even greater scandal, leading people to doubt the Church's commitment to the full dignity and personhood of human embryos. Sarah-Vaughan Brakman and Darlene Fozard Weaver, "Embryo Adoption before and after *Dignitas Personae*: Defending an Argument of Limited Permissibility," in *Contemporary Controversies in Catholic Bioethics*, ed. Jason T. Eberl (New York: Springer, 2017), 147–168. Brakman and Weaver conclude that embryo adoption is permissible if done with the right intentions. They argue that this requires welcoming the embryos regardless of quality (164). I completely agree with this requirement, if understood as a condition on how adoptive parents treat the embryos *after* they have been adopted (i.e., after going through the matching process and finalizing their contract with the placing family). However, if they mean this to be a condition requiring that prospective adoptive parents be willing to adopt *any* embryos, regardless of what is known about their medical history or likelihood of health and survival, I believe that this is too stringent, for this is not required of postnatal adoptive parents. As noted above, embryo adoption as practiced by Snowflakes already allows for less selection than postnatal adoption.

Thus, the child adopted as an embryo does not suffer from the primal wound of separation from his birthmother and is, therefore, saved from what some believe to be the lifelong psychological effects of that wound.[36]

This analysis shows that, while the ideal for children is to be conceived, gestated, and raised within marriage, embryo adoption does not violate that ideal any more than postnatal adoption does. For in neither scenario is the adoptive couple responsible for the nonideal circumstances. If anything, embryo adoption comes closer to the ideal scenario than postnatal adoption, because it at least allows for continuity between gestational and social parenthood.

Is there anything else about HET that might be morally suspect in relation to the child's dignity and rights? The thawing process involves risks to the embryo, but cryopreservation is itself a state contrary to the dignity of the child, and thawing is the only way to allow the child to resume her normal trajectory of development. There is also a risk that the embryo will not implant and will thus die after being transferred to the woman's body, but embryo transfer protocols are designed to minimize this risk (by, for instance, testing to ensure that that the woman's uterine lining is healthy and sufficiently thick to allow for implantation), and this is a risk even for embryos conceived naturally.[37] At any rate, given that the risk is not intended as an end or as a means but is merely accepted as a side effect, and that accepting the risk is proportionate (for this is the only way for the embryo to even have a chance at growing to maturity), the criteria of the principle of double effect are satisfied in this case.

There thus seems to be no plausible reason to think that embryo adoption—either inherently or in the way it is practiced by the Snowflakes program—involves any *new* injustice or failure to respect the dignity and

---

36. Nancy Newton Verrier, *The Primal Wound* (Baltimore: Gateway Press, 1993).
37. While accurately determining the rate of early embryo loss in natural conception is difficult, analysis of the available data estimates that there is a 10–40 percent rate of pre-implantation embryo loss in healthy women. Gavin E. Jarvis, "Early Embryo Mortality in Natural Human Reproduction: What the Data Say," *F1000 Research* 5 (November 25, 2016): 2765, doi: 10.12688/f1000research.8937.2. For a recent overview of the research on embryo transfer protocols, see Sezcan Mumusoglu et al., "Preparation of the Endometrium for Frozen Embryo Transfer: A Systematic Review," *Frontiers in Endocrinology* 12 (July 9, 2021): 688237, doi: 10.3389/fendo.2021.688237.

rights of the child. If, as I argued in the previous section, any act that dissociates procreation from marital union inherently violates the dignity of nascent human life, then it would seem that embryo adoption must not involve any dissociation of procreation from marital union, for if it did, then it would necessarily violate the dignity of the child. Further, if the *reason* why it is wrong to separate procreation from marital union is that such a separation violates the dignity of the child, then the fact that embryo adoption involves no such violation is a strong reason to be skeptical of the claim that the norm prohibiting that separation includes a prohibition on seeking *pregnancy* (narrowly defined as the implantation of an already-existing embryo) apart from the marital act. To further support this claim, in the next section I will directly address several recent arguments claiming that seeking pregnancy apart from the marital act is an inherent violation of conjugal fidelity.

Response to Counterarguments

Earlier I noted that arguments against HET relying on *Donum vitae*'s statement that "the child has the right to be conceived, carried in the womb, brought into the world and brought up within marriage" are problematic, because they prove too much, implying that postnatal adoption is also impermissible. This same problem of proving too much plagues the various arguments made in defense of the claim that the inseparability of the unitive and procreative aspects of marriage should be taken to include pregnancy (narrowly defined), such that seeking to become pregnant apart from the marital act would be intrinsically immoral for the same reason as seeking to procreate apart from the marital act.[38]

Rev. Nicanor Austriaco, who has argued most explicitly for this extended inseparability thesis, claims that "having sex, making a baby, and becoming pregnant are teleologically linked and should therefore be understood as one movement that actualizes the full potency of the conjugal act."

---

38. In a previous essay, I responded to several arguments against HET on the grounds that it violates conjugal fidelity, insofar as it makes a woman a mother apart from her husband or results in a lack of parity between husband and wife with regard to the child being gestated (Moschella, "Gestation Does Not Necessarily Imply Parenthood," 21–48). Thus, I here limit myself to responding to more recent arguments not addressed in the previous essay.

He further explains this point by arguing, "In the natural order, having sex leads to making a baby, which then leads to becoming pregnant. All of these reveal the fruitfulness of the act of self-giving that occurs in marriage in all its perfection."[39] Yet why stop the sequence at pregnancy? For clearly the teleological linkage extends biologically to include (at least) nursing the child, and (if the teleology is not conceived of in a narrow biological fashion) it extends also to raising the child to maturity. For indeed, all of these things—procreating, gestating, nursing, and raising the child—"reveal the fruitfulness of the act of self-giving that occurs in marriage in all of its perfection." Thus, Austriaco's argument, if taken to its logical conclusion, would imply that nursing another woman's child and perhaps even postnatal adoption are morally impermissible.

Similarly, Charles Robertson argues that the uterus is part of the generative faculty and thus that HET is wrong, because it involves "directing the activity of one's generative faculty to someone who is not one's spouse."[40] Once again, however, this argument proves too much. For the biological purpose of a woman's breasts is clearly to provide nourishment for her children, and thus the breasts and the act of nursing should also be seen as part of the generative faculty according to this logic. And if that is the case, then Robertson's view would imply that nursing another woman's child is an illicit use of that faculty to feed another man's child.

Alexander attempts to respond to this wet-nursing objection from the perspective of her argument that the rationale for the inseparability norm is the importance of respecting conjugal agency in union and procreation. She claims that wet-nursing does not usurp the husband's causal agency, for "the husband does not have a causal role in the act of breastfeeding, whereas he does have a very important and morally significant causal role in being an agent cause of his own wife's impregnation."[41] Yet this argument is flawed. First, her claim is only biologically true because she appears to define *impregnation* as conception inside of the woman's body and thus as occurring

---

39. Austriaco, "Embryo Adoption and the Extended Inseparability Argument," 33, 34.
40. Robertson, "Thomistic Analysis," 695.
41. Alexander, "Is Artificial Impregnation Opposed to the Unity of Marriage?," 53, 79–80.

prior to *implantation*.⁴² This definition of impregnation is highly idiosyncratic. Even if we accept her definition, however, we then still need to explain why there is a problem seeking pregnancy (understood as *implantation*) apart from the direct causal role of the husband. Biologically, the direct agent of *implantation* is the embryo. Alexander might argue that by causing impregnation through sexual intercourse, the husband begins a causal series that then makes possible the embryo's causal agency in implantation. But if one extends the husband's causality to implantation via his more direct causality in conception, why not extend it also to lactation, which is also an effect of the causal series begun by sexual intercourse? Thus, if we consider only the husband's *direct* causal role, then Alexander's claims fail to show why *implantation* apart from the marital act is problematic. However, if we include *all* the effects of the causal sequence initiated by sexual intercourse, then her argument would imply that wet-nursing is impermissible.

Alexander might respond that what she objects to is not the implantation as such, but the impregnation of the woman, understood as placing the embryo inside the woman's uterus. For she might see this as failing to respect the husband's causal agency. But this would change the definition of impregnation to isolate it from conception, and her argument for the moral relevance of impregnation hinges on its connection to conception. At any rate, if what she objects to is the placing of the embryo inside the woman's uterus apart from the husband's causal agency, then her view would seem to imply that even *homologous* embryo transfer—that is, the transfer of embryos created through IVF into the uterus of the genetic mother—would be wrong. Yet this seems implausible. For once the embryos have been created, it would seem that the genetic mother has an *obligation* to gestate them if she is able to. Further, the argument would seem to imply that HET could be permissible if the husband were to insert the embryo into his wife's uterus. Yet it seems implausible that the morality of HET would turn on who the technician is.

These fundamental flaws in the arguments claiming that HET involves some inherent violation of marital fidelity lend further support to my claim

---

42. I say "appears to define," because she never gives a precise definition of what she means by the term. I have constructed this definition on the basis of her claim that "it is *only* in natural conjugal relations that 'impregnation' is a reality simultaneous with conception." Alexander, "Is Artificial Impregnation Opposed to the Unity of Marriage?," 63, emphasis original.

that we should understand the norm forbidding procreation apart from marital intercourse as fundamentally about protecting the dignity of the child and thus as safeguarding the *procreative* aspect of the dual good of marriage. Arguments like Austriaco's, Robertson's, and Alexander's go astray by analyzing HET solely from the perspective of marital unity, understood in a way that tends toward physicalism. In doing so, they ignore the inseparable connection between marital norms and the protection of the dignity and rights of children, a connection which is abundantly clear in *Donum vitae*.

Concluding Thought Experiment

Let us return to where we started, with *Donum vitae*'s statement that "the fundamental values connected with the techniques of artificial human procreation are two: the life of the human being called into existence and the special nature of the transmission of human life in marriage." Since embryo adoption involves a situation in which human life has *already* been transmitted, it would seem that the only value directly implicated in the embryo adoption debate is the life of the child. If, as I have argued, embryo adoption can be done in a way that fully respects the dignity of the child, then it should be praised and encouraged, just as postnatal adoption is.

It is, in fact, hard to imagine that there would be any debate if we found ourselves in an analogous situation with children whose humanity and dignity are more obvious to us. Imagine, for instance, the following scenario: There is an (unjust) experiment in which large numbers of embryos are created in a lab and then gestated in artificial wombs, perhaps with a view toward completely eliminating the natural process of procreation and gestation. When the children reach about five months' gestation, the experiment begins to fail, and the children will all die if nothing is done. The scientists believe that the children can be saved by connecting each child temporarily to a woman's uterus via an external artificial placenta and that this procedure would involve no greater risks to the woman than normal pregnancy. Who would argue that it is wrong for a woman to volunteer for this task—which we might call heterologous external gestation (HEG)—in order to save a child or for a woman and her husband to decide to adopt that child, knowing that the first stage of caring for the child will require HEG? There would obviously be no general obligation to do so, just as there is no general obligation for someone to donate a kidney in order to save the life of a person with kidney failure or for someone to adopt an abandoned infant. But it seems unlikely to me that, in such a scenario, Catholic ethicists would deem HEG impermissible on the grounds that this is a misuse of the generative faculty or otherwise contrary to marital unity. For these claims seem absurd when applied to a case in which the children are at five months' gestation rather than at the embryonic stage and in which the children will be *externally* connected to the woman's uterus rather than being gestated *inside* her body. Yet none of these differences—the age or exact location of the child—has any plausible relevance to the moral permissibility of the act. What this thought experiment suggests is that, if we really took seriously the fact that embryos are *complete* (though immature) human beings, equal in dignity to more mature human beings, there would be no debate about the inherent permissibility of embryo adoption, just as there are no debates about the inherent permissibility of postnatal adoption.

The concluding words of *Donum vitae* invite all, "like the good Samaritan, to recognize as a neighbor even the littlest among the children of men." Cryopreserved embryos are, indeed, the littlest and most vulnerable among us, and embryo adoption is a morally praiseworthy response to their plight.

13

Adoption as a Spiritual Status and a Social Practice

Contextualizing the Catholic Practice of Prenatal and Postnatal Adoption

John Berkman

In the literature on how the Catholic tradition should ethically evaluate adopting prenatal orphans, the lack of careful attention to the theological and moral meanings of adoption and parenthood is striking. For example, some commentators presume that adoptive parenthood is a morally questionable or even dubious practice, one that is at best an unfortunate substitute in comparison to lineal (i.e., biological or generative) parenthood.[1] This presumption is most common among philosophers who, in giving rightful attention to the importance of the natural law, fail to recognize that any adequate Catholic theological judgment must be equally attentive to the requirements of the New Law of Christ.

Thus, this paper begins by discussing the importance of adoption for Catholic Christianity, both historically and at present, as both a spiritual reality and a social practice. As a spiritual reality, every Christian, as a Christian, is a spiritual adoptee. I will say more about this in the next section.

---

1. For my critique of one interlocutor who, early on in the debate, went so far as claim that adoptive parents are not really parents, see John Berkman, "Response to Tonti-Filippini on 'Gestating the Embryos of Others,'" colloquy, *National Catholic Bioethics Quarterly* 3.4 (Winter 2003): 660–664, doi: 10.5840/ncbq2003341.

Part 3: Defenses of Embryo Adoption

As a social practice, since adoption of children typically arises as a response to tragedy or human sin, some ideal-focused theologians and philosophers attempt to marginalize the practice. But this is both a theological and a moral error. As Pope Francis and others have noted, the Church is a field hospital, not a country club.[2] The Gospel of Jesus Christ must not be confused with middle class bourgeois respectability.

The practice of adoption and all it entails constitute a great good that the Church has long recognized. Throughout history, there have always been orphans who needed homes, and the Church at its best has stepped forward to facilitate care for such children.[3] The scriptural imperative to care for widows and orphans and those whom Matthew's Gospel refers to as "the least of these" is as urgent today as ever (25:45; Exod. 22:22). A loving adoption of an orphan is one of the most remarkable gifts that one human being can give another.

Although the task to care for the orphaned is age-old, it seems especially daunting in modern philo-technical societies, which are adept—whether through war, social engineering, or biotechnology—at orphaning children most efficiently. Thus, the decision by some Catholics and other people of good will to adopt prenatal orphans is, on one level, nothing particularly new. If much of contemporary society fails to recognize a class of orphans in their midst, then it is the special duty of the Christian to witness to the dignity of those prenatal lives.

With the case of prenatal orphans, the situation may appear so overwhelming and hopeless that some will throw up their hands, concluding that little or nothing can be done, even if they notionally acknowledge the claim such orphans have on us. If some think that nothing (morally speaking) can be done to aid these orphaned prenatal children, then their reasons must be truly decisive; they must clearly and unequivocally demonstrate

---

2. Deborah Castellano Lubov, "Pope Francis: Church a 'Field Hospital for Vulnerable,'" Vatican News, May 14, 2022, https://www.vaticannews.va/en/pope/news/2022-05/pope-francis-audience-village-of-francis.html.
3. On this question, see John Boswell, *The Kindness of Strangers: The Abandonment of Children in Western Europe from Late Antiquity to the Renaissance* (Chicago: University of Chicago Press, 1998); and Darrel W. Amundsen, *Medicine, Society, and Faith in the Ancient and Medieval Worlds* (Baltimore: Johns Hopkins University Press, 1996), 50–69.

that to aid these orphans is truly a sin. Otherwise, those who proclaim that the Christian community may not attend to "the least of these" in our contemporary society are engaged in a rejection of Christ himself.

This paper thus proceeds in two parts: The first part is on the moral and theological significance of adoption as a spiritual reality and a social practice. Having established the great importance of adoption for the Catholic theological and moral tradition, the second part challenges the cogency of arguments claiming that prenatal adoption is somehow intrinsically wrong.

Adoption and Catholic Identity

Subordination of Kinship to Adoption in a Catholic Theology of the Family

What many Westernized Catholic Christians have forgotten (or simply fail to realize) is that, compared with almost any other religion or traditional culture, the Catholic tradition throughout its history has challenged and undermined the centrality of traditional bonds of kinship and has relativized the loyalty the Christian owes to her kin.[4] Jesus did not tell his followers to leave him and go fulfill their familial responsibilities. Rather, "You cannot be my disciple, unless you love me more than you love your father and mother, your wife and children, and your brothers and his sisters. You cannot follow me unless you love me more than you love your own life" (Luke 14:26 CEV).

While not negating the moral and spiritual significance of the family into which a person is born, Jesus clearly subordinates the loyalty a person owes to her natural family to the loyalty she owes to Christ and to her spiritual family, which is found in Christ's Church. Christ speaks of this new loyalty as beginning with a *spiritual* birth: "Truly, truly, I say to you, unless one is born anew, he cannot see the kingdom of God ... unless one is born

---

4. Christianity was arguably the greatest enemy to the traditional bonds of kinship up until the industrial revolution. Then came Adam Smith's version of capitalism, predicated on the rule of law and the mobile workforce, which first allowed and then required the breakup of extended families to maximize economic productivity.

of water and the Spirit." (John 3:3, 3:5). While the Christian's origin lies in her natural family, the Christian's destiny lies with her spiritual family.

In his letter to the Galatians, St. Paul highlights the language of adoption for understanding the Christian's identity and spiritual destiny: "We also, when we were children, were enslaved to the elementary principles of the world. But when the fullness of time had come, God sent forth his Son, born of woman, born under the law, to redeem those who were under the law, so that we might receive adoption as sons. And because you are sons, God has sent the Spirit of his Son into our hearts, crying, 'Abba! Father!' So you are no longer a slave, but a son, and if a son, then an heir through God" (Gal. 4:3–7).

When, a few years later, Paul writes to the Christians in Rome, he repeats his understanding of the Christian's identity as an adopted child of God: "For all who are led by the Spirit of God are sons of God. For you did not receive the spirit of slavery to fall back into fear, but you have received the spirit of sonship. When we cry, 'Abba! Father!' it is the Spirit himself bearing witness with our spirit that we are children of God" (Rom. 8:14–16). In these letters, Paul's description of a Christian's identity is compared to a child's status under Roman law. On the one hand, in both cases, it is the will of the father who grants status as an adopted child. On the other hand, whereas under Roman law the child becomes heir to material wealth, theologically the child becomes heir to spiritual wealth.

In light of Christianity's relativizing of the family, it might seem odd that, in giving us the Lord's Prayer, Jesus teaches his followers to call God *Father* (Matt. 6:9–14). But in doing so, Jesus uses familiar natural realities to point to spiritual realities. There is no natural analog that can more adequately point to God's love for human beings than the love and concern of parents for their children. While a Christian's loyalty to God transcends any earthly loyalties, there remains the appropriate response of gratitude to the properly ordered love of parents for their children. While the fourth commandment requires filial piety, this must be ordered to the requirements of the first commandment, not vice versa.

Primacy of Adoption for Christian Self-Identity

On a spiritual level, the Church has recognized an analogous tension between familial and ecclesial bonds in at least two different ways. First, by its use of familial language, the Church presupposes an understanding of well-functioning familial roles, for example, using familial titles in religious orders. The Church also employs familial language to point to a set of relationships even more fundamentally important than those in earthly families. For example, Christians are given a new identity at Baptism. While the child's familial identity is by no means negated, it becomes, spiritually speaking, secondary to one's status as a member of the family of God. This claim is not a metaphorical nicety; when Christians are adopted as children of God, a fundamental ontological change occurs in them. Second, while Christians are to respect and honor their earthly parents and are to love their families, the Catholic tradition has recognized the penultimate status of these bonds. Both in the Gospels and in the lives of the saints, we are shown that, when a fundamental conflict arises between familial and ecclesial fidelity, the spiritual has priority over the earthly.

Implications for Christian Parents

So what are the theological implications for Christian parents when they realize that their baptized children belong primarily to God as his adopted children? First, the Christian family will have a different understanding of its primary ends. Lisa Cahill puts the matter well, noting that while "the Christian family may be seen as a biologically-based sphere of special affections ... if the family is truly a community of disciples, then it reflects the transforming power of kingdom life. ... The specifically Christian contribution of the family is sublimation of kinship loyalty into identity with all those who suffer or are in need, as 'God's children' or our 'brothers and sisters in Christ.'"[5] In other words, while Christian parents naturally and rightly care for their biological offspring, their mission as a family is oriented outward in hospitality. Understanding themselves as adopted children, they will welcome those in need into their midst, including, when appropriate, being open to adopting as they have been adopted.

At its heart, Christian parenting lies not in a biological function (although that is certainly a good) but in receiving the gift of children rightly, which lies in honoring the moral commitment demanded of parents. The view that a Christian parent's real children are her biological children cannot be justified theologically. The mission of the Christian parent lies primarily in the raising of her children, regardless of their biological origin. As Germain Grisez puts it, "Parenthood is far more a moral than a

---

5. Lisa Cahill, *Sex, Gender and Christian Ethics* (Cambridge: Cambridge University Press, 1996), 210.

biological relationship: its essence is not so much in begetting and giving birth as in readiness to accept the gift of life, commitment to nurture it, and faithful fulfillment of that commitment through many years."[6] That acceptance of the gift of life, the long-term moral commitment to nurture a child to adulthood, is what is key. Whether that commitment occurs at the conception of a child or at the adoption of a child, at whatever stage of development, is morally irrelevant.

This judgment—that parenthood ultimately lies in honoring a moral commitment—is almost always corroborated by the experience of those most capable of recognizing the difference between types of parenthood, namely, those who have been adopted. When one speaks to these people, some of whom have known or been reunited with their genealogical parents, almost all consider those who adopted them to be their true parents. This is because their parents not simply adopted them but rather lived out the long-term commitment to parent them. This is not a phenomenon to be explained away.

Moral Significance of Kinship Relationships in Christianity

Now, the fact that the goodness of the family lies in the natural order does not mean it has no moral significance. Far from it. The Church recognizes the family's profound importance as the most basic natural social reality, as the natural forum for the nurturing of children, which must be safeguarded, for example, against claims which substitute the state for the family.[7] On this count, the Church will always argue for the prima facie and fundamental right and duty of parents to raise their children and for children to be raised by their parents.

However, as should be obvious, this right cannot be absolute (e.g., an orphan obviously cannot have a right to be raised by his or her parents). Every assertion of human rights functions within particular contexts outside of which such assertions make no sense. The right of parents to raise their children is also limited to those contexts in which the parents are at least minimally capable of doing so. In a variety of circumstances when

---

6. Germain Grisez, *The Way of the Lord Jesus*, vol. 2, *Living a Christian Life* (Quincy, IL: Franciscan Press, 1993), 689.
7. Pontifical Council for Justice and Peace, *Compendium of the Social Doctrine of the Church* (Rome: Libreria Editrice Vaticana, 2004), n. 214.

parents (or, more typically, a single parent) recognize that trying to raise their child is not what is best, the Church or some other social agency may find foster or adoptive parents. These are almost always tragic circumstances, where it may be very difficult to know what is really in the best interests of the parent and the child, both immediately and in the long term. Catholic teaching strongly recognizes the inherent and natural goodness of the bond of kinship between parent and child, which is to be given great weight as a fundamental natural good. Nevertheless, there have always been instances where this good cannot be achieved, such as when it becomes tragically obvious that parents' raising their biological child ultimately will not be conducive to the good of that child.

Justifying Prenatal Adoption

With the above account of the centrality of adoption for Christian identity and its importance as a Christian social practice, I now turn to the question of prenatal adoption. On one level, providing a justification for prenatal adoption is superfluous, if indeed it is a form of adoption, for the reasons outlined above. As I noted above, throughout most of the Church's history, her institutions have been involved in the rescue and placement of foundlings, orphans, and relinquished children. The good of finding loving and stable homes for infants and children whose parents are, for whatever reason, unable or unwilling to raise them is not questioned.[8] In general, the willingness of married couples (or, in some cases, single relatives or other single persons) to take in orphans typically constitutes a good for the child, for the adoptive parents, and for the society, though in reality a wide variety of motives may be present.

In the literature on prenatal adoption, occasionally an author criticizes the motives of persons seeking to adopt a child, claiming that their desire is not primarily for the good of the child but for some ulterior motive. On the

---

8. Of course, this is not to deny that particular instances or kinds of adoption (e.g., some international or interracial adoptions) have been questioned morally. These questions are usually raised because of perceived or actual injustices done to the birth parents, the child, or both. That such concerns should arise is not at all surprising, considering that the very necessity of adoption arises from a preexisting evil (i.e., the child cannot be raised by its birth parents because of some tragedy like death or disability, because of irresponsibility, or in due consideration of the best interests of the child).

one hand, since it is possible for human beings to do almost any otherwise good thing from perverse motives, I have no doubt that on occasion people may well adopt with bad motives.[9] On the other hand, any generalized suspicion regarding the motives of people who wish to adopt is in itself deeply suspect, assuming as it does a false opposition between the good of a child needing a permanent family and the good of the potential adoptive parent. The desires to aid an orphan and find fulfillment in the raising of a child are perfectly compatible when rightly ordered. In fact, it could very well be argued that a potential adoptive parent who has purely altruistic motives, who foresees no personal fulfillment in raising a child, is precisely the kind of person who should not be raising a child.[10] In summary, I see no need to generate a systematic defense of the good of adoption or a generalized moral justification for those who wish to adopt.

Now, many well-meaning persons have naïve or one-sided views about what is involved in adopting either a prenatal or a postnatal child. It is also common for people to make unfounded generalizations about the intentions or character of prospective adoptive parents. Thus, it is important to recognize

---

9. See L. M. Montgomery, *Anne of Green Gables* (Boston: L. C. Page and Co., 1908). Historically, one can very well question how often adoption was done per se for the good of the child. Anne Shirley, arguably the most famous adopted child of early twentieth-century fiction, was adopted not out of Matthew Cuthbert's desire to assist a needy child, but to get help on the farm. We see no reason to believe that Cuthbert's motives, though fictional, were atypical in that time.

10. See Immanuel Kant, *Groundwork of the Metaphysics of Morals*, ed. M. Gregor (Cambridge: Cambridge University Press, 1997), 11–12. Such a person is reminiscent of Kant's grieving philanthropist: "Suppose then, that the mind of this philanthropist were overclouded by his own grief, which extinguished all sympathy with the fate of others, and that while he still had the means to benefit others in distress their troubles did not move him because he had enough to do with his own; and suppose that now, when no longer incited to it by any inclination, he nevertheless tears himself out of this deadly insensibility and does the action without any inclination, simply from duty; then the action first has its genuine moral worth." While it is by no means clear that Kant thought that any *inclination* toward an action detracts from its moral worth, many interpret him this way. Regardless, Kant's quest to differentiate and isolate motives and criticize those that fail the so-called duty test resonates with the kind of moral viewpoint we are here critiquing.

the complexity of intentions in those adopting (or relinquishing) prenatal children. When one begins to read the literature on adoption, one quickly discovers that, on the one hand, some commentators idealize the prospective adoptive parents, waxing poetic as to how they will be acting sacrificially and displaying unparalleled charity. On the other hand, other commentators are inordinately suspicious of those adopting children, sometimes accusing them of shopping for a child and engaging in an egotistical quest to accessorize their lives. One can find similarly extreme viewpoints by commentators when discussing those parents who choose to relinquish their prenatal children for adoption. Some unduly praise their compassionate gift of life to others, while others harshly criticize their abandonment of their children.

With regard to both prospective adoptive parents and those considering relinquishing their prenatal children for adoption, in the vast majority of cases the truth lies somewhere in the middle. While prenatal adoption has an aspect of charity in many cases, that neither is nor should be the primary motivation for adoption. Why is that? Any prospective adoptive parent who understands her relationship to her child as one of charity will be necessarily problematic over the long term. More significantly, adoptive children should be received by Christians as all children should be received, that is, as gifts from God. That is the fundamental norm for Christian parenthood. But developing a theology of parenthood belongs elsewhere.

Current Impasse on Prenatal Adoption

In his 2021 article on the topic, Rev. Nicanor Austriaco speaks of the debate over prenatal adoption as being at an impasse.[11] I think he is correct, although I think the impasse has existed almost as long as the debate has gone on. For instance, in an issue of the *National Catholic Bioethics Quarterly* published in the summer of 2003, I presented the first overview of the contours of the debate about prenatal adoption, outlining what I took to be the three different conceptual paradigms through which the debate was being seen by those reflecting on the question through the Catholic moral tradition.[12]

---

11. Nicanor Pier Giorgio Austriaco, "Embryo Adoption and the Extended Inseparability Argument," *National Catholic Bioethics Quarterly* 21.1 (Spring 2021): 29–35, doi: 10.5840/ncbq20212114.
12. See John Berkman, "Gestating the Embryos of Others: Surrogacy? Adoption? Rescue?," *National Catholic Bioethics Quarterly* 3.2 (Summer 2003): 309–329,

Part 3: Defenses of Embryo Adoption

Two decades later, I believe my original analysis holds up. It required relatively little modification, which I undertook in a 2006 article.[13] In the scholarly literature that has followed in the last twenty or so years, there continue to be three paradigmatic moral descriptions of the kind of act chosen by the woman who decides to gestate an abandoned or relinquished prenatal child.[14] First, her action is analogous to a *rescue* of a human being

---

doi: 10.5840/ncbq20033256. In the previous year, I had written two other articles on prenatal adoption. One of these articles analyzed *Donum vitae* to find out which viewpoints were ruled out and which were not. The other article focused on the empirical realities of prenatal adoption: To what extent was it going on? For what reasons? Who was adopting prenatal children? To what political ends was the moral question of prenatal adoption being instrumentalized? John Berkman, "The Morality of Adopting Frozen Embryos in Light of *Donum Vitae*," *Studia Moralia* 40 (2002): 115–141; and John Berkman, "Adopting Embryos in America: A Case Study and an Ethical Analysis," *Scottish Journal of Theology* 55.4 (November 2002): 438–460, doi: 10.1017/S0036930602000455.

13. John Berkman, "Virtuous Parenting and Orphaned Embryos," in *Human Embryo Adoption: Biotechnology, Marriage, and the Right to Life*, ed. Thomas V. Berg and Edward J. Furton (Philadelphia: National Catholic Bioethics Center, 2006), 13–36.

14. The following articles are early examples of the various positions. For prenatal rescue, see Geoffrey Surtees and William Smith, "Adoption of a Frozen Embryo," *Homiletic and Pastoral Review* 96.11–12 (1996): 7–17; Germain Grisez, *The Way of the Lord Jesus*, vol. 3, *Difficult Moral Questions* (Franciscan Press: Quincy, IL, 1997), 244; and William E. May, *Catholic Bioethics and the Gift of Human Life* (Huntington, IN: Our Sunday Visitor, 2000), 106–108. For prenatal adoption, see Helen Watt, "Are There Any Circumstances in Which It Would Be Morally Admirable for a Woman to Seek to Have an Orphan Embryo Implanted in Her Womb?," part 2, in *Issues for a Catholic Bioethic*, ed. Luke Gormally (London: Linacre Centre, 1999), 347–352; Berkman, "Adopting Embryos in America," 438–460; and Mary Jo Iozzio, "It Is Time to Support Embryo Adoption," *National Catholic Bioethics Quaterly* 2.4 (Winter 2002): 585–593, doi: 10.5840/ncbq2002242. For surrogacy, see William B. Smith, "Rescue the Frozen?," *Homiletic and Pastoral Review* 96.1 (October 1995): 72–74; Mary Geach, "Are There Any Circumstances in Which It Would Be Morally Admirable for a Woman to Seek to Have an Orphan Embryo Implanted in Her Womb?," part 1, in Gormally, *Issues for a Catholic Bioethic*, 341–346; and Nicholas Tonti-Filippini, "The Embryo Rescue Debate: Impregnating Women, Ectogenesis, and Restoration from

in a life-threatening or demeaning situation. Second, her action is analogous to a postnatal adoption. Third, her action is analogous to adultery, but it is *procreative* (rather than sexual) *infidelity*. While these three paradigmatic descriptions are distinct, they are not all mutually exclusive. For example, those who advocate for the rescue paradigm usually would consider it morally good for a woman to adopt the prenatal child.

These alternative ways of describing a woman's decision to gestate an abandoned or a relinquished prenatal child are integral to its moral evaluation, as, for example, one's description of a military rebel alternatively as a terrorist or a freedom fighter also shapes or reflects one's moral evaluation of that rebel. Because moral description is so important, a couple of early contributors to the debate proposed "heterologous embryo transfer" as a neutral characterization of the phenomenon.[15] However, others rightly pointed out that there is no neutral way to describe what is going on.[16] While the term "heterologous embryo transfer" may seem more neutral because it is so abstract, it obscures the agency of the woman who receives the prenatal child into her womb, and it ignores the fact that she is entering into a relationship with that prenatal child. In fact, the term ignores agency altogether, without which no moral evaluation can proceed. In contrast, as we have seen in the years since the early part of the debate, *prenatal adoption* has been the most intuitive and accessible and, thus, the most common characterization of the reality.

Suspended Animation," *National Catholic Bioethics Quarterly* 3.1 (Spring 2003): 111–137, doi: 10.5840/ncbq20033181. For procreative infidelity, see Geach, "Orphan Embryo Implantated in Her Womb," 341–346; Francis M. de Rosa, "On Rescuing Frozen Embryos," *Linacre Quarterly* 69.3 (August 2002): 228–260, doi: 10.1080/20508549.2002.11877649; and Helen Watt, "Becoming Pregnant or Becoming a Mother? Embryo Transfer with and without a Prior Maternal Relationship," in Berg and Furton, *Human Embryo Adoption*, 55–67.

15. Tonti-Filippini, "Embryo Rescue Debate," 111–137; and William E. Stempsey, "Heterologous Embryo Transfer: Metaphor and Morality," in *The Ethics of Embryo Adoption and the Catholic Tradition: Moral Arguments, Economic Reality and Social Analysis*, ed. Sarah-Vaughan Brakman and Darlene Fozard Weaver (Cham, CH: Springer, 2007), 25–41.

16. Sarah-Vaughan Brakman and Darlene Fozard Weaver, "Introduction," in *Ethics of Embryo Adoption*, 3–23.

Part 3: Defenses of Embryo Adoption

Advocates of prenatal rescue are not opposed to prenatal adoption but argue that the characterization of adoption leads to overly restrictive moral conclusions about gestating prenatal children. Those who take the procreative infidelity viewpoint and consider prenatal adoption to be intrinsically wrong typically do not deny that the woman's motivation to transfer the prenatal to her womb and gestate it may well be adoption. But they add that, whatever the woman's good ends may be, the intention (or, technically, the object) of her act involves an intrinsically wrong means. Thus, to call the practice prenatal adoption does not per se rule out the possibility of making a further allowance for non-adoptive rescues, nor does it preclude the view that prenatal adoption may be intrinsically morally wrong. It also allows for the possibility that, while prenatal adoption may not be intrinsically wrong, a variety of other moral objections may rule it out in many, most, or all practical situations.

Prenatal Adoption Is Not Intrinsically Wrong

Having presented the obvious and compelling importance of adoption for Catholics as both a spiritual reality and a defining social practice for Christian parents, the one remaining task is to show that there is nothing inherently problematic about prenatal adoption. The best way for me to do this is to address the most subtle critiques made by those who see the practice as intrinsically wrong. However, to understand the perspective of opponents, we should first ask how the question of a woman's decision to gestate abandoned embryos came to be described most commonly as prenatal adoption. To answer this question, we do well to go back to the earliest programmatic arguments about prenatal adoption.

Prenatal Adoption

Not long after the earliest writers on this question proposed the paradigm of *embryo rescue*, Helen Watt challenged it, arguing that an adequate characterization of the woman's choice, morally speaking, required the focus to be on the nature of the relationship into which she was entering. Claiming that a woman, once pregnant, is always already a mother, Watt defended the centrality of adoption for the discussion, arguing that the analogy of adoption best characterizes a gestational relationship into which a woman might be justified in entering. Watt was arguing that the gestational relationship had both an inherent and a specific kind of *moral* significance. In choosing to gestate a prenatal child, a woman necessarily initiates a parental relationship which she ought to be acknowledging. In initiating a parental relationship, the woman takes on the moral responsibilities associated with parenthood. In response to the objection that it would be surrogacy for a woman to rescue a prenatal child, Watt maintained that "it is therefore wrong to *plan in advance* of conception (or, if one is not the genetic mother, in advance of gestation) to bear a child who will be brought up by others."[17]

Here we see the fundamental difference between the advocates of the rescue view and those of the adoption view. The former do not see the gestational relationship as necessarily parental, whereas the latter see pregnancy as inherently parental. According to the former, the choice to gestate a prenatal child with the intention to relinquish her at birth is simply part of the nature of a rescue; for the latter, to make such a choice reflects a failure to understand one of the fundamental moral requirements of parenthood.

That there would be disagreement on this point is not surprising. After all, until recently, Catholic ethicists had not had to seriously think through the moral significance of the gestational relationship independent of the lineal relationship (e.g., Catholic ethicists rejected surrogacy without the need to seriously consider this issue). When the question of prenatal adoption arose, for the first time there was a plausible moral scenario in which gestational and lineal motherhood could be separated.

As is evident, while rescue advocates and adoption advocates differ on the moral significance of the gestational relationship, they agree that it can be morally acceptable to separate the gestational and lineal relationships. In other words, both viewpoints consider it morally acceptable for a woman to initiate a relationship (whether it is foster parenting or adopting) at the point of gestation as well as at conception or after birth.[18] However, as we

---

17. Watt, "Orphan Embryo Implantated in Her Womb," 347, emphasis added.
18. Another way of characterizing the difference is as follows: Both the rescue view and the adoption view recognize that, with abandoned frozen prenatal children, the normative link between the three elements of motherhood (i.e., genetic, gestational, and social) has already been severed, and a woman legitimately can choose to become a gestational mother even if she is not the genetic

shall see in the next section, this viewpoint—shared by rescue and adoption advocates alike—is at the heart of one of the main objections of those who see prenatal adoption as intrinsically morally wrong.

Procreative Infidelity

The end of a couple or an individual who wishes to adopt a prenatal child abandoned after conception—to give her an opportunity to develop and be born—is clearly laudable.[19] Within the debate, this is generally agreed, for the fundamental good of unimpeded human development from conception to birth and onward is clear. The objections to prenatal adoption are typically about the *means*—that they involve some kind of sin. Christians may not sin to bring about some end, as laudable as the end might be. So if the means necessarily involves sin, then there is no morally permissible means to bring about this end. However, naming the sin involved in the choice to adopt a prenatal child is the burden of those who object in principle to prenatal adoption.

---

mother of a child. They differ in that rescue advocates argue that a woman can choose to become a gestational mother fully intending not to be the social mother of the child, whereas adoption advocates argue that one should never intend to separate the gestational and social aspects of motherhood.

19. In discussions of the morality of adoption, concerns are raised that parents may wish to adopt not primarily for the good of the child but to fulfill needs or desires in their own lives. For an interesting discussion of legitimate and illegitimate motives for adoption, see Timothy P. Jackson, ed., *The Morality of Adoption: Social-Psychological, Theological, and Legal Perspectives* (Grand Rapids, MI: Eerdmans, 2005), esp. Don S. Browning, "Adoption and the Moral Significance of Kin Altrusim," 52–77, Lisa Sowle Cahill, "Adoption: A Roman Catholic Perspective," 148–171, Stephen G. Post, "Adoption: A Protestant Agapic Perspective," 172–187, and Brent Waters, "Adoption, Parentage, and Procreative Stewardship," 32–51. Additionally, arguments which liken prenatal adoption to adultery or procreative infidelity ignore the fact that there are cases all around the world in which single persons rightly postnatally adopt children in need. Since it can be appropriate for a single woman to postnatally adopt a child, would advocates of this viewpoint object to single women's adopting prenatal children, acknowledging that arguments based on procreative infidelity are limited to spouses?

Defective Marital Act

In the earliest days of the debate over prenatal adoption, the sin was thought to be surrogacy, something condemned in *Donum vitae*.[20] Prenatal adoption was seen in terms of the relationship between the woman and the prenatal child and necessarily involved the former sinning against the latter. However, that charge failed to stick and was quickly abandoned.[21] At this point, there was a fundamental shift in the nature of the objection. Those who claim that a woman sins in adopting a prenatal child now focus on the relationship between the woman and her husband, namely, that adopting a prenatal child is a form of marital infidelity. The earliest version of this argument was that a married woman may become pregnant only as the fruit of a conjugal act and that becoming pregnant in any other way constitutes adultery. It was quickly recognized that the bald claim that it was adultery would not do. While some tried to sexualize the physician's act in transferring the prenatal child to the woman's uterus—speaking of it as impregnating the woman—this claim got little traction, since adultery refers to a married person's having sexual intercourse with a partner other than one's spouse.[22] Leaving aside sexist assumptions that the physician would be male, accusing a woman who adopts a prenatal child of being an adulterer revealed more about equivocal uses of *impregnate* than about sexual sin.

A more sophisticated attempt to name the sin that is committed by a woman who prenatally adopts a child is to draw an analogy to adultery. Mary Geach argues that since any act of marital infidelity is intrinsically immoral, and since prenatal transfer of the child is a marital act by the wife without her husband, prenatal transfer (and thus prenatal adoption) constitutes a marital infidelity and is, thus, intrinsically immoral.[23] But the

---

20. Congregation for the Doctrine of the Faith (CDF), *Donum vitae* (February 22, 1987), II.A.3 and III.
21. See Berkman, "Morality of Adopting Frozen Embryos," 115–141; and Berkman, "Gestating the Embryos of Others" (Summer 2003), 309–329.
22. Geach, "Orphan Embryo Implanted in Her Womb," 341–346; and Tonti-Filippini, "Embryo Rescue Debate," 111–137.
23. Mary C. Geach, "Rescuing Frozen Embryos," in *What Is Man, O Lord? The Human Person in a Biotech Age*, ed. Edward J. Furton and Louise A. Mitchell (Boston: National Catholic Bioethics Center, 2002), 217–230.

argument that transferring the prenatal child is intrinsically immoral fails, because there are clearly contexts where this would not be the case.[24] The most obvious one is if a newly pregnant woman were shown to have a cancer that required radiation, which would very probably kill the prenatal child. If technically possible, it would clearly be a good act to transfer the prenatal child out of her womb while she underwent radiation and then, when the uterine environment was again safe, to transfer the child back.[25] This is a prenatal transfer and is clearly not intrinsically immoral. To argue the contrary seems clearly wrong. Again, Geach's objection needs to be contextualized and qualified.

A second counterexample is the situation where a husband and wife undergo in vitro fertilization and have some embryos cryopreserved. While the embryos are frozen, the couple have a moral conversion, repent of their creating prenatal children in vitro, but want to give their children an opportunity for a full human life. Far from being intrinsically immoral, it would seem that these parents have an obligation to gestate their cryopreserved prenatal children.

But if we set aside the overly generalized claim that the very transfer of a prenatal child is intrinsically immoral and, thus, a sin, does Geach provide a more restricted claim about the *kind* of act being done, which necessitates it being considered a sin? Her argument is that a wife, in initiating a pregnancy, is engaging in a marital infidelity. This argument also fails, since it depends on the false premise that the transfer of a prenatal child is a marital act by the wife without her husband. For this depends on erroneously defining a marital act as *any act by a woman which is apt to lead to her becoming pregnant.*[26] This definition is false, because it excludes cases that clearly are marital acts and includes cases that clearly are not marital acts. For instance, the definition excludes marital acts that are not apt to lead to pregnancy, such as marital acts by a postmenopausal, pregnant, or sterile woman. The definition also includes nonmarital acts, like taking a

---

24. I will leave aside the error of defining the transfer of a prenatal child as a defective marital act, because a single woman who has a prenatal child transferred to her womb is clearly not engaged in a *marital* act, however else one might describe it.
25. See CDF, *Donum vitae*, I.3. The CDF approves of such therapeutically beneficial treatment for a prenatal child.
26. See Geach, "Orphan Embryo Implanted in Her Womb," 341–346.

medication after coitus that induces ovulation. What is the reason for the erroneous definition? Geach confuses a marital act (i.e., an act of sexual intercourse with particular conditions and circumstances prevailing) with one of its possible effects (i.e., aptness for conception or pregnancy).

Once one understands that, in the Catholic tradition, marital acts are acts of sexual intercourse under certain conditions (i.e., the couple is married, consenting, and open to the procreation of new life), it becomes clear that the choice to adopt an orphaned prenatal child and the attendant means of transferring the child are in no way at all a kind of marital act, much less licit or illicit.[27] Whereas marital acts are oriented toward the unitive and procreative goods of marriage, the transfer of a prenatal child involves neither of these goods.[28]

Neither Natural nor Conventional

Whereas Geach focuses on conjugal acts, Watt approaches procreative infidelity from the perspective of the morally acceptable means of becoming a mother: via the natural means of conjugal acts or the conventional means of postnatal adoption.[29] The nature of conjugal acts is that they do not enable a woman to become pregnant and thus a mother by fiat; but they only enable

---

27. Cf. Mary Geach, "Motherhood, IVF, and Sexual Ethics," in *Fertility and Gender: Issues in Reproductive and Sexual Ethics*, ed. Helen Watt (Oxford: Anscombe Bioethics Centre, 2011), 169. In fairness to Geach, it should be noted that, in this later essay, she says, "An act that does not contain both [unitive and procreative] meanings is not a marriage act." Geach argues that prenatal adoption can be considered an imitative or defective marriage act, because it "[shares] with the marriage act a description which is specific to it." The question remains: What is the legitimate shared description that renders the act of prenatal adoption intrinsically wrong?
28. Geach says that the woman is perversely participating in the procreative good, which is properly ordered to bringing about new life. However, the choice the woman makes in transferring the prenatal child to her womb is to nurture an already existing human life.
29. Watt, "Becoming Pregnant or Becoming a Mother," 61. Watt says that since adoption has nothing to do per se with a woman's fertility, it does not contravene the necessary respect for conjugal acts and the natural limits of her fertility. Watt changed her position on embryo adoption. In 1999, her view was for embryo adoption, and by 2005 her view is more or less the infidelity view, although with qualifiers, as I have tried to indicate.

it, rather, according to the contingencies of her (and her spouse's) fertility.[30] In contrast, the nature of an act of adoption is that the woman does become a mother by fiat, through a direct choice and commitment by the spouses. Since adopting has nothing per se to do with conjugal acts, it in no way contravenes the morally appropriate respect for such acts.

Watt rejects acts that seek to overcome the contingency of the couple's fertility, enabling them to become natural parents by conventional means or fiat.[31] According to Watt, the choice of prenatal adoption is this kind of choice, whereby the woman becomes a mother by direct choice once a prenatal child is transferred to her body. Becoming pregnant through such means requires a manipulation of a woman's natural fertility by transferring a prenatal child to her body. Like Geach, Watt concludes that procreative infidelity is morally wrong in a way analogous to sexual infidelity.

Watt diverges from Geach by claiming that her approach to sexual ethics generally and views on prenatal adoption specifically derive from concerns for the good of children. Watt claims that the long-term good of children is best safeguarded when they are conceived by conjugal acts, that is, acts of a couple who are expressing a life-long commitment to each other and to their potential children.[32] She argues that it is hugely important for the welfare of children that their parents are in a committed, reasonably well-functioning marital relationship, both for their actual security and for their sense of security. For only in such a context can children begin their lives with a sense that they are completely accepted and cared for.

Watt's emphasis on the good of children is laudatory and consonant with the emphases of the historic Christian tradition. While one might quibble with details of her child welfare analysis, her approach finds extremely

---

30. Helen Watt, "Becoming Pregnant or Becoming a Mother," 60. Watt's argument for restricting natural means of becoming a mother to conjugal acts is that these "express the marital relationship in which the child is best nurtured." She goes on to make the stronger claim that, for the good of the child, lineal and gestational (what Watt together calls biological) motherhood should be initiated in conjugal acts which come to their natural fulfillment in pregnancy and birth.
31. Watt, "Becoming Pregnant or Becoming a Mother," 61.
32. Watt puts it as follows: "Pre-natal adoption also fails to respect the crucial social role of pregnancy in 'placing' a child in the world in terms of the child's origin"(personal correspondence to author).

wide support in the social science literature, particularly her claim that her focus is to give a social rather than a psychological analysis.[33]

However, the relevance of her concern for child welfare to prenatal adoption is confounding. Does Watt have any evidence that children who are adopted prenatally are loved or socially provided for less than children born naturally or adopted postnatally? While there is no evidence, one can reasonably imagine that the social situation of children adopted prenatally would generally be better, in terms of child welfare, than that of either the general population of children born naturally or those children adopted postnatally. But one way or the other, this is surely not the basis for considering prenatal adoption a sin.

Beyond this, there is a fundamental problem with both Geach's and Watt's arguments. Geach's starting point is what is normative for marital sexual (conjugal) acts—that they have indissoluble unitive and procreative meanings. While the telos, or orientation, of conjugal acts is, as Geach puts it, the "one flesh union" and the "begetting" of children, neither of these is present in prenatal adoption, where the spouses become parents conventionally, like in postnatal adoption.

Similarly, Watt's explicit objection to prenatal adoption is that "if it truly is the case that a woman becomes a mother in becoming pregnant," then those who accept prenatal adoption "need to explain why another 'technical' way of becoming a mother—prenatal adoption—is not also a harmful supplanting of a deeply significant interpersonal act as a way of entering on parenthood."[34] Watt here forgets her basic distinction between the two ways of becoming a mother. When a woman becomes a mother via a conjugal act, Watt is correct that she becomes a mother by virtue of becoming pregnant. However, when a woman becomes a mother via adoption, she becomes a mother by shared choice and commitment. So with prenatal adoption, she is a mother prior to being impregnated via embryo transfer and does not become a mother by technical means any more than one who adopts postnatally. Thus, prenatal adoption does not supplant conjugal acts, because, as Watt herself tells us, adoption has nothing to do with the conception of children.

---

33. Helen Watt, *The Ethics of Pregnancy, Abortion and Childbirth: Exploring Moral Choices in Childbearing* (New York: Routledge, 2016), 112–114.
34. Watt, *Ethics of Pregnancy*, 114.

Part 3: Defenses of Embryo Adoption

Counter Objections

While the above in-principle objection to the adoption of prenatal children has significant internal problems, its silence on what seems to me to be an obvious concern is also troubling: one has to at least acknowledge that these orphans have some claim on us as a society. Where is the sense of justice and of what is owed to them? Some of the writing against prenatal adoption tends to wax poetic and at great length on the beauty of marital love, and yet these authors do not acknowledge that there have always been children who, through tragedy or sin, need parents and homes. While this is not the ideal, the world is typically not ideal, especially for orphaned children.

Furthermore, some who declare that prenatal adoption is intrinsically immoral emphasize the ugliness of the transfer of a prenatal child and make generalized criticisms of biomedical technology, so that the fundamental objection sometimes appears to be more aesthetic than ethical. Again, too often opponents of prenatal adoption trivialize or simply ignore the Christian commitment to the care of orphans and the deep importance of adoption in Christian theology and tradition. Yes, of course, we wish that all children were conceived, gestated, and raised by one and the same mother and father. But the Catholic tradition has never thrown up its hands in despair, nor has it ever turned its back on helpless orphans. Rejecting orphans of low birth or dubious stock has been the stance of a variety of pagan and post-Christian societies, but it has never been the Christian stance. We must not allow prenatal children who are orphaned to become the proverbial bastards of the century, from whom we turn away in horror because of their parents' sins.

In arguing that the adoption of an orphaned prenatal child in no way involves a (married) woman in a marital infidelity, I am aware that I have addressed only the main intrinsic objection to prenatal adoption. Concerns that it might encourage some to create even more prenatals, that it would lead to inappropriate cooperation with the in vitro fertilization industry, and that it would be a cause of scandal are all legitimate. However, since these are not intrinsic objections but, rather, may be larger or smaller problems depending on circumstances, they must be addressed in the individual contexts where prenatal adoption might be practiced. Of course, there are a variety of contexts where prenatal adoption currently goes on; some of it is laudatory, and some is morally problematic. If the practice is to be done well, in ways consonant with Catholic faith, it will require significant vigilance and care.

Catholic Social Teaching and Adoption

A full defense of prenatal adoption will include a vision of the good of prenatal adoption in relationship to Catholic social teaching. What fundamental principles should underlie the efforts of a Catholic institution which would facilitate prenatal adoptions? Four particularly relevant principles are the sanctity of human life and the dignity of the human person, the common good, the preferential option for the poor, and subsidiarity. Their importance lies in orienting an institution toward fundamental elements of the human good and in ruling out certain activities as incompatible with the true human good.

However, while such principles serve as important referents, in themselves they do not lead to a flourishing process of prenatal adoption unless those persons operating it possess virtues which enable them to perform certain kinds of tasks well. For example, those persons facilitating prenatal adoption will need to appropriately apply the above principles and to make wise decisions in the multiplicity of possible situations and contexts. Furthermore, the virtuous application of these principles does not produce a minimalist ethic (e.g., merely avoiding the intentional killing of prenatal persons) but, rather, produces one which seeks the true good of all those involved in the process, without, at the same time, requiring a high level of virtue from all of them.[35] The virtue possessed by the person who lives Catholic social principles is that of solidarity.[36] So in presenting the above four principles as the moral basis for a Catholic institution that might participate in prenatal adoptions, the point is not simply that these principles are to be held up as exemplary, but that those who make decisions about situations

---

35. However, it is by no means adequate to simply appeal to such principles—Catholicism has traditionally held a kind of minimalism with regard to moral principles. This is a matter not just of avoiding killing embryos but of expressing a constructive concern for them—an aspirational ethic with an interest in contributing to the cultural transformation. A particularly important statement of this goal through institutional action from a Catholic perspective can be found in the final chapter of Pope St. John Paul II's *Evangelium vitae* (March 25, 1995).
36. See *Catechism of the Catholic Church*, 2nd ed. (Washington, DC: US Conference of Catholic Bishops / Libreria Editrice Vaticana, 2018 update), nn. 1939–1942.

Part 3: Defenses of Embryo Adoption

in which prenatal adoption is to be considered appropriate embody the virtue of solidarity. The virtuous applications of the above principles—shaped by the virtue of solidarity—always function in specific contexts and thus require an extended causuistry which is beyond the scope of this paper.

However, for an institution dedicated to prenatal adoption, the virtue of solidarity will shape its understanding of two principles. First, it will shape such an instituions' understanding the preferential option for the poor to embryos, especially in recognizing the relevance of the scriptural injunction to care for "the least of these" (Matt. 25:40, 25:45). Abandoned frozen embryos qualify as some of "the least of these." Second, it will shape that institutions' understanding of the relevance of the principle of the common good to the adoption of cryopreserved embryos.

14

The Annunciation and Embryo Adoption
Francis Etheredge

In view of Pope Francis's saying that the question of the personhood of the embryonic child is still being debated,[1] I begin this chapter by explaining briefly why this author advocates human personhood from the first instant of human fertilization, and insofar as this question is open to debate, it follows that I am free to advocate a position not formally advocated by the magisterium of the Catholic Church. I advocate this position, of the reality of human personhood from the first instant of fertilization, both because I argue it is true in itself and because it is completely relevant to this chapter on the Annunciation and embryo adoption. Thus, there will be a brief defense of this position, a discussion on the Annunciation and embryo adoption, and a reply to the objection that the Incarnation is not relevant to the discussion of embryo adoption.

The first instant of human personhood is integral to the incarnational union between Christ and all who come into existence. The identity of the human embryo is no less relevant to the identity of Mary, who was miraculously conceived without original sin and, it is argued elsewhere, could not be conceived without original sin if she were not one in body and soul from the first instant of fertilization.[2] While the Immaculate Conception

---

1. Editors, "Exclusive: Pope Francis Discusses Ukraine, U.S. Bishops and More," *America*, November 28, 2022, https://www.americamagazine.org/faith/2022/11/28/pope-francis-interview-america-244225.
2. See Vatican Council II, *Gaudium et spes* (December 7, 1965), nn. 14, 22; and Francis Etherege, *Mary and Bioethics: An Exploration* (St. Louis, MO: En Route Books and Media, 2020), chap. 5.

of Mary and the Incarnation of Christ are unique acts of God, echoing in a new way the original creation of Adam and Eve, God nevertheless acts at the beginning of each one of us. No sooner does the body exist than it is ensouled and, from then on, is a whole, if nascent, person. The moment most characteristic of an action of God is when there is an outward sign of an inward act, namely, the first instant of fertilization whereby the human embryo is encased, so to speak, in his or her embryonic skin.

In a word, Francis has not said that a human being is not a person, and if there is uncertainty, then it entails acting in accordance with the good of human life. But according to the foregoing arguments, we need to address the injustice of the frozen and frustrated unfolding of a human person.[3]

Does the Annunciation, the divine fecundation of Mary with Jesus Christ without her husband's involvement, make embryo adoption morally acceptable? The discussion on embryo adoption takes place in the context of salvation history: we live in a fallen world, but the Resurrection of Jesus Christ is timelessly beneficial to the human race and so stretches throughout the ongoing work of redemption. In other words, it is not enough to speak of living in a fallen world, because the fallen world is embraced, from the beginning, in Christ's work of redemption.[4] We draw upon the Annunciation for inspiration in view of a whole history of God's action, which not only makes the infertile fertile but also entails that the Son of God take human flesh and enter wholly into the humanity of embryonic

---

3. See John Paul II, *Evangelium vitae* (March 25, 1995), n. 60; Francis Etheredge, *The Human Person: A Bioethical Word* (St. Louis, MO: En Route Books and Media, 2017), chap. 7; and John Berkman, "Adoption as a Spiritual Status and a Social Practice," in *Human Embryo Adoption: Catholic Arguments For and Against*, ed. Kent Lasnoski and Trent Horn (Broomall, PA: National Catholic Bioethics Center, 2025), 219–240.
4. See Francis, *Humana communitas* (January 6, 2019), introduction. See also Benedict XVI, general audience, Vatican City, July 7, 2010. Just as Duns Scotus argued that the grace of Christ was effective for Mary's Immaculate Conception, calling it "preventive Redemption," so the whole history of salvation is imbued with the salvific beneficence of Christ's redeeming work.

personhood.[5] For as was recognized, the Son of God did not enter into union with an animal or a plant, but with a human being. Therefore, entering wholly into human development, He redeemed us from the first instant of conception—from the first instant of his own existence as a human being, which, embracing us all, constitutes a saving contact with all who come to exist.[6] Thus, Baptism actuates the saving contact that the Incarnation establishes with each one of us.

There is, then, a threefold logic to this chapter. First, the Son of God has entered wholly into human nature, beginning from the first instant of being conceived by the Holy Spirit. Therefore, everyone, from conception onward, is entered into this union with Christ.[7] Second, the word of God is ever alive and active and is suitable for any good work (Heb. 4:12). Therefore, as the frozen embryo is embraced within the framework of redemption, the word of the Lord can both inspire our understanding of and help to bring about our love of neighbor. Third, truth will not contradict truth, nor faith and science conflict, where each identifies what is relevant to the benefit of the frozen human embryo. Therefore, where reason and evidence

---

5. See Francis Etheredge, "Embryo Adoption and Reciprocal Human Relationships," colloquy, *National Catholic Bioethics Quarterly* 17.2 (Summer 2017): 196–198, doi: 10.5840/ncbq201717219; and the summary of Kent Lasnoski's position in Teofilo Giovan S. Pugeda III, "An Overview of the Embryo Adoption Debate," *Philippiniana Sacra* 57.173 (May–August 2022): 208–209. See also Etheredge, *Mary and Bioethics*, chap. 7; and Joseph Ratzinger, *Daughter Zion: Meditations on the Church's Marian Belief*, trans. John M. McDermott (San Francisco: Ignatius Press, 1983), 48.
6. See Francis Etheredge, *Conception: An Icon of the Beginning* (St. Louis, MO: En Route Books and Media, 2019), 220–221; and John Saward, *Redeemer in the Womb: Jesus Living in Mary* (San Francisco: Ignatius Press, 1993), 8–13.
7. See Thomas Aquinas, ed., *Catena aurea: Commentary on the Four Gospels, Collected out of the Works of the Fathers*, English ed. John Henry Newman, vol. 3, *St. Luke*, trans. Thomas Dudley Ryder (Oxford: John Henry Parker, 1841; London: J. G. F. and J. Rivington, 1841), Luke 1:30–33 (pp. 28–31). See specifically Aquinas's citation to Serverus Antiochenus (p. 29): "For the Divine Word came to purify man's nature and birth, and the first elements of our generation. And so without sin and human seed, passing through every stage as we do, He is conceived in the flesh, and carried in the womb for the space of nine months." See also Vatican Council II, *Gaudium et spes*, n. 22.

proclaim the first instant of human fertilization to be the first instant of being a person, there is an obligation on all of us to both ensure the good of completing human embryological development and end the profoundly unjust practices experienced by human embryos, including multiple fertilizations, destruction, experimentation, and freezing. What follows, therefore, is a closer examination of the text of the Annunciation, a theological commentary on certain elements of it, a discussion on embryo adoption in the light of the Annunciation, and three conclusions.

The Verb *to Know* and the Presence of the Blessed Trinity

Pope St. John Paul II speaks of Mary and Joseph as being married and her remaining a virgin, "because the child conceived in her at the Annunciation was conceived by the power of the Holy Spirit."[8] Without going too far into comparative texts or translations, the significance of procreation as fundamentally a cooperation in God's creative act reveals the relevance of the Annunciation for human procreation generally. St. Luke's text is a natural choice in view of both his detailed account of Christ's conception and the use, as we shall see, of particular words which have a relevant Old Testament allegory:

> "And behold, you will conceive in your womb and bear a son, and you shall call his name Jesus. He will be great, and will be called the Son of the Most High; and the Lord God will give to him the throne of his father David, and he will reign over the house of Jacob for ever; and of his kingdom there will be no end." And Mary said to the angel, "How can this come about, since I have no husband?" And the angel said to her, "The Holy Spirit will come upon you, and the power of the Most High will overshadow you; therefore the child to be born will be called holy, the Son of God." (Luke 1:31–35)

The Jerusalem Bible, however, takes up the theme of virginity, even that of perpetual virginity, saying, "But how can this come about, since I am a virgin?" The Catholic Revised Standard Version is more interpretative, and in answer to the possibility of her becoming pregnant, Mary says, "How can this be, since I have no husband?" The New Jerusalem text follows the

---

8. John Paul II, *Redemptoris custos* (August 15, 1989), n. 2.

Greek words *ou ginwskw* more closely, rendering the verb *to know* in a more ancient, biblical sense of not having sexual relations with a man: "But how can this come about, since I have no knowledge of man?"[9] Indeed, more than that, the Greek text and the New Jerusalem text echo the description of Eve, Mary's precursor as it were: "Now Adam *knew* Eve his wife, and she conceived and bore Cain" (Gen. 4:1, emphasis added). The Hebrew word is *ya-da*, which *The Brown-Driver-Briggs Hebrew and English Lexicon* takes to mean, in the context, to "*know a person* carnally, of sexual intercourse." In another context, it makes sense to understand this to mean to "know by experience,"[10] and we can take the more embracing sense that Adam and Eve have experienced an intimate knowledge of each other rather than the more reductive sense of sexual relations. Indeed, as the *Navarre Bible* commentary on the Pentateuch says, "The Bible uses the term 'to know,' thereby signalling the human depth of that relationship: although it takes place via the body, it does so in a context of mind and will."[11]

At the same time, Eve goes on to say emphatically, without direct reference to Adam, "I have gotten a man *with the help of the Lord*" (Gen. 4:1, emphasis added). Thus, Luke takes up the theme of the action of God in bringing about the existence of the human being, and it is almost as if Mary is saying that, while she does not know man, through the experience of the *Annunciation* she knows God through his action in her life. On the one hand, then, there is this intimate knowledge of God concerning the Incarnation of the Son of God. On the other hand, with respect to our theme of the relationship between the Annunciation and embryo adoption, there is both the ancient perception of the action of God at the beginning of human life and a radically new understanding of it in the light of the conception of

---

9. Alfred Marshall, *The Interlinear NRSV-NIV Parallel New Testament in Greek and English* (Grand Rapids, MI: Zondervan, 1994).
10. Francis Brown, Samuel Rolles Driver, and Charles Augustus Briggs, *The Brown-Driver-Briggs Hebrew and English Lexicon: Coded with Strong's Concordance Numbers*, Biblesoft unabridged electronic database ed. (Biblesoft, 2006), s.v. "yada," Bible Hub, accessed September 20, 2023, https://biblehub.com/hebrew/3045.htm.
11. University of Navarre, *The Navarre Bible: Pentateuch*, ed. José María Casciaro et al., trans. Michael Adams, ed. James Gavigan, Brian McCarthy, and Thomas McGovern (Dublin: Four Courts Press, 1999), 58.

Christ. We receive, then, from this discussion a kind of priority of the action of God in the conception of human beings.

Moreover, we can see that the Blessed Trinity, the Father, the Son, and the Holy Spirit, are present and active in the mystery of Christ's conception and also in the conception of every human being: "The angel announced to her not just the incarnation but fundamentally the entire mystery of the Trinity: 'The Lord is with you'—that is Yahweh, the Father-God, whom she knows. Then to her wondering what sort of greeting this might be: 'You will conceive a son' who at the same time will be the son of David. To her question how she should behave, since this son could not come from a man: 'The Holy Spirit.' The Trinity is therefore included in what befell her."[12] If this is the work of re-creation, as it were, echoing the very first Trinitarian act of creation,[13] then it follows that we, too, are conceived in the active presence of the Blessed Trinity: "Before creating man, the Creator withdraws as it were into himself, in order to seek the pattern and inspiration in the mystery of his Being, which is already here disclosed as the divine 'We.' From this mystery the human being comes forth by an act of creation: '*God created man in his own image*, in the image of God he created him; male and female he created them.'"[14] In particular, "the Second Adam stamped his image on the first Adam when he created him. That is why he took on himself the role and the name of the first Adam, in order that he might not lose what he had made in his own image."[15]

In other words, drawing on the adage "activity manifests being," there is a clear relationship between the mystery and action of God as the Blessed Trinity. Even if this was not too explicit in the history of salvation, the disclosure of it transcends the time of discovery and, therefore, applies to the whole of creation's relationship to God. In particular, then, we can consider

---

12. Hans Urs von Balthasar, *Mary for Today*, trans. Robert Nowell (Slough, UK: St. Paul Publications, 1987), 35.
13. See Francis Etheredge, *Scripture: A Unique Word* (Newcastle upon Tyne, UK: Cambridge Scholars, 2014), chap. 8; and John Paul II, *Familiaris consortio* (November 22, 1981), n. 11.
14. John Paul II, *Gratissimam sane* (February 2, 1994), n. 6, citing Gen. 1:27, emphasis original.
15. *Catechism of the Catholic Church*, 2nd ed. (Washington, DC: US Conference of Catholic Bishops / Libreria Editrice Vaticana, 2018 update), n. 359, internal quotation marks omitted.

there to be a relationship between the coming into existence of the human person and the Blessed Trinity. As *Dignitas personae* says, "*The acts that permit a new human being to come into existence*, in which a man and a woman give themselves to each other, *are a reflection of trinitarian love.* 'God, who is love and life, has inscribed in man and woman the vocation to share in a special way in his mystery of personal communion and in his work as Creator and Father.'"[16]

On the one hand, then, it could be argued that when the "acts that permit a new human being to come into existence" in the instance of the reciprocal self-giving of husband and wife are clearly absent, there is no "reflection of trinitarian love." On the other hand, while not disagreeing with the embodied sign language of human, reciprocal self-giving, what is of concern here is the divine-human *act of each child's coming to exist* entailing a relationship to the Blessed Trinity, just as the act of the Incarnation of the Son of God did. Moreover, just as each human person is not a being-in-isolation but a being-in-relationship, it follows that *we* are in a relationship to the Blessed Trinity *through* each other. Thus, our response to each other entails, as it were, a response to the presence of God, who brings each of us to exist in relationship to his redeeming love. Each human embryo, however conceived, is conceived in relationship to the creative-redeeming love of the Blessed Trinity. This relationship between God and each other implies an imperative that we act for the benefit of each other, an imperative already expressed in the natural law as *do good and avoid evil.*

Moreover, the particular challenge of the uncertainty of what to do with frozen embryos is graced by the dialogue between Mary and the angel Gabriel. Mary suffered all the spiritual and psychological uncertainty of being pregnant from the mysterious action of the Holy Spirit before she came to live with Joseph, and although her spouse accepted this truth in a dream (Matt. 1:18–25)—and Elizabeth and her child in the womb, John the Baptist, responded under the influence of the Holy Spirit (Luke 1:41–45)—there were still those who "gave their tongues free rein" about the circumstances of her pregnancy.[17] Similarly, there is a whole psychological and spiritual suffering entailed in welcoming into a marriage a child who both

---

16. Congregation for the Doctrine of the Faith (CDF), *Dignitas personae* (September 8, 2008), n. 9, quoting CDF, *Donum vitae* (February 22, 1987), introduction, 3, emphasis original. See also *Catechism*, 238–248, 290–292.
17. Von Balthasar, *Mary for Today*, 13.

came to exist outside the body and has no relation, beyond that of being human, to either the mother or the father who have adopted him or her as an embryonic infant child.

In other words, there is sometimes a dark night wherein nothing is particularly clear, but at the same time, all the anguish and angst which embryo-adopting parents experience is within their relationship to God. Therefore, just as Mary experienced "the most stripped down faith that finally enabled her to look on the horror of her child being crucified,"[18] perhaps there is an element of this "stripped down faith" involved in accepting the threefold uncertainty of adopting an embryonic child. First, there is uncertainty about the welfare of the children being thawed for adoption, who, at any time, may not make the transition from frozen to unfrozen. In a poignant example of this uncertainty, Hannah Strege, the first child to be adopted as a human embryo, was the only one of her nineteen frozen siblings to survive.[19] Second, there is the whole uncertainty for the adopting parents, particularly for the adopting mother, as it is she who is undergoing, in a decisive way, the welcoming of the thawed children. Finally, there is the moral uncertainty and, indeed, anguish that, understandably, people pass through in the course of determining, as best they can, that this is an upright course of action.

In view of the discussion of there being a dark night, it is rather striking that John and Marlene Strege, the first parents to adopt a frozen embryo, wrote, "They were complicated questions only to us. The answers came without a great deal of difficulty, again an early indication to us that God had his own plan for us—that we needed to 'walk by faith, not by sight,' as Paul noted in his second letter to the Corinthians, and that God was working in our lives."[20] Nevertheless, prayer and spiritual counselling are not in themselves totally reliable, especially in view of the possibility of an erroneous or mistaken conscience. However, where counsel has been

---

18. Von Balthasar, *Mary for Today*, 15.
19. John Strege, *A Snowflake Named Hannah: Ethics, Faith, and the First Adoption of a Frozen Embryo* (Grand Rapids, MI: Kregel Publications, 2020), 54.
20. Strege, *Snowflake Named Hannah*, 35. See also Francis Etheredge, *Unfolding a Post-Roe World* (St. Louis, MO: En Route Books and Media, 2022), chap. 10; and Francis Etheredge, *Human Nature: Moral Norm* (St. Louis, MO: En Route Books and Media, 2023).

sought, there is clearly an intention to be open and obedient, insofar as the truth is known, to the grace of God. Therefore, while they are not of the Catholic faith, there is every reason to accept that John and Marlene acted in accordance with both reason and Christian faith—seeking prayerful advice, recognizing the action of God in their lives, and acknowledging that "these boys and girls are not spare parts."[21] Just as we trust in the Gospel account of Mary's radical experience of being shown the possibility of participating freely and more fully in the will of God, so we can accept a different but related testimony of passing through a challenging uncertainty about whether adopting an embryonic child is also in accord with the will of God.[22]

Theological Commentary on Certain Elements of the Annunciation

On the one hand, the Annunciation presupposes Mary's Immaculate Conception, a human conception identical with our own except for sin.[23] Thus, Mary is conceived without original sin and, therefore, transmits the flesh of the redeemed to her son, Jesus Christ. On the other hand, as we know from *Gaudium et spes*, "by His incarnation the Son of God has united Himself in some fashion with every man."[24] It is possible, then, to understand a threefold mystery. First, the Son of God has entered into a relationship with the whole human race in such a way that this relationship is the divine-human prerequisite of the grace of redemption for all. Therefore, any salvific divine-human act builds upon the foundational relationship that Christ entered into on being incarnate of the Virgin Mary. Second, Mary herself

---

21. George W. Bush, speech on stem cell research policy, cited in Strege, *Snowflake Named Hannah*, 185.
22. See John Paul II, general audience, Vatican City, September 16, 1998, n. 2. Clearly, *different* refers to the fact that Luke's account is the word of God, whereas John and Marlene's is their honest account. However, Aquinas says that all truth is of the Holy Spirit. So there is an element of commonality between the two accounts.
23. See Etheredge, *Mary and Bioethics*, chap. 5. Clearly, however, I am not including the creation of Adam and Eve, who were also created without original sin.
24. Vatican Council II, *Gaudium et spes*, n. 22.

is intimately implied in this relationship both from the very first instant of her own conception and, if this is possible, through the explicit expression of this in the Incarnation of the Son of God, which concretely entails his graced union with her. Third, each human being comes into existence "united ... in some fashion" to Jesus Christ.

This is not proposing that anyone is with grace on coming into existence, except Adam, Eve, Mary, and of course Christ himself. Rather, we all come into existence *in relationship* to the Incarnation of the Son of God. This said, it is clear that the ontological relationship into which we enter on coming into existence is established as a gift of God, which is both totally gratuitous and foundational for our salvation. This relationship to the Son of God, established in the very act of the Incarnation as it were, is the very vehicle of grace, whether communicated through the sacrament of Baptism or in whatever way God pleases. This calls to mind the vine in the Gospel to which we are attached and through which God acts with us or we act with God (John 15:1–11). At the same time, this is the ontological foundation for Christ's identification with us: "Truly, I say to you, as you did it to one of the least of these my brethren, you did it to me" (Matt. 25:40).

Embryo Adoption in Light of the Annunciation

Adoption through Baptism, first of all, follows on the ontological relationship God established through the Incarnation with each one of us, arising as it does out of the mystery that Christ "has united Himself in some fashion with every man." This reality is reflected in the New Testament, where "from the lips of Jesus to the pen of Paul, the radical notion that God adopts us as true sons and daughters through baptism has been a core belief."[25] Each person is *caused* to exist by God, which is to be caused to exist in relationship to the Incarnation of the Son of God. The human embryo, then, in whatever way he or she comes to exist, comes to exist in relationship to Jesus Christ and, if in relationship to Jesus Christ, then to Mary and to the rest of us. Baptism is both a development and a fruit of Christ's redeeming

---

25. Whitney E. Anderson, "Justice for the Orphan: The Ethics of 'Embryo Adoption,'" master's thesis (University of St. Thomas, Minnesota, 2019), 44. Anderson references Matt. 6:9–13 and Rom. 8:15 in relation to this statement.

love through which the intention of God is already made manifest in that He "has united Himself in some fashion with every man."

This love of God, which ascends, as it were, from the beginning of each one of us, is a superabundant love, a love ever seeking to reclaim what was lost, deficient, and unrecoverable by our own efforts or intention. In the perspective of the redeeming action of God, then, the frozen human embryo is the exemplary beneficiary of a divine love of the lost—being the most unreachable in the human terms of arrested development. What is striking here, however, is that the act of the Incarnation is not a potentiality. Rather, the Incarnation brings to exist a potentiality that is there because of it. In other words, because of the Incarnation, because of the reality of the relationship between Christ and each person that comes into existence, there is a relationship to be developed, which seeks, in its own inimitable way, to be developed. The frozen human embryo, having come to exist from the first instant of human fertilization, is in relationship to Christ, and by implication Christ is not in relationship to a stage of human development, a prehuman entity of some kind. Rather, Christ is in relationship to you or me from the beginning of our being begotten, one in soul and body: a whole human person, a being-in-relationship.[26] The act of embryo adoption, not without its risks, is an act of gratuitous love in the perspective of the divine-human adoption of man by God.

If, as it has been argued, a spiritual experience in the process of adopting an embryo parallels that of Mary's agreeing to the Incarnation of the Son of God, are there also significant differences? Is it significant that Mary is alone when she accepts the possibility of the Incarnation of the Son of God? Is it significant that Joseph had no say in Mary's acceptance of becoming the Mother of the Lord? Mary is betrothed to Joseph but decides independent of him, or so it seems, to cooperate with God and accept conceiving the Son of God in the flesh.[27] However, what seems to be independent of Joseph is only superficially so. It is the will of God that Mary and Joseph are betrothed but do not come together as man and wife and that Mary remains a virgin while conceiving the Son of God in her flesh. It is not a betrayal of her marriage to Joseph that she has accepted this singular but complex

---

26. See Vatican Council II, *Gaudium et spes*, n. 14.
27. Anderson, "Justice for the Orphan," 35. See also John 1:14.

vocation. Indeed, this is confirmed by God's revealing to Joseph that the child she has conceived is uniquely of the Holy Spirit and that, therefore, he can accept Mary, pregnant as she is, into his home (Matt. 1:18–25). In other words, Mary's action, insofar as it is in the perspective of the will of God, is neither contrary to the nature of marriage nor an offence to Joseph in reality. Therefore, what enables Joseph's acceptance of this mysterious conception is the fact that he has undertaken his own vocation to be betrothed to Mary in the same perspective of the will of God.

The question here with respect to the adoption of the frozen embryo is the following: Is it within the will of God that this embryo adoption is a good, moral act? In other words, independent of all the external signs—including the child's being conceived outside the body of his or her mother, frozen, thawed, and then transferred to the womb of a woman willing to mother this child independent of the husband's paternal contribution to the child's existence—is the question of the will of God. Ordinarily, one might say, there is the husband's intention to be open to life, which, in the case of Joseph, is evident in his acceptance of Christ's conception within his marriage.[28] However, even more ordinarily in the case of a husband and wife's being open to life, there is no certainty that a child will be conceived. Therefore, both the husband and the wife are in the same reality relationship, as it were, as were Mary and Joseph—namely, that all children are an unmerited gift to their parents, but within the mystery of the will of God, those children nevertheless are loved into existence by him and entrusted to the parents as a love gift.

In reality, then, the very dependence of parents on God's gift of a child puts all parents on an equal relationship to both each other and to Mary and Joseph. Therefore, in the perspective of the child-as-gift, the child conceived, frozen, thawed, and transferred to the womb of the woman who is willing to be a mother is no less a gift than any other child—a gift both to the originating couple and in the nature of being-in-existence through a gratuitous act of God. In other words, irrespective of how a child comes to exist, this is

---

28. See Francis Etheredge, "A Reflection on the Language of the Body," *Communio* 24.2 (September 1997): 406–407. For further discussion of marital unity and the Annunciation, see Christopher Kaczor, "Artificial Wombs and Embryo Adoption," in *The Ethics of Embryo Adoption and the Catholic Tradition: Moral Arguments, Economic Reality and Social Analysis*, ed. Sarah-Vaughan Brakman and Darlene Fozard Weaver (Cham, CH: Springer, 2007), 313–314.

always and everywhere a gratuitous act of God's generous giving of existence and, as such, an expression of the person's being an irrevocable end in himself or herself: "Man, who is the only creature on earth which God willed for itself, cannot fully find himself except through a sincere gift of himself."[29]

If the nature of person as self-gift is inscribed in the very existence of the person-as-gift, then it follows that the nascent nature of the child calls out, as it were, to complete the cycle of being given existence by making a gift of his or her existence to God. Parents, then, who are themselves ministers and not masters of the gift of children, are both cocreators and cooperators with the work of God.[30] Therefore, this natural appeal, characteristic of the very nature of the person, to make a gift of himself or herself is a vocational appeal to the human family—first to the natural parents but also, in and through them, to the whole human family. Whosoever answers this appeal, whether it be the natural parents or others, answers the call of being-in-relationship to which all are called—both in the very nature of human reality as an expression of the Blessed Trinity and in the incarnation of this reality in the human nature of the family.

Overall, then, while there are significant differences with respect to the Incarnation of the Son of God and embryo adoption, there are both a language of the person-gift of the child and an orientation of parents to the acceptance of the child-as-gift, which surprisingly seems to suggest that embryo adoption falls within the logic of salvation history. In other words, the very different reality of the Incarnation led to a reflection in favor of embryo adoption.

On the basis of the previous discussion, even human fatherhood, like motherhood, rests on the gratuitous gift of God, and while there are factors which can facilitate human conception, there is a primary dependence on the act of God which brings a person to exist: infertile couples can truly be parents, because "parenthood is far more a moral than a biological relationship: its essence is not so much in begetting and giving birth as in readiness to accept the gift of life."[31] However, defining parenthood as a "readiness to

---

29. Vatican Council II, *Gaudium et spes*, n. 24. The document references Luke 17:33 in relation to this statement.
30. Paul VI, *Humanae vitae* (July 25, 1968), n. 13.
31. Berkman, "Adoption as a Spiritual Status and a Social Practice," 223–224, citing Germain Grisez, *The Way of the Lord Jesus*, vol. 2, *Living a Christian Life* (Quincy, IL: Franciscan Press, 1993), 689.

accept the gift of life" is the natural, psychological foundation of parenthood and, therefore, preexists whether a husband or wife will become an ontological parent. In other words, there is not just a moral but a moral-psychological origin to parenthood, in that a "readiness to accept the gift of life" is inscribed in the being of man and woman.[32] Thus, both St. Joseph and John Strege, neither of whom were involved in the conception of the child carried by their respective wives, the Blessed Virgin Mary and Marlene Strege, still stand in the same relationship to the parents of a child conceived through the acts of marriage, namely, that the child is a gratuitous gift. Moreover, both Joseph and John Strege were united with their spouses in their prayerful relationship to God. Neither man was a passive partner in either the Incarnation of the Son of God or the adoption of a human embryo; both were active participants through the power of prayer.

It could be that Joseph was of a noble if not a kingly line,[33] which, if true, exalts him to the extent that it remained hidden. Bearing in mind the scriptural exhortation that "he who humbles himself shall be exalted" (Luke 14:11), it is fitting not only that Joseph does humble himself but that his humility befits his vocation as guardian of the Redeemer (the title of John Paul II's apostolic exhortation *Redemptoris custos*). At the same time, just as Joseph humbles himself, it is true, too, that he acts as parent to Jesus, "who, though he was in the form of God, did not count equality with God a thing to be grasped. ... He humbled himself and became obedient unto death, even death on a cross" (Phil. 2:6, 8). Moreover, according to John Paul II, the father is called to the service of "the Gospel as Truth,"[34] which, in the case of Joseph, is literally true of his love of Christ, who is "the way, and the truth, and the life" (John 14:6).

Thus, despite the uniqueness of the Incarnation and the uncommon circumstances of embryo adoption, the examples of Joseph and John Strege

---

32. It will take us too far outside the scope of this chapter to discuss what happens to this natural orientation to children because of fallen human nature. For a further examination, see Etheredge, *Human Nature*.
33. Tracey Rowland, "St Joseph the Man, the Knight, the Prince, the Saint," *Catholic Weekly*, August 14, 2022, https://www.catholicweekly.com.au/st-joseph-the-man-the-knight-the-prince-the-saint/.
34. John Paul II, *The Way to Christ: Spiritual Exercises*, trans. Leslie Wearne (San Francisco: Harper, 1994), 53.

nevertheless share similarities with the responsibility that all fathers have in service to the truth and their families, especially their responsibility to teach their children about God: "As I was preparing to marry, my father defined a husband as a servant of his wife and family. I read, too, an address to male students by Bishop Karol Wojtyla, later to become Pope John Paul II; he said that when Christ instructed the apostles to 'make disciples of all nations' (Mt 28: 19): This means, 'Go and teach,' which in turn means that we must take responsibility for the Gospel as Truth! In contemporary terms it means that, in accordance with our specific characteristics as men, we must take responsibility for the Gospel as *Weltanschauung* and idea."[35]

We Are Taken Up into a "Marian Relationship" to Christ

Although this is a biblical answer to the question of the morality of embryo adoption, the text is not separable from the reality it depicts but rather expresses the realities to which it refers.[36] Furthermore, relationality speaks, as it were, to the wider understanding of conceiving a child.[37] To begin with, then, there seems to be a starting point with the action of God, which from ancient times has been understood to be present in the conception of a human being and, in view of the perfection of God, has no other object than the good of the person who exists for his or her own sake.[38] Just, then, as God's embracing love of his creation includes the redemption and sanctification of human beings, so spousal love unfolds in the different but complementary parental love of their children. Thus, human beings love

---

35. Etheredge, *Scripture: A Unique Word*, 108. *Weltanschauung* translates as "worldview or philosophy of life." See also John Paul II, *Way to Christ*, 53–56; and Francis Etheredge, *Lord, Do You Mean Me? A Father-Catechist!* (St. Louis, MO: En Route Books and Media, 2023).
36. See Vatican Council II, *Dei verbum* (November 18, 1965), n. 8. Further discussion of the nature of Scripture is beyond the remit of this chapter. For more information, see Etheredge, *Scripture: A Unique Word*, which is dedicated to this investigation.
37. See "Family Global Compact," accessed September 21, 2023, https://familyglobalcompact.org/family-global-compact-home-eng/.
38. See Melissa Moschella, "Protecting the Dignity of the Child," in Lasnoski and Horn, *Human Embryo Adoption*, 195–218; and Vatican Council II, *Gaudium et spes*, n. 24.

in their totality, like God, and not just in a functional sense, as if offering the hospitality of the woman's womb can, in reality, be separated from her total identity as a person called to love.[39] In the same spirit of recognizing the generosity of the reality of a woman's self-gift, let all concerned be fully aware, as was Tobit, of the risks that a woman takes in doing the good she does: "Remember, my son, that she faced many dangers for you while you were yet unborn" (Tobit 4:4).[40]

Thus, we can see that there is a natural emphasis on the relationship of the child to the mother—not only a maternal emphasis but almost a salvific relationship in that the woman is particularly capable of recognizing that she is in relationship to God, the Author of life (see John 19:25-29; 2 Macc. 7:1, 20-31, 39-42). Furthermore, the Incarnate Word takes the flesh of the Virgin Mary, whereas the adopted embryo, already formed as an embryonic human being, nevertheless shares a common characteristic with Jesus in that both, however incompletely identical, are ordered to the mother: the Son of God preexists but receives human form from Mary, and the embryonic child receives hospitality and the whole human, mothering relationship from his or her mother.

What has emerged, however, is not so much a discussion about the details of embryonic existence or transfer,[41] but rather a kind of embracing circularity by which embryo adoption, in its holistic reality, contributes to the reciprocal gift of personhood to which each of us is called and from which, in a dramatically real way, the frozen embryo is excluded—both the naturally dynamic engagement as integral to his or her living response to life and the mother's recognition of her vocation as taken up into a relationship with the Author of life to whom, as it were, she will introduce her child. In other words, the mother stands in a certain more direct relationship to the action of God at conception than does the man, and in view of this, she introduces him to that action, so that together they can bring the child up in

---

39. For a more explicit discussion of the totality of the person implicated in parental love, see Christopher Tollefsen, "The Procreative Dimension of Marital Union and Embryo Transfer," in Lasnoski and Horn, *Human Embryo Adoption*, 173-193.
40. See Cara Buskmiller, "Medical Aspects of Embryo Adoption," in Lasnoski and Horn, *Human Embryo Adoption*, 15-16.
41. See Anderson, "Justice for the Orphan, 35."

the perspective of the relationship to God which his action at the child's conception has established. Just, then, as God acted in the life of Eve after the fall, drawing the good of life from Adam and Eve's knowledge of each other, so God draws the good of human life out of the real, however imperfect, beginning of human conception: "St. Thomas explains that ... 'God allows evils to be done in order to draw forth some greater good. Thus St. Paul says, "Where sin increased, grace abounded all the more" (Rom 5: 20); and the *Exultet* sings, "O happy fault ... which gained for us so great a Redeemer.""[42]

Therefore, whatever the circumstances of our origin, and however clearly it is contrary to our being "the minister of the design established by the Creator,"[43] God strives to bring about the whole relationship to him and others to which each one of us is called in virtue of being a member of the human race. While we are not, then, caught up in the specifics to which these discussions tend, it seems that Mary's Annunciation, her resounding yes to the will of God, enables us to appreciate a salvific vision which embraces wholeheartedly the embryonic adoption of human beings—enabling human beings-in-relationship to continue uninterrupted the interrupted path to both the manifestation of the person present from the first instant of fertilization and the unfolding of their relationship to God and to others.

Francis's address for the thirty-seventh World Youth Day, "Mary Arose and Went with Haste," reveals another connection between the Blessed Virgin and women who adopt frozen embryos. The Pope says that Mary

> got up and went forth, into the world of life and movement. Even though the astonishing message of the angel had caused a seismic shift in her plans, the young Mary did not remain paralyzed, for within her was Jesus, the power of resurrection and new life. Within herself, Mary already bore the Lamb that was slain and yet lives. She arises and sets out, for she is certain that God's plan is the best plan for her life. Mary becomes a temple of

---

42. Thomas Aquinas, *Summa theologiae* III.1.3 ad 3, quoted in University of Navarre, *Pentateuch*, 55.
43. Paul VI, *Humanae vitae*, n. 13.

Part 3: Defenses of Embryo Adoption

God, an image of the pilgrim Church, a Church that goes forth for service, a Church that brings the good news to all![44]

Mary, then, was touched by the needs of her elderly cousin to whom God granted a child in her later years, and therefore she "arose and went with haste." Thus, the question for us is this: Do we arise and go with haste concerning the needs of the frozen human embryo? Are we doing everything we can to resolve this question of whether it is right to intervene on behalf of these forgotten children, some of whom have been frozen for thirty years and lived? Are we advancing the charity necessary to save the world and advertising the organizations which help to make known the possibility of adopting a frozen embryo—even if the Church's uncertainty is, at the very least, only a window of opportunity? Perhaps we need to let the plight of unborn, aborted, experimented upon, or frozen human embryonic persons reach us, to let it be like a sword through our hearts (Luke 2:34–35) that helps humanize us and focus us on "going out to the other"—reaching out to our brothers or sisters who implicate us, as it were, in their suffering.[45]

All in all, then, it is fitting to call this account of the Annunciation and embryo adoption Marian, as it focuses on the existence of the child first and foremost, and it is about seeing the person with our hearts. In a word, when a mother mourns the loss of a child through miscarriage, it is not meaningless—it is precisely because she sees with the heart the loss of a person, her son or daughter, and, at the same time, remembers that he or she has gone before her to the Father. There cannot be a full account of a mother and father's experience without the recognition, in all the highways and byways of bioethics, that it is not *what* begins but *who* begins at conception.[46] Without a who, he or she is not "united ... in some fashion" to the Incarnation of Christ.[47] Therefore, whether frozen or not, if Christ "has united Himself in some fashion" with each human being at conception, then we need to follow

---

44. Francis, Message for the Thirty-Seventh World Youth Day (August 15, 2022).
45. See Joshua Hordern, "'A Knife into My Heart': Cries, Compassion and Ethical Life," *New Bioethics* 29.3 (September 27, 2022): 279–295, doi: 10.1080/20502877.2022.2124604.
46. See Francis Etheredge, *The Prayerful Kiss* (St. Louis, MO: En Route Books and Media, 2019), chap. 4, especially the prose introduction, "An Unexpected Joy: An Unprecedented Pain," 49–54, and the poem, "Indelible," 54–56.
47. See Vatican Council II, *Gaudium et spes*, n. 22.

his lead to the depths of human existence and the completion of human development which follows on embryo adoption.

Answer to Three Objections

Charles Robertson objects that appealing to the Incarnation in the defense of embryo adoption "seems to pit faith against reason."[48] If there is a settled conclusion from evidence, and if the argument that flows from it is that embryo adoption is wrong, then it follows that to advance a contrary argument from Scripture is to "pit faith against reason." However, just as there is no settled doctrine on the first instant of human personhood, there is no settled conclusion on whether it is right to adopt an embryonic child. Consequently, it behoves us to consider the variety of sources which are open to us and which, in view of Catholicism, draw on faith and reason. Alternatively, given that truth cannot contradict truth, it follows that if an argument can be sustained from Revelation and demonstrated as true, then reason, albeit proceeding from a different starting point, can nevertheless be helped to come to the same conclusion.[49]

Robertson questions the proposition "[if] Mary could licitly consent to be acted on by God in order to attain to a miraculous pregnancy, so can a woman consent to be acted on by a technician in order to attain to a technologically miraculous pregnancy."[50] It must be said that there is no comparison between an act of God bringing about the Incarnation, expressing the unique relationship between the eternal generation of the Son of God, and that of a technician whose action of fertilizing a woman's ovum is without reference to the natural order established by God or Revelation. In other words, Robinson is not comparing like with like. Rather, there is a specific act of embryo transfer in the case of a human embryonic child's critical need.[51] Nevertheless, before we continue the discussion, there is

---

48. Charles Robertson, "Embryo Adoption and the Incarnation," colloquy, *National Catholics Bioethics Quarterly* 17.3 (Autumn 2017): 382, doi: 10.5840/ncbq201717339. Robertson's arguments are responding to Etheredge, "Embryo Adoption and Reciprocal Human Relationships," 196–198.
49. See John Paul II, *Fides et ratio* (September 14, 1998), nn. 12–23.
50. Robertson, "Embryo Adoption and the Incarnation," 383.
51. See Elizabeth Bothamley Rex, "The Magisterial Liceity of Embryo Transfer: A Response to Charles Robertson," *National Catholic Bioethics Quarterly*

more to be said by way of clarification, namely, that there are two acts of God. While each is different, both bring to exist what did not exist. On the one hand, there is the single act of the Incarnation, whereby the Son of God was embodied in the whole of human flesh, one in body and soul, bringing about the indivisible unity of the God-Man (John 1:14). On the other hand, there is a single act of God which brings about the unity of the human person, one in body and soul.

First, then, this discussion entails a specific event, namely, the transfer to a married woman's womb of a human embryo who, through no fault of his or her own, has been conceived outside the body and the reality of spousal union. If he or she remains frozen, existing in an uncertain state, at the very least there is a frustration of the natural development of the child's dynamic growth, and over time there is an increasing risk of death by deterioration. Thus, there is a specific action, an embryo transfer, being considered in the light of the Incarnation of Christ. Second, the specific action is the rescue of an abandoned human embryo, a rescue which is comparable to the Incarnation of Christ on the grounds that each person is welcomed by the mother in view of it being the will of God. Thus, this is not a generalized case; it is a specific help to a specific child. Third, if "God allows evils to happen in order to bring a greater good therefrom,"[52] then what is the greater good? Generally, from the sin of Adam and Eve came the redemptive mission of Jesus Christ. In the case of a thawed, hitherto frozen embryo, the greater good is the lifesaving action of a welcoming, married woman.

Robertson further contends, "By arguing in this manner, [Etheredge] implicitly shows that we do not so much draw a conclusion about the liceity of embryo transfer from the account of the Incarnation as see in it an illustration of the way in which a woman can will to be artificially impregnated apart from intercourse."[53] Again, this point misses the salvific nature of an act of God, insofar as the logic of the Incarnation applies, which instructs

---

15.4 (Winter 2015): 701–722, doi: 10.5840/ncbq201515471. The good of embryonic transfer is simply that it is required for a legitimate help to a human embryo.

52. Thomas Aquinas, *Summa theologiae*, trans. Fathers of the English Dominican Province (1920; New Advent, 2017), III.1.3 ad 3, https://www.newadvent.org/summa/4001.htm.

53. Robertson, "Embryo Adoption and the Incarnation," 383.

us as to the possibility of a married woman's participation in a redemptive act. Although we must bear in mind the utter injustice, vulnerability, and frustration of the frozen embryo's normal development, there cannot be a redemptive act without the presence of the grace of God, for as Christ says, "Apart from me you can do nothing" (John 15:5). Therefore, owing to the redemptive act of the Incarnation by which "the Son of God has united Himself in some fashion with every man," it follows that a married woman can collaborate with a redemptive act of God in this way.

Robertson's third objection could be related to his view that, although "God does not contradict the moral law He has created, I do not see how this view entails that whatever can be done by God without contradicting that law can also be done by us without contradicting that law." "God could directly inspire some individual woman to undergo embryo transfer in order to further his designs for the continuation of the species. However, the possibility of such an essentially extraordinary and supernatural commission serves as no basis for a general rule permitting or counselling embryo adoption or rescue."[54] On the one hand, the continuation of the species involves specific individuals and is not, therefore, a kind of indifferent generic goal of the action of God. On the other hand, what is the difference between the possibility of a graced act of a mother's rescue of a thawed frozen embryo and Robertson's admission that "God could directly inspire some individual woman to undergo embryo transfer in order to further his designs for the continuation of the species"? In other words, Robertson concedes the possibility of what I argue in this chapter.

Furthermore, the possibility that God's command changes an otherwise immoral act to a moral one seems incoherent, especially as it draws on examples which allow of a different interpretation.[55] The object of Samson's act was bringing down the temple to which he was tied in order to kill the enemies of his people. However, it does not follow that his own death was the deliberate object of his act, but rather a foreseeable possibility that he did not intend, in that, if the pillars had collapsed in a different way, his

---

54. Robertson, "Embryo Adoption and the Incarnation," 383, 384.
55. See Anthony Hollowell, "Virgin Suicide and Vital Conflicts," *National Catholic Bioethics Quarterly* 21.2 (Summer 2021): 87–102, doi: 10.5840/ncbq202121227.

own life could have been spared. As regards God's commanding Abraham to kill his son, in that God sees his own end, namely, that of testing the heart of Abraham, God's intention was to test Abraham, not command the death of Isaac. As with the case of Pelagia, who jumped off a roof and died rather than let herself be taken prisoner, it does not follow that God commanded her to kill herself. It is possible that the girl did not intend her death. Rather, she intended to escape possible capture. In other words, the argument that God contradicts his own law that forbids murder or suicide cannot be adequately answered with respect to events susceptible to other interpretations. Therefore, we cannot exclude either our use of reason or the wisdom of the Church in forming and discerning the possibility that God can contradict his own law. Moreover, we cannot exclude the possibility of an erroneous conscience which acts as if God commands it but does not in fact do so. In this discussion, it is far from clear that God can command embryo adoption if it were, in reality, a moral wrong.[56] Nor, in view of embryo adoption's being a disputed question, can it be claimed that the person who adopts or advocates the adoption of a thawed, frozen embryo is necessarily subject to an erroneous conscience.

Implicit Definition of Human Conception

If we adapt a comment from Aquinas, the question of human conception can be put like this: Is the soul embodied at "the end of the process of human generation" or at the beginning?[57] As it happens, this comment helps bring to a conclusion the question of when human ensoulment takes place. It can be argued that "a new human life begins at the moment when the genetic information contributed by the sperm from the father is combined with the genetic information contributed by the ovum (egg cell) from the mother.

---

56. Furthermore, the expression of an opinion by one of the Fathers of the Church or an authoritative theologian like Aquinas does not guarantee in itself the truth of that opinion. Aquinas was mistaken about the possibility of Mary's being free from original sin. Further discussion of this point is beyond the remit of this chapter. See Aquinas, *Summa theologiae*, III.27, https://www.newadvent.org/summa/4027.htm.
57. Thomas Aquinas, *Summa Theologiae: A Concise Translation*, ed. Timothy McDermott (London: Methuen, 1991), I.118.2.

As soon as fertilization is completed, a new human being begins its life."[58] In other words, if ensoulment entails the fusion of the nuclear content of the sperm and the ovum, then it follows that ensoulment cannot be the first instant of fertilization. However, as I have argued elsewhere, if the first instant of fertilization originates the embryonic life of the child and if the human soul is the life of the body, then it follows that the first instant of fertilization is the first instant of human personhood.[59] This is because the first instant of the new human life is expressed by the closure of the embryonic wall and the fact that this is the first moment of the existential existence of the human embryonic person (and all that event entails).

This conclusion is relevant to the whole discussion, because it is this moment of human beginning which founds Mary's conception and the unity between each human person and the Incarnation. Thus, the adopted human embryo is taken up into Christ's redemptive act as expressed by the Incarnation's uniting, in a certain way, with each human being. Therefore, the married woman who accepts an embryonic child transferred to her womb is acting in accordance with the graced good to be done to the thawed, nascent embryonic human life.

---

58. Dicastery for Laity, Family and Life and Jérôme Lejeune Foundation, "Keys to Bioethics," Dicastery for Laity, Family and Life, accessed October 19, 2023, https://laityinvolved.org/project/keys-to-bioethics/.
59. See Etheredge, *Scripture*, chap. 12; and *Catechism*, n. 363.

15

The Theology of the Body and the Morality of Embryo Adoption

What Does the Magisterium of the Catholic Church Teach?

Elizabeth Bothamley Rex

Preface

Perhaps the single greatest magisterial challenge facing the Catholic Church today is the seemingly "absurd fate" of millions of abandoned and orphaned frozen embryos languishing in cryostorage tanks around the world.[1] Is prenatal adoption an acceptable moral option for them? Sacred Scripture, Tradition, and the magisterium of the Catholic Church, including the magisterial teachings developed by Pope St. John Paul II in his Theology of the Body, biblically and theologically defend the inviolable dignity of the human person from the very first instant of his or her conception. Included in this preface are important magisterial teachings that defend the human embryo as a person—*and as a patient*—like any other human being.

---

1. Congregation for the Doctrine of the Faith (CDF), *Donum vitae* (February 22, 1987), I.5.

Part 3: Defenses of Embryo Adoption

The Catechism of the Catholic Church

The embryo must be defended, cared for, and healed, like any other human being.

> Since it must be treated from conception as a person, the embryo must be defended in its integrity, cared for, and healed, as far as possible, like any other human being.[2]

Embryos are patients, and therapeutic medical interventions must be upheld as licit.

> One must uphold as licit procedures carried out on the human embryo which respect the life and integrity of the embryo and do not involve disproportionate risks for it but are directed towards its healing, the improvement of its condition of health, or its individual survival.[3]

The Church condemns heterologous artificial fertilization, not heterologous embryo transfer.

> Techniques that entail dissociation of husband and wife, by the intrusion of a person other than the couple (donation of sperm or ovum, surrogate uterus), are gravely immoral. These techniques (heterologous artificial insemination and fertilization) infringe on the child's right to be born of a father and mother known to him and bound to each other by marriage. They betray the spouses' "right to become a father and a mother only through each other."[4]

Instruction Donum Vitae on Respect for Human Life in Its Origin and on the Dignity of Procreation: Replies to Certain Questions of the Day

Embryos conceived in vitro must not be deliberately exposed to death.

> *It is therefore not in conformity with the moral law deliberately to expose to death human embryos conceived "in vitro."*[5]

---

2. *Catechism of the Catholic Church*, 2nd ed. (Washington, DC: US Conference of Catholic Bishops / Libreria Editrice Vaticana, 2018 update), n. 2274.
3. *Catechism*, n. 2275, citing CDF, *Donum vitae*, I.3.
4. *Catechism*, n. 2376, citing CDF, *Donum vitae*, II.1.
5. CDF, *Donum vitae*, I.5, emphasis original.

Cryopreservation exposes embryos to risks of death or harm and deprives them of gestation.

> *The freezing of embryos,* **even when carried out in order to preserve the life of the embryo—cryopreservation—***constitutes an offense against the respect due to human beings* by exposing them to grave risks of death or harm to their physical integrity, and **depriving them, at least temporarily, of maternal shelter and gestation**, thus placing them in a situation in which further offenses and manipulation are possible.[6]

In vitro fertilization (IVF) embryos are living gifts of divine goodness and must be brought up with love.

> Although the manner in which human conception is achieved with IVF and ET cannot be approved, every child that comes into the world must in any case be accepted as a living gift of the divine Goodness and must be brought up with love.[7]

Instruction Dignitas Personae on Certain Bioethical Questions

The majority of cryopreserved embryos are orphans, and their parents do not ask for them.

> The majority of embryos that are not used remain "orphans." Their parents do not ask for them and at times all trace of the parents is lost. This is why there are thousands upon thousands of frozen embryos in almost all countries where in vitro fertilization takes place.[8]

Cryopreservation kills, harms, and deprives embryos of maternal reception and gestation.

> Cryopreservation is *incompatible with the respect owed to human embryos*: it presupposes their production in vitro; it exposes them the serious risk of death or physical harm, since a high percentage does not survive the process of freezing and thawing; it **deprives them at least temporarily of maternal reception**

---

6. CDF, *Donum vitae*, I.6, emphasis in italics original, emphasis in bold added.
7. CDF, *Donum vitae*, II.B.5.
8. CDF, *Dignitas personae* (September 8, 2008), n. 18.

and gestation; it places them in a situation in which they are susceptible to further offense and manipulation."[9]

The Gospel according to Matthew

Jesus heals on the Sabbath.

> And they asked him, "Is it lawful to heal on the sabbath?" so that they might accuse him. He said to them, "What man of you, if he has one sheep and it falls into a pit on the sabbath, will not lay hold of it and lift it out? Of how much more value is a man than a sheep!" (12:10–11)

Jesus desires mercy and does not condemn the guiltless.

> And if you had known what this means, I desire mercy not sacrifice, you would not have condemned the guiltless. (12:7)

Introduction

In his preface to a book titled *The Miracle of Life*, Pope Francis invites "everyone around the world" to reflect upon "the wonder and joy of each one's coming into the world. It shows the beauty of looking at unborn life as the holder of the highest right that belongs to everyone: that of existing. Beauty, yes, because the spectacle of nature taking its course instills wonder and calls for care, protection, and welcome." Then, in a unique and profound way, Francis recommends

> "listening" to the voice of the embryo, questioning us about his or her nature, his or her singularity, on how he or she faces every threat that stands between him or her and their own existence. ... In this regard, I renew my appeal to all those who, faced with unborn life, do not stop and do not give in to a tragic and definitive solution, such as abortion, but feel they can offer the unborn child and the mother the help of a society that is finally dedicated to defending the dignity of all, starting with the most vulnerable. It is a society that, in short, rejects the "throwaway culture" in every area and at every stage of existence. On behalf of so many innocent victims, may God bless all those who

---

9. CDF, *Dignitas personae* (September 8, 2008), n. 18, emphasis in italics original, emphasis in bold added.

are willing to discuss and reflect together on this "miracle" that is life."[10]

This chapter is dedicated to following Francis's inspiring and heartfelt invitation to listen to "the voice of the embryo," who can and does speak to us through the voice of the magisterium of the Catholic Church, which is inspired and guided by the outpouring of the Holy Spirit, who, in the words of St. Thomas Aquinas, "interiorly perfects our spirit, communicating to it a new dynamism so that it refrains from evil for love."[11]

The first section of this chapter will begin with a brief overview of the magisterial teachings in the Theology of the Body, which provide the solid biblical and theological foundation for understanding and defending not only *Humanae vitae*, for which it was written, but also all the Church's subsequent magisterial teachings in *Donum vitae*, *Dignitas personae*, and the *Catechism*. The magisterial teachings of Pope John Paul II, Pope Benedict XVI, and Pope Francis continue to promote and defend, above all else, the life and the dignity of every human person from the moment of conception, because each embryo not only is created by God and in God's own image and likeness but reveals the mystery of God.

After reviewing the Theology of the Body, the second and third sections of this chapter will highlight the magisterial teachings that are frequently ignored or omitted and that clearly defend the licitness of embryo transfer, which confirms the implicit morality of embryo adoption. The adoption of orphaned frozen embryos fulfills virtually all the corporal and spiritual works of mercy. What we do for the least of our brothers and sisters, we do unto Jesus, who himself was once a one-cell embryo, just like every one of us. As the Theology of the Body teaches, the human body, beginning with the body of the human zygote, speaks the language of the body.

---

10. Francis, "Pope: May We Hear the Voice of the Unborn through Science," Vatican News, May 21, 2023, https://www.vaticannews.va/en/pope/news/2023-05/pope-may-we-hear-the-voice-of-the-unborn-through-science.html; working translation of Francis, preface to Gabriele Sempreton, Luca Crippa, and Arnoldo Mosca Mondadori, *Il miracolo della vita: Riscoprire oggi l'avventura di nascere* (Milan: Piemme, 2023).
11. Thomas Aquinas, *Commentary on the Second Epistle to the Corinthians*, chap. 3, lect. 3, trans. Peter John Cameron, *Novenas for the Church Year* (Huntington, IN: Our Sunday Visitor, 2012), 94.

Part 3: Defenses of Embryo Adoption

In conclusion, this chapter argues that the Church is telling us to listen to the voices of millions of frozen embryos who must be therapeutically transferred, maternally sheltered, and gestated until birth by their own natural parents. If the parents do not fulfill this duty, then embryo adoption is a praiseworthy moral solution and "a *great 'yes' to the recognition of the dignity and inalienable value of every single and unique human being called into existence.*"[12]

Theology of the Body: A Defense of Marriage and the Procreative Meaning of the Marital Act

The Magisterial Teachings in the Theology of the Body

John Paul II's magnificent Theology of the Body provides the abundant biblical and magisterial foundations that defend the perennial teachings of the Catholic Church regarding the sacredness of marriage and the inseparability of the procreative and unitive meanings of the marital act, through which the two spouses are called to procreate, with God, a *third person*, a new human being, a child who is equally made in the image and likeness of God and who has the equal dignity of a human person from the first moment of conception.

Some authors who are opposed to embryo transfer and to embryo adoption attempt to claim that their moral arguments can be found in the Theology of the Body. Nothing could be further from the truth. The Theology of the Body was originally written and prepared for publication as a book by Karol Wojtyla *prior* to his election as Pope on October 16, 1978, and its primary purpose was to respond to the immediate and widespread dissent and disobedience within the Catholic Church to the magisterial teachings in *Humanae vitae*, which was promulgated in 1968. The Theology of the Body was never intended to justify abandoning "spare" cryopreserved human embryos who were illicitly conceived during IVF and left to an "absurd fate."[13] In fact, Louise Brown, the world's first IVF baby, was not even born until July 25, 1978, just three months before John Paul II was elected Pope; and Hannah Strege, the world's first adopted frozen embryo,

---

12. See CDF, *Dignitas personae*, n. 37, emphasis original.
13. CDF, *Dignitas personae*, n. 19.

was not even born until December 31, 1998, twenty years later and twelve years *after* the promulgation of *Donum vitae* in 1987.[14]

The Theology of the Body Defends the Dignity of the Body as Inseparable from the Dignity of the Person

In his extraordinary work, *Man and Woman He Created Them: A Theology of the Body*, John Paul II repeatedly emphasizes the inseparable connection between the dignity of the person and the dignity of the body. This teaching was publicly delivered to the Church through his weekly catechesis between 1979 and 1984. In his Theology of the Body, John Paul II argues that the human body, in its masculinity and femininity, is integral to each unique person's identity and personal dignity: "[Christ] assigns to each—both to the man and to the woman—his or her own dignity, *in some sense the 'sacrum' of the person, specifically with respect to* the person's femininity or masculinity, *with respect to the 'body.'*"[15] The inseparability of the dignity of the body from the dignity of the person is clearly a fundamental principle of the Theology of the Body and of all the Pope's later magisterial teachings on the sanctity of human life, on marriage, on the family, and on the sexual ethics of both artificial contraception and artificial procreation.

Biblical and Magisterial Foundations of the Dignity of the Human Person

The concept of the dignity of the human person in Catholic teaching is deeply rooted in Sacred Scripture, particularly in the creation narrative of Genesis 1:27: "God created man in his own image, in the image of God he created him; male and female he created them." This divinely revealed truth regarding the inherent dignity of every human being constitutes the biblical and theological foundation of the magisterium's teaching on the dignity of the human person.

---

14. See John Strege, *A Snowflake Named Hannah: Ethics, Faith, and the First Adoption of a Frozen Embryo* (Grand Rapids, MI: Kregel Publications, 2020), 54.
15. John Paul II, *Man and Woman He Created Them: A Theology of the Body*, trans. Michael Waldstein (Boston: Pauline Books and Media, 2006), 100.6, emphasis original.

Part 3: Defenses of Embryo Adoption

As far back as the first century, the Catholic Church has constantly upheld the principle of the inviolable dignity of the human person—including human embryos and newborns—based upon man's direct creation by God in his own image and likeness. Therefore, the Church always has condemned all acts of violence and death against them: "You shall not kill the embryo by abortion and shall not cause the newborn to perish."[16]

One of the more recent and highly influential Church documents to articulate the dignity of the human person was the Pastoral Constitution on the Church in the Modern World *Gaudium et spes* from the Second Vatican Council. This document emphasizes that human life and the dignity of the person must be respected and protected from conception, and it teaches that "God, the Lord of life, has conferred on men the surpassing ministry of safeguarding life in a manner which is worthy of man. Therefore from the moment of its conception life must be guarded with the greatest of care."[17] This foundational teaching would later serve as the basis for all of the post-conciliar documents that focus on the dignity of the human person from the moment of conception until natural death.

The Theology of the Body Defends the Primacy of the Dignity of the Person

John Paul II's Theology of the Body represents a truly significant theological development in understanding the importance of the dignity of the human person as the very foundation of the Church's defense of human life, marriage, the marital act, and the dignity of procreation: "The analysis of the *personalistic aspects* contained in this document has an existential meaning for establishing what *true progress* consists in, that is, the development of *the human person*."[18]

John Paul II offers a profoundly personalistic exploration of the human body as a reflection of God's own image by the intimate relationship between man's body and his soul as a single unity, a person who reflects and reveals the very mystery of God: "The body, in fact, and only the body, is

---

16. *Catechism*, n. 2271, quoting the Didache. This paragraph of the *Catechism* also references the following early Church sources: the Epistle of Barnabus, the Epistle to Diognetus, and the writing of Tertullian.
17. Vatican Council II, *Gaudium et spes* (December 7, 1965), n. 51.
18. John Paul II, *Man and Woman He Created Them*, 133.3, emphasis original.

capable of making visible what is invisible: the spiritual and the divine. It has been created to transfer into the visible reality of the world the mystery hidden from eternity in God, and this to be a sign of it."[19]

In his general audience on November 28, 1984, which marks the end of the Theology of the Body, John Paul II discusses his pastoral concern about the importance of defining and defending the essential dignity of the person as well as the authentic development of the human person. His final recommendation to the faithful is to face and define the difficult moral and ethical questions and then to seek answers in the "biblical, theological sphere" where the truth will prevail in defending the dignity of the person:

> In contemporary civilization as a whole—especially in Western civilization—there exists, in fact, a hidden and at the same time rather explicit tendency to measure this progress [of man] with the measure of "things," that is, material goods.
>
> The analysis of the personalistic aspects of the Church's teaching contained in Paul VI's encyclical highlights a resolute appeal to measure man's progress with the measure of the "person," that is, of that which is a good of man as man, which corresponds to his essential dignity.
>
> The analysis of the *personalistic aspects* leads to the conviction that *the fundamental problem* the encyclical presents is the viewpoint of the *authentic development of the human person;* such development should be measured, as a matter of principle, by the measure of ethics and not only of "technology." ...
>
> ... Still, the most important aspect seems to be the essential aspect that, in the whole of the reflections carried out, one can specify as follows: to face the questions raised by *Humanae Vitae* above all in theology, to formulate these questions, and to look for an answer to them, one must find *that biblical, theological sphere* to which we allude when we speak about the "redemption of the body and the sacramentality of marriage." It is in this sphere that one finds the answers to the perennial questions of our contemporary world concerning marriage and procreation.[20]

---

19. John Paul II, *Man and Woman He Created Them*, 19.4.
20. John Paul II, *Man and Woman He Created Them*, 133.3, 133.4, emphasis original.

Part 3: Defenses of Embryo Adoption

Donum Vitae Defends Human Life and the "Dignity of the Person" at Conception

The importance of protecting human dignity from the moment of conception was subsequently reaffirmed in the instruction *Donum vitae* (The Gift of Life) that was issued in 1987 by the Congregation for the Doctrine of the Faith (CDF) during the pontificate of John Paul II and under the guidance of its prefect, Cardinal Joseph Ratzinger, who later became Benedict XVI. This magisterial document addresses the philosophical, theological, and magisterial implications of artificial reproductive technologies, particularly IVF, and it reaffirms the Church's strong moral opposition to the many gravely illicit methods of artificial contraception and artificial procreation that separate procreation from the sexual act within marriage.

Donum vitae unequivocally states, "*The human being must be respected—as a person—from the very first instant of his existence.*"[21] It emphasizes that the dignity of the person is present from conception and that any treatment or manipulation of human embryos that fails to respect their dignity violates the natural moral order. The instruction categorically rejects any practice that can physically harm or kill embryos—such as freezing, nontherapeutic experimentation, and selective (eugenic) abortions—based upon the biblical and theological grounds that these acts gravely violate the dignity of the human person.

Donum vitae develops its own important theological teachings based on the theological arguments that were previously used in both *Humanae vitae* and the Theology of the Body. In fact, *Donum vitae*'s arguments in many ways are a mirror image of *Humanae vitae*'s arguments, given the technical methods of *artificial contraception* (various pharmaceuticals and other devices) and the technical methods of *artificial procreation* (artificial insemination, artificial fertilization, and the artificial use of a surrogate uterus) that effectively separate the unitive and procreative meanings of the marital act.[22] In other words, *Donum vitae* condemns artificial procreation

---

21. CDF, *Donum vitae*, I.1, emphasis from CDF, *Instruction Donum Vitae* (Washington, DC: Libreria Editrice Vaticana / US Conference of Catholic Bishops, 2013), 7.
22. CDF, *Donum vitae*, II.5. By "'artificial procreation' or 'artificial fertilization' are understood here the different technical procedures directed towards obtaining

by further developing the theological arguments used in *Humanae vitae* and the Theology of the Body to condemn artificial contraception.[23]

In addition, by defending the primacy of the dignity of the human person, John Paul II's Theology of the Body prepared the way for *Donum vitae*'s deepest theological discussions regarding the moral licitness of using therapeutic procedures on embryos in order to heal them and to save their lives because they have the dignity of persons and patients from the first moment of their conception and, therefore, equally deserve to be healed and saved like all other human beings.

---

a human conception in a manner other than the sexual union of man and woman. This Instruction deals with fertilization of an ovum in a test-tube (*in vitro* fertilization) and artificial insemination trough transfer into the woman's genital tracts of previously collected sperm." Note that embryo transfer is not mentioned.

23. Note that the paragraphs in the *Catechism* that address artificial procreation also do not mention embryo transfer or embryo adoption: "Techniques that entail the dissociation of husband and wife, by the intrusion of a person other than the couple (donation of sperm or ovum, surrogate uterus) are gravely immoral. These techniques (heterologous artificial insemination and fertilization) infringe the child's right to be born of a father and mother known to him and bound to each other by marriage. They betray the spouses' 'right to become a father and a mother only through each other'" (n. 2376, quoting CDF, *Donum vitae*, A.2). "Techniques involving only the married couple (homologous insemination and fertilization) are perhaps less reprehensible, yet remain morally unacceptable. They dissociate the sexual act from the procreative act. The act which brings the child into existence is no longer an act by which two persons give themselves to one another, but one that 'entrusts the life and identity of the embryo into the power of doctors and biologists and establishes the domination of technology over the origin and destiny of the human person. Such a relationship of domination is in itself contrary to the dignity and equality that must be. common to parents and children.' 'Under the moral aspect procreation is deprived of its proper perfection when it is not willed as the fruit of the conjugal act, that is to say, of the specific act of the spouses' union. ... Only respect for the link between the meanings of the conjugal act and respect for the unity of the human being make possible procreation in conformity with the dignity of the person'" (n. 2377, quoting CDF, *Donum vitae*, II.1, II.5).

Taken together, the Theology of the Body and *Donum vitae* provide a seamless doctrinal foundation for understanding the moral responsibilities of the embryos' parents, health care providers, lawmakers, and religious leaders of every denomination—especially within the Catholic Church—to legally protect and care for human embryos as persons and patients, regardless of the how they were conceived or the circumstances of their *absurd* and *unjust* cryostorage in fertility clinics.

Dignitas Personae Defends Human Embryos and Their "Dignity as Persons"

Twenty years later, in 2008, the CDF issued a follow-up instruction, *Dignitas personae* (The Dignity of the Person), during the pontificate of Benedict XVI. The document chose as its very title the principle of the dignity of the person that must continue to guide the Catholic Church when she seeks faithful moral answers to difficult questions involving the use of any new biotechnology in the field of assisted reproductive techniques.

Dignitas personae was written to address and provide answers to "certain bioethical questions" regarding new advancements—or old unresolved problems—in biotechnology, including the staggering problems of cryopreservation, genetic manipulation, cloning, and stem cell research. From its very first sentence, *Dignitas personae* reaffirms *Donum vitae* and all its magisterial teachings that proclaim and defend the inviolable dignity of the human person.

The growing problem of hundreds of thousands of frozen embryos appears to have been one of the major concerns considered by the CDF and by Benedict XVI himself. It is highly significant that the CDF expanded its discussion of the immorality of the freezing of surplus embryos from just one paragraph in *Donum vitae* to eight paragraphs in *Dignitas personae*.[24] After condemning the various immoral uses of the surplus frozen embryos, *Dignitas personae* compassionately refers to them as orphans and laments the fact that their parents have not returned for them. The instruction even

---

24. CDF, *Donum vitae*, I.6; and CDF, *Dignitas personae*, nn. 18–19. See also Teofilo Giovan S. Pugeda III, "An Overview of the Embryo Adoption Debate," *Philippiniana sacra* 57.173 (May–August 2022): 191, doi: 10.55997/2001pslvii173a.

goes so far as to recognize the tragic reality that, for so many of them, "all trace of the parents is lost."[25]

Like *Donum vitae*, *Dignitas personae* emphasizes the need to protect embryos from further exploitation and harm, particularly in the context of destructive research and experimentation. The instruction distinguishes between *technical interventions* that are illicitly used to harm and kill frozen embryos and *medical interventions* that are therapeutic and licitly used to heal and save the life of an embryo who must be treated like any other patient. Given that embryo transfer to a maternal womb must be considered a therapeutic medical intervention to heal and save the life of the embryo,[26] embryo transfer is, therefore, morally licit and can also be therapeutically used in prenatal adoption to transfer the adopted frozen embryo into the maternal womb of the adoptive mother. If the object of the act (*finis operis*) is good and the intention of the act (*finis operantis*) is good, then the act of embryo transfer and the intention of embryo adoption ethically confirm and establish the morality of embryo adoption.[27]

The Magisterium Praises the Adoption of Orphans and Condemns Cryopreservation

Built upon the biblical and theological principle of the dignity of the human person so strongly articulated in the Theology of the Body and subsequently in both *Donum vitae* and *Dignitas personae*, the practice of embryo adoption is now increasingly understood as a moral and even heroic work of mercy in response to the orphaning of surplus frozen embryos, regardless of how they were immorally conceived using IVF. When frozen embryos are abandoned by their biological or genetic parents—whether because of a decision to avoid their implantation, gestation, and birth or because of any other

---

25. CDF, *Dignitas personae*, n. 18.
26. See *Donum vitae*, I.3.
27. See Mónica López Barahona, Ramón Lucas Lucas, and Salvador Antuñano Alea, "The Moral Licitness of Adopting Frozen Embryos, with Answers to Objections," in *Human Embryo Adoption: Biotechnology, Marriage, and the Right to Life*, ed. Thomas V. Berg and Edward J. Furton (Philadelphia: National Catholic Bioethics Center, 2006), 273–295; and Glenn Breed, "The Only Moral Option Is Embryo Adoption," *National Catholic Bioethics Quarterly* 14.3 (Autumn 2014): 441–447, doi: 10.5840/ncbq20141436.

factors—frozen embryos are ontological nascent human beings who have the same inalienable human rights and inviolable human dignity as any other person. The moral defense of embryo adoption rests primarily on the recognition that these frozen embryos, even though they have been immorally conceived and then rejected and abandoned by their biological parents, are still persons, created directly by God and in the image and likeness of God, and they fully deserve the same respect, care, and medical treatment as any other person.

The Church's unchangeable doctrine on the dignity of the human person makes clear that the responsibility to protect frozen embryos from harm and death is not just a secondary concern but rather a moral imperative. Embryo adoption, in this context, should be officially recognized by the Catholic Church as a biblically, theologically, and morally based option to rescue orphaned embryos from the intrinsically evil—and utterly inhumane—endangerment of cryopreservation that the magisterium condemned in both *Donum vitae* I.6 and *Dignitas personae* n. 18. It should be noted that the Church has never condemned or prohibited embryo transfer or embryo adoption, but it has absolutely condemned cryopreservation, even temporarily. Recommending cryopreservation as a permanent solution is tantamount to an unjust death sentence and therefore could potentially "fall within the *sin of abortion*."[28]

Concerned and loving adoptive families are undoubtedly, therefore, the only moral solution to the seemingly absurd fate of and grave injustice that has been done to orphaned frozen embryos, who have the inviolable dignity of human persons. Embryo adoption is increasingly understood and accepted by theologians, ethicists, and citizens of every denomination as an exceptionally loving act of mercy that fulfills the moral and magisterial

---

28. See CDF, *Dignitas personae*, nn. 18–19. See also *Dignitas personae*, n. 23, quoting John Paul II, *Evanglium vitae* (March 25, 1995), n. 58: "As is known, abortion is 'the deliberate and direct killing, by whatever means it is carried out, of a human being in the initial phase of his or her existence, extending from conception to birth.' Therefore, the use of means of interception and contragestation fall with the *sin of abortion* and are gravely immoral. Furthermore, when there is certainty that an abortion has resulted, there are serious penalties in canon law" (emphasis original).

obligation to care for and protect vulnerable and endangered human beings, especially those in the earliest stages of life.

Furthermore, embryo adoption can be seen as a praiseworthy way to uphold not only the dignity of the adopted children but also the dignity of their adoptive parents, who thereby participate in the divine work of bringing new life into the world. It is not simply a matter of rescuing a life but also an act that affirms the personal dignity of the embryo, a person who must not be deprived of maternal shelter, gestation, birth, and the loving parental care of a family—a communion of persons—that has been constantly defended in the Theology of the Body and by the magisterium.

Summary

The Catholic Church has consistently upheld the dignity of the human person from the moment of conception, recognizing that every human being—regardless of his or her age, stage of development or condition of health—is just like any other person. This fundamental magisterial teaching has been most recently proclaimed in such important Church documents as *Gaudium et spes*, John Paul II's Theology of the Body, *Donum vitae*, *Dignitas personae*, and the *Catechism*. These major magisterial teachings define the ethical treatment of embryos and form a coherent moral framework that defends the sanctity of life at conception, the dignity of the human person at conception, and the moral imperative of protecting, healing, and caring for every human embryo from the first moment of conception. Embryos are the most vulnerable human beings within the Body of Christ. The very least of our brethren are millions of abused, frozen, and abandoned human beings who deserve to be licitly transferred into the womb of their mother—or into the maternal womb of an adoptive mother—to be raised by a loving family who will recognize and protect the inviolable dignity that every newly conceived person deserves.

In sum, the only moral options for parents who have surplus frozen embryos is to practice what the Theology of the Body has called "responsible parenthood."[29] It is the duty of the parents who have frozen embryos to responsibly decide whether to (1) lovingly raise their own children or (2) lovingly place their frozen embryos for adoption by a married couple

---

29. John Paul II, *Man and Woman He Created Them*, 121.5.

longing to start a family or increase their family by means of adoption. The *Catechism*—under the heading of "The gift of a child"—eloquently praises adoption and encourages married couples to "give expression to their generosity by adopting abandoned children."[30]

Donum Vitae, Dignitas Personae, and the *Catechism of the Catholic Church*

On November 28, 1984, John Paul II finished delivering his 129 weekly audiences on the Theology of the Body. Just fifteen months later, on February 22, 1987, the Pope approved the promulgation by the CDF of the *Instruction on Respect for Human Life and on the Dignity of Procreation: Donum vitae*, which begins with these words: "The gift of life which God the Creator and Father has entrusted to man calls him to appreciate the inestimable value of what he has been given and to take responsibility for it: this fundamental principle must be placed at the center of one's reflection in order to clarify and solve the moral problems raised by the artificial interventions on life as it originates and on the processes of procreation."[31]

Just as the Theology of the Body focuses on explaining why *Humanae vitae* condemns every form of *artificial contraception*, *Donum vitae* builds on the solid foundation of the Theology of the Body to explain why the Catholic Church also condemns every form of *artificial procreation*. The instruction begins with an introduction followed by three parts with an overall magisterial emphasis on respecting human life in its origin:

- "The first part will have as its subject *respect for the human being from the first moment of his or her existence*."
- "The second part will deal with the moral questions raised by technical interventions on human procreation" (in vitro fertilization and insemination).
- "The third part will offer some orientations on the relationships between moral law and civil law in terms of the *respect due to human embryos* and foetuses and as regards the legitimacy of techniques of artificial procreation."[32]

---

30. *Catechism*, n. 2379.
31. CDF, *Donum vitae* (February 22, 1987), introduction, 1.
32. CDF, *Donum vitae*, forward, emphasis added.

The introduction of *Donum vitae* revisits and promotes the fundamental magisterial teachings of the Theology of the Body:

> God, who is love and life, has inscribed in man and woman the vocation to share in a special way in his mystery of personal communion and in his work as Creator and Father. For this reason marriage possesses specific goods and values in its union and in procreation. ... Such values and meanings are of the personal order and determine from the moral point of view the meaning and limits of artificial interventions on procreation and on the origin of human life. These interventions are not to be rejected on the grounds that they are artificial. ... But they must be given a moral evaluation in reference to the dignity of the human person, who is called to realize his vocation from God to the gift of love and the gift of life.[33]

The second part of *Donum vitae* further expands and develops the Theology of Body:

> The parents find in their child a confirmation and completion of their reciprocal self-giving: the child is the living image of their love, the permanent sign of their conjugal union, the living and indissoluble concrete expression of their paternity and maternity. By reason of the vocation and social responsibilities of the person, the good of the children and of the parents contributes to the good of civil society; the vitality and stability of society require that children come into the world within a family and that the family be firmly based on marriage. The tradition of the Church and anthropological reflection recognize in marriage and in its indissoluble unity the only setting worthy of truly responsible procreation.[34]

Given the significance of the parent-child relationship, *Donum vitae* also issues a very grave warning to spouses to never "destroy directly an innocent human being" and to procreate responsibly:

> From the moment of conception, the life of every human being is to be respected in an absolute way because man is the only creature on earth that God has "wished for himself" and the spiritual soul of each man is "immediately created" by God;

---

33. CDF, *Donum vitae*, introduction, 3.
34. CDF, *Donum vitae*, II.A.1.

his whole being bears the image of the Creator. Human life is sacred because from its beginning it involves "the creative action of God" and it remains forever in a special relationship with the Creator, who is its sole end. God alone is the Lord of life from its beginning until its end: no one can, in any circumstance, claim for himself the right to destroy directly an innocent human being. Human procreation requires on the part of the spouses responsible collaboration with the fruitful love of God; the gift of human life must be actualized in marriage through specific and exclusive acts of husband and wife, in accordance with the laws inscribed in their persons and in their union.[35]

Just as *Humanae vitae* and the Theology of the Body specifically defended marriage and the procreative meaning of the marital act, it is also abundantly clear that *Donum vitae* II.A.1 is specifically defending marriage and how "a truly responsible procreation" *should take place*:

Every human being is always to be accepted as a gift and blessing of God. However, from the moral point of view a truly responsible procreation vis-à-vis the unborn child must be the fruit of marriage.

For human procreation has specific characteristics by virtue of the personal dignity of the parents and of the children: the procreation of a new person, whereby the man and the woman collaborate with the power of the Creator, must be the fruit and sign of the mutual self-giving of the spouses, of their love and of their fidelity. The fidelity of the spouses in the unity of marriage involves the reciprocal respect of their right to become a father and a mother only through each other. The child has the right to be conceived, *carried in the womb*, brought into the world and brought up within marriage: it is through the secure and recognized relationship to his own parents that the child can discover his own identity and achieve his own proper human development.[36]

Far from condemning embryo transfer or embryo adoption, this magnificent passage in *Donum vitae* magisterially defines what "*a truly respon-*

---

35. CDF, *Donum vitae*, introduction, 5.
36. CDF, *Donum vitae*, II.A.1, emphasis original in the first paragraph; emphasis in the last paragraph added.

sible procreation" should be for all unborn children. This definition applies equally to all unborn children who are conceived either *outside of marriage* or *outside of the marital act*. How many countless millions of children have been immorally conceived *outside of marriage* as the result of fornication, adultery, rape, and incest? The purpose of *Donum vitae* II.A.1 is to protect *every* human life *in its origin* and to defend *the dignity of procreation in general*. Its purpose is to magisterially define and defend marriage, the unitive and procreative meanings of the marital act, and, especially, the inviolable rights of each and every unborn child, whose human and civil rights *should never* be violated by the immoral sexual and reproductive sins of *the child's own parents!*

As carefully discussed above, *Donum vitae* strictly prohibits artificial fertilization and artificial insemination, and it would be erroneous to argue that *Donum vitae* II.A.1 is in any way *prohibiting* the adoption of a child, at any stage of development, simply because he or she was immorally conceived either *outside of marriage* or *outside of the marital act*. The Catholic Church has always praised adoption as a loving work of mercy whenever a child is unplanned, unwanted, or has been abused or abandoned by his or her own parents.

Donum vitae II.A.1 explicitly states, "*Every human being is always to be accepted as a gift and blessing of God.*" This passage does not in any way condemn embryo adoption. On the contrary, it condemns the many grave procreative sins that are so often committed against the child by *the child's own parents*. Over one million frozen embryos are being deprived of maternal shelter and gestation. *Dignitas personae* cries out against the parents who have abandoned their children: "The majority of embryos that are not used remain 'orphans.' Their parents do not ask for them and at times all trace of the parents is lost. This is why there are thousands upon thousands of frozen embryos in almost all countries where *in vitro* fertilization takes place."[37] Since even *Dignitas personae* is decrying the absurdity and the injustice of "thousands upon thousands of frozen embryos" who have been abandoned and are "orphans," this magisterial statement is in effect advocating for the adoption of these abandoned embryos who are "orphans."

---

37. CDF, *Dignitas personae*, n. 18.

Part 3: Defenses of Embryo Adoption

The adoption of abused and abandoned children has always been praised by the Catholic Church and by Jesus himself: "Whoever receives one such child in my name receives me" (Mark 9:37). In addition, the *Catechism* beautifully recommends that spouses who suffer from infertility "can give expression to their generosity by adopting abandoned children."[38] So many abandoned frozen embryos are waiting for adoption by a forever family!

Finally, *Donum vitae* unequivocally defends the fundamental rights of each person: "The inalienable rights of the person must be recognized and respected by civil society and the political authority. These human rights depend neither on single individuals nor on parents; nor do they represent concessions made by society and the State: they pertain to human nature and are inherent in the person by virtue of the creative act from which the person took his or her origin."[39]

In my opinion, one of the most powerful passages in *Donum vitae* explains to the parents who have frozen embryos that their children "*must in any case be accepted*" and "*brought up with love*," and if the parents are unable or unwilling to do so, then they must find adoptive parents to do so: "Although the manner in which human conception is achieved with IVF and ET cannot be approved, every child that comes into the world must in any case be accepted as a living gift of the divine Goodness and must be brought up with love."[40]

Both Cryopreservation and Artificial Wombs Are Condemned by the Magisterium

Before this chapter begins its formal defense of the magisterial licitness of embryo transfer and the morality of embryo adoption in the third section, it is important to closely examine, in this second section, why the magisterium of the Catholic Church condemns the intrinsic evil of cryopreservation and any proposals for the future use of artificial wombs:

> *The freezing of embryos*, even when carried out in order to preserve the life of the embryo—cryopreservation—*constitutes an*

---

38. *Catechism*, n. 2379.
39. CDF, *Donum vitae*, III.
40. CDF, *Donum vitae*, II.B.5, emphasis added.

offense against the respect due to human beings by exposing them to grave risks of death or harm to their physical integrity and **depriving them, at least temporarily, of maternal shelter and gestation**, thus placing them in a situation in which further offenses and manipulation are possible.[41]

Cryopreservation *is incompatible with the respect owed to the human embryos*; it presupposes their production *in vitro*; it exposes them to the serious risk of death or physical harm, since a high percentage does not survive the process of freezing and thawing; it **deprives them at least temporarily of maternal reception and gestation**; it places them in a situation in which they are susceptible to further offense and manipulation.

The majority of embryos that are not used remain "orphans." Their parents do not ask for them and at times all trace of the parents is lost. This is why there are thousands upon thousands of frozen embryos in almost all countries where *in vitro* fertilization takes place.[42]

The Catholic Church has absolutely condemned as an intrinsically evil act the cryopreservation of human embryos because cryopreservation kills and harms them, and it also deprives them—*even temporarily*—of maternal shelter and gestation. Clearly, since the freezing of surplus embryos is an intrinsically evil technical procedure, it cannot be used or recommended as an evil means in order to achieve the good intention of preserving the life of the embryo.

Increasingly, moral theologians and ethicists, including Rev. Tadeusz Pacholczyk, have been advising married couples that they should not transfer their own frozen embryos into their own mother's womb, recommending instead that their only option is to keep their children frozen indefinitely, thereby continuing to deprive them of maternal shelter and gestation by a state that has been absolutely condemned by the Catholic Church. The following quote is taken from a June 2009 Making Sense of Bioethics article, titled "What Should We Do with the Frozen Embryos?":

---

41. CDF, *Donum vitae*, I.6, emphasis in italics original, emphasis in bold added.
42. CDF, *Dignitas personae*, n. 18, emphasis in italics original, emphasis in bold added.

Part 3: Defenses of Embryo Adoption

In fact, however, the decision to continue cryopreserving an embryo in liquid nitrogen is not likely an instance of using extraordinary means, since the burdens and costs associated with taking care of embryonic children in this way are actually minimal. When we have children, we have a duty to clothe, feed, care for, and educate them, all of which costs plenty of money. When our children are frozen, we don't need to clothe, feed, or educate them; our care for them can only be expressed by paying the bill each month to replenish the liquid nitrogen in their storage tanks. This way of caring for our children is obviously unusual, but it does not seem morally extraordinary in terms of achieving the desired end of safeguarding their physical integrity.

In my opinion, parents have an obligation to care for their children in this way until some other option becomes available in the future (maybe a sophisticated "embryo incubator" or "artificial womb" of some kind), or until there is a reasonable certainty that they have died on their own from decay or "freezer burn," which may occur whenever frozen embryos are stored for extended periods. Perhaps after a few hundred years, all the stored embryos would have died on their own, and they could finally be thawed and given a decent burial. This approach would not involve us in the direct moral agency of ending their lives by withdrawing their life-sustaining liquid nitrogen.[43]

These statements are deeply troubling on many levels, and they clearly contradict the magisterium of the Catholic Church. Except in exceptional medical situations, the freezing of embryos has been legally sanctioned with fines and imprisonment in Germany and other countries.[44] There is no question that cryopreservation should be universally banned around the world and included in the Nuremburg Code as a crime against humanity.

---

43. Tadeusz Pacholczyk, "What Should We Do with the Frozen Embryos?," Making Sense of Bioethics 48 (June 2009): 2.
44. Kelly Buchanan, "New Law Library Report on the Legal Treatment of Embryos Created through IVF," *Law Library* (blog), Library of Congress, April 4, 2024, https://blogs.loc.gov/law/2024/04/new-law-library-report-on-the-legal-treatment-of-embryos-created-through-ivf/.

In addition, Pacholczyk recommends that the parents of frozen embryos continue to pay their monthly cryostorage bills to the fertility clinics in order to "care for" their children. He has even suggested that parents set up a trust to continue paying the cryostorage bills after they die.[45] This, too, is simply unconscionable. It not only prolongs the intrinsically evil sin of cryopreservation but constitutes an ongoing direct cooperation with evil by financially supporting the very fertility clinics that are manufacturing, killing, harming, and even eugenically aborting countless human embryos.

Finally, it must be pointed out that Pacholczyk and many others have been advocating for the development of artificial wombs to gestate human embryos until birth. However, since 1987 the CDF has categorically condemned any proposals for constructing artificial wombs—or using animal wombs—to gestate human embryos:

> Techniques of fertilization *in vitro* can open the way to other forms of biological and genetic manipulation of human embryos, such as attempts or plans for fertilization between human and animal gametes and the gestation of human embryos in the uterus of animals, or **the hypothesis or project of constructing artificial uteruses for the human embryo**. *These procedures are contrary to the human dignity proper to the embryo, and at the same time they are contrary to the right of every person to be conceived and to be born within marriage and from marriage.*[46]

The Magisterial Liceity of Embryo Transfer Defends the Morality of Embryo Adoption

The preface of this chapter includes many scriptural and magisterial teachings, including *Catechism* n. 2275 that authoritatively defends the magisterial liceity of embryo transfer, because it is a therapeutic medical procedure that must be considered licit when used to heal and save the lives of embryos. In addition, *Donum vitae* I.3, which is cited in *Catechism* n. 2275, also authoritatively defends human embryos as being patients: "As with all medical interventions on patients, *one must uphold as licit procedures carried out*

---

45. Tadeusz Pacholczyk, "Orphans in Liquid Nitrogen," Making Sense of Bioethics 137 (November 2016): 1.
46. CDF, *Donum vitae*, I.6, emphasis in italics original, emphasis in bold added.

on the human embryo which respect the life and integrity of the embryo and do not involve disproportionate risks for it but are directed towards its healing, the improvement of its condition of health, or its individual survival" (emphasis original).[47]

Embryo transfer clearly satisfies this magisterial definition of being a therapeutic medical intervention or procedure that can be licitly and therapeutically used to heal and to save the lives of human embryos, especially when it is necessary to transfer an embryo to a woman's womb for its implantation and gestation. Similar reasoning would apply in a medical emergency, including, if possible, an ectopic pregnancy. The principle of double effect in an ectopic pregnancy requires attempting to save the child's life, if possible, by transferring the ex utero human embryo to the womb for implantation and gestation: "The death of the child is not willed and should be avoided if at all possible—if, for example, re-implantation in the womb were reasonably possible."[48] This lifesaving medical intervention should soon be made possible.

---

47. See Elizabeth Bothamley Rex, "The Magisterial Liceity of Embryo Transfer: A Response to Charles Robertson," *National Catholic Bioethics Quarterly* 15.4 (Winter 2015): 715–721, doi: 10.5840/ncbq201515471. Rex provides an analysis of the magisterial liceity of therapeutic embryo transfer as authoritatively taught in *Donum vitae* I.3 (and *Catechism* n. 2275) that simply and faithfully resolves the problematic statements in *Donum vitae* I.5 and *Dignitas personae* n. 19. For further works by Rex published in the *National Catholic Bioethics Quarterly*, see "IVF, Embryo Transfer, and Embryo Adoption: A Response to Repenshek and Delaquil," *National Catholic Bioethics Quarterly* 14.2 (Summer 2014): 227–234, doi: 10.5840/ncbq201414226; "Embryo Adoption and Conscience," colloquy, *National Catholic Bioethics Quarterly* 11.4 (Winter 2011): 622–623, doi: 10.5840/ncbq20111141; "Embryo Adoption and the Bodily Relationship of Biological Mother and Child," colloquy, *National Catholic Bioethics Quarterly* 15.2 (Summer 2015): 208–209, doi: 10.5840/ncbq201515224; and "Impregnation versus Implantation in the Embryo Adoption Debate," colloquy, *National Catholic Bioethics Quarterly* 17.3 (Autumn 2017): 385–386, doi: 10.5840/ncbq201717339.
48. Charles Grondin, "Ectopic Pregnancy and Double Effect," Catholic Answers, accessed March 12, 2024, https://www.catholic.com/qa/ectopic-pregnancy-and-double-effect.

Embryo Transfer Licitly Resolves the "Absurd Fate" in Donum Vitae 1.5 and the "Situation of Injustice" in Dignitas Personae n. 19

John Haas, Tadeusz Pacholczyk, and many others usually defend their opposition to embryo transfer by citing *Donum vitae* I.5,[49] which states that "those embryos which are not transferred into the body of the mother and are called 'spare' are exposed to an absurd fate, with no possibility of their being offered safe means of survival which can be licitly pursued," as well as *Dignitas personae* n. 19, which also deplores the plight of abandoned embryos:

> All things considered, it needs to be recognized that the thousands of abandoned embryos represent a *situation of injustice which in fact cannot be resolved*. Therefore John Paul II made an 'appeal to the conscience of the world's scientific authorities and in particular to doctors, that the production of human embryos be halted, taking into account that there seems to be no morally licit solution regarding the human destiny of the thousands and thousands of 'frozen' embryos which are and remain the subjects of essential rights and should therefore be protected by law as human persons."[50]

These are indeed perplexing passages, but as I have extensively explained in my 2015 article "The Magisterial Liceity of Embryo Transfer," there is indeed a morally licit solution that can be discovered by carefully analyzing every word and then applying the clear magisterial teachings of the Church: "IVF and ET are two scientifically distinct acts, just as [fertilization] and implantation are two distinct acts. Without ET the newly conceived (or frozen) IVF embryo would be exposed to death. A clear moral principle that is taught in *Donum vitae* I.5 states that 'it is not in conformity with the moral law deliberately to expose to death human embryos conceived

---

49. See, for example, John Haas and Tadeusz Pacholczyk, "Moral Contraindications to the Adoption of Abandoned, Frozen Human Embryos," *Linacre Quarterly* 90.2 (May 2023): 139–144, doi: 10.1177/00243639231165252.
50. CDF, *Dignitas personae*, n. 19, citing John Paul II, Address to the Participants in the Symposium on "*Evangelium Vitae* and Law" and the Eleventh International Colloquium on Roman and Canon Law (May 24, 1996), n. 6.

in vitro.' This would explain why *Donum vitae* always includes the term ET immediately after every reference to IVF. ET prevents the death of embryos after IVF."[51] And since embryo transfer must be upheld as a morally licit therapeutic medical intervention, it can indeed be licitly used as a "safe means of survival" that, in turn, can morally resolve the "absurd fate" of the spare embryos by licitly transferring them into their mother's womb for implantation and gestation.

First of all, both of these texts are referring *only* to the frozen embryos "which are *not* transferred into the body of the mother and are called 'spare'" (emphasis added). In other words, these passages *do not* apply to the IVF embryos, albeit conceived illicitly, who were immediately transferred, using a therapeutic, lifesaving medical procedure, into the body of the mother. All of the millions of IVF embryos that have already been *licitly transferred* are *not* being exposed to an "absurd fate." Neither are they among the thousands of abandoned frozen embryos who are facing a "situation of injustice which cannot be resolved." Why? Because embryo transfer, which is a morally licit medical intervention and a lifesaving medical procedure, was used to heal and save them.

The magisterium's use of the words "deprives [the frozen embryos] *at least temporarily* of maternal reception and gestation" (emphasis added) *speaks volumes*. An abandoned or orphaned cryopreserved embryo must not be deprived of its natural right to maternal shelter, gestation, and birth, even for a single moment, much less indefinitely.

The millions of abandoned embryos, currently facing an "absurd fate" and a "situation of injustice," are only the *unwanted* "spare" frozen embryos that have *not* been *licitly transferred* into the mother's womb. All of the *wanted* IVF embryos have already been *licitly transferred* to the mother's womb for maternal shelter, gestation, and birth. Therefore, embryo transfer is a therapeutic medical intervention that can licitly save embryos' lives.

John Paul II, as cited in *Dignitas personae* n. 18, states that "there *seems to be* no morally licit solution" (emphasis added). The Pope did not say that *there is no morally licit solution*. He made this statement on May 24, 1996, in his Address to the Participants in the Symposium on "*Evangelium Vitae* and Law" and the Eleventh International Colloquium on Roman

---

51. Rex, "Magisterial Liceity of Embryo Transfer," 708.

and Canon Law. Hannah Strege, the world's first adopted frozen embryo, would not be born until December 31, 1998, two years and seven months later. John Paul II was looking for a "morally licit solution" for thousands of "orphaned" embryos that was completely unknown and unheard of at that time, *because, in fact, prenatal adoption would not happen—for the very first time—until nearly three years later!*

Should IVF be banned? Yes. Should cryopreservation also be banned? Yes. But until new civil laws are enacted, prenatal adoption is a *morally licit* solution that can be pursued for "thousands and thousands of 'frozen' embryos which are and remain the subjects of essential rights and should therefore be protected by law as human persons."[52]

To the question posed in *Dignitas personae* n. 19—"What to do with them?"—there *is* a morally licit answer. Embryo transfer is a magisterially licit, therapeutic medical intervention and procedure that can in fact be used to transfer any spare or orphaned embryos into the womb of an adoptive mother for maternal shelter, gestation, and birth in order to save their lives. Prenatal adoption is the only moral solution for millions of orphaned embryos.

Conclusion

In the concluding paragraph of *Donum vitae*, the CDF invites the faithful to heed Jesus's parable of the Good Samaritan: "In the light of the truth about the gift of human life and in the light of the moral principles which flow from that truth, everyone is invited to act in the area of responsibility to each and, like the good Samaritan, to recognize as a neighbor even the littlest among the children of men (cf. Lk 10:29–37). Here Christ's words find a new and particular echo: 'What you do to one of the least of my brethren, you do unto me' (Mt 25:40)."[53]

Does not this magisterial conclusion, inviting the faithful to see the face of Jesus in the "littlest among the children of men," poignantly and compellingly *imply* the licitness of embryo transfer and the morality of embryo adoption, which save these orphaned embryos from death and welcome them into loving *adoptive* families, regardless of how their conception happened?

---

52. CDF, *Dignitas personae*, n. 19, citing John Paul II, Address, n. 6.
53. CDF, *Donum vitae*, conclusion.

Part 3: Defenses of Embryo Adoption

Citing some of the final words of *Dignitas personae* as my chapter's own conclusion, I wish to humbly and faithfully implore the Holy See to open wide the doors of the Catholic Church and joyfully welcome *into* the very Body of Christ the millions of orphaned frozen human embryos—who are indeed the very least of our brothers and sisters—by officially proclaiming the magisterial morality of embryo adoption as "a *great 'yes' to the recognition of the dignity and inalienable value of every single and unique human being called into existence.*"[54]

---

54. CDF, *Dignitas personae*, n. 37.

16

The Rescue of Embryonic Persons and Organ Transplants

Corporal Works of Mercy

Janet Smith

Among the many persuasive arguments for the moral permissibility of the rescue of embryonic persons, an important fact is often missed, namely, that such rescue is best understood as a corporal work of mercy justified by the principle of charity. This fact is illustrated by reviewing a similar debate that occurred during the mid-twentieth century: the moral permissibility of organ transplants from living donors (LOT). In important ways, LOT is similar to the rescue of embryonic persons: both are corporal works of mercy justified by the principle of charity. In fact, in both cases, the word *corporal* points in two directions: it is the loving gift of a part of one's own body for the benefit of another's body. In respect to both issues, it has been challenging to determine which moral principles should determine the moral evaluation of the actions.

Should it be determined that the rescue of embryonic persons is not intrinsically evil, and even that it is an important good, we need to anticipate and take steps to minimize the ways that this work of mercy may be harmful to individuals and to society at large. The negative consequences may be sufficiently horrendous that the procedure, even if morally licit, should be discouraged and highly regulated or even forbidden. On the other hand, if the Church determines the rescue of embryonic persons to be morally permissible and promotes this practice in the correct fashion, it may

Humanizing the Terminology

reduce some of the more egregious offenses against life that arise from the artificial production of human life much more than contribute to them.

Perhaps the most technical term for what we are talking about is "heterologous embryo transfer of excess embryos" (HET), a term that, in my view, serves almost no useful purpose. *Heterologous*, a rarely used and largely unknown word, is somewhat off-putting. A more serious problem is that *embryo* is used for any organism that reproduces by means of a fertilized egg and rather dehumanizes the tiny human person by speaking of him or her only in terms of gestational stage. *HET* does not capture the reality that the issue of the rescue of embryonic persons concerns the transfer of a tiny, helpless, vulnerable embryonic person that has been subjected to the indignity of having been made in a petri dish rather than having been conceived by an act of marital intercourse. Then, because it is an excess little human person who will not be gestated by his or her mother, it has been frozen. *Donum vitae* speaks of the "absurd fate" of these little persons,[1] which refers to the fact that they may be used for purposes of experimentation and die in the process, may remain frozen until they disintegrate, or may be discarded when they are deemed no longer useful. Here we are examining if being gestated and adopted by someone other than their mother is also an absurd and immoral fate.

However we speak of these precious creatures, we must keep in mind that they are fully human, and thus they possess all the rights that belong to human persons by virtue of their nature, by virtue of their being made in the image and likeness of God. We should refer to them by terms that reflect their nature and not use words such as *embryo* and *fetus* in unqualified ways, since they refer to stages of gestation.

Analogously, I have long thought that, in the fight for the rights of the unborn, the word *abortion* has nearly become an abstraction that hides the reality of what really goes on. As often as possible, I believe we should not use the word *abortion*. We need to use a variety of phrases, such as "the procedure that dismembers a tiny human person in his or her mother's womb" or "the choice that destroys the life of the unborn child" or "the legal killing

---

1. Congregation for the Doctrine of the Faith (CDF), *Donum vitae* (February 22, 1987), I.5.

of our youngest citizens." These descriptions are much more powerful in capturing the reality of abortion than is the word *abortion* and help people more immediately grasp what is at stake. (Additionally, using the same term repeatedly can dull our awareness of the reality we are considering.) When such language is used, argumentation can sometimes become unnecessary, since it is a rather obvious truth that we should not be dismembering, destroying, or killing tiny human persons, unborn children, or our youngest citizens. Those who promote abortion will object, but these terms are in fact accurate, and we should not be pressured into sanitizing what is happening.

For similar reasons, I think we should use many descriptions of the procedure we are considering here: rather than speaking of *excess embryos*, we should speak of "unborn children produced artificially and then abandoned by their mothers" or "tiny human persons stuck in a freezer who need to be gestated and need suitable people to love and raise them." We should not confine ourselves to *HET* or even the terms *embryo adoption* and *embryo rescue*, although they are efficient ways of speaking. We should never lose sight of the fact that we are speaking of very small human persons who are trapped in freezers and are unlikely to ever reach full development or even see the light of day.

Thus, I will speak of "the rescue of embryonic persons" rather than *embryo adoption*. I do this to reinforce to the reader that the embryos of which we speak are indeed human beings, persons. I do not use an acronym for the same reason. I use the word *rescue* rather than *adoption*, since not all those gestating the embryonic persons will necessarily be their adoptive mothers: some may gestate embryonic persons who will subsequently be adopted by others. Some may object that the phrase is prejudicial or biased toward the acceptance of the rescue of embryonic persons. There may be a measure of truth to that objection, but it seems to me to be an important description. Indeed, even if the rescue of embryonic persons is eventually judged by the Church to be intrinsically evil or so problematic that it should not be permitted, I do not think that judgment would invalidate the description.

Using the term *embryo donation* to describe the act of a woman who has frozen her excess unborn babies and has decided to let another woman gestate one or more quite seriously misrepresents what she is doing. To make a donation is generally understood as a generous act. It is, however, hardly generous for a mother to arrange to have some of her own offspring manufactured in a petri dish and then be willing to have other women gestate and raise the children she does not want or cannot gestate. While her decision not to have her children destroyed is laudable, it is not truly generous. She is properly speaking an *abandoning mother* or, most innocently, "a mother allowing another woman to gestate her embryonic children."

Responding to Usual Objections

In this section, I am going to briefly explain my reasons for rejecting the arguments against the practice of women's gestating babies conceived in a petri dish and then abandoned and stored in freezers. Although others very ably defend the position that the rescue of embryonic persons can be a moral action, it is important to present the foundations of my thinking, especially since they revolve around the merciful act of rescuing precious embryonic persons from destruction.[2]

Gestation

The primary argument against the rescue of embryonic persons in principle is that a woman who gestates a frozen embryonic person is violating the right of her husband to be the source of her motherhood and the right of a child "to be conceived, carried in the womb, brought into the world and brought up within marriage."[3]

---

2. I have sketched out my views in "Adopting Embryos: Why Not?," *National Catholic Register*, March 27, 2009, https://www.ncregister.com/commentaries/adopting-embryos-why-not. I believe my views are virtually identical to those in John Finnis, "Understanding *Dignitas Personae* on Embryo Adoption," in "Symposium on *Dignitas Personae*," ed. Christian Brugger, *National Catholic Bioethics Quarterly* 9.3 (Autumn 2009): 474–477, doi: 10.5840/20099333.
3. CDF, *Donum vitae*, II.A.1. A foremost advocate of this position is Rev. Tadeusz Pacholczyk. See "On the Moral Objectionability of Human Embryo Adoption," in *The Ethics of Embryo Adoption and the Catholic Tradition: Moral Arguments, Economic Reality and Social Analysis*, ed. Sarah-Vaughan Brakman and Darlene Fozard Weaver (Cham, CE: Springer, 2007), 69–83. A response to Pacholczyk's argument appears in the same volume: Christopher O. Tollefsen, "Could Human Embryo Transfer Be Intrinsically Immoral?," 85–101. A report of an interaction between Pacholczyk and me on the issue can be found in Editorial, "Top Catholic Ethicists Duel over Frozen Embryo Adoption," LifeSite News, August 2, 2011, https://www.lifesitenews.com/news/top-catholic-ethicists-duel-over-frozen-embryo-adoption/.

I do not believe that *Donum vitae* is addressing, in any way, the question of the rescue of embryonic persons. Rather, it makes the claim that a wife should not conceive a child with, and thus become a mother by, anyone other than her husband. Such an act would be a kind of adultery. In the rescue of embryonic persons, there is no violation of the marital bond as such; the wife has not *conceived* a child with anyone other than her husband; neither of them has a biological relationship with the child the wife gestates. Gestation is very different from conception, which is the union of the unique gametes of a specific male and female. As the Church teaches, all children should be conceived by a natural act of marital intercourse engaged in by his or her parents. Gestation is not such an intensely personal action as is conception; it is basically providing shelter and food to another person and is altogether separable existentially from conception. In my view, offering one's uterus as a home and conduit for nutrition is nearly morally identical to breastfeeding another woman's child; both the woman breastfeeding and the woman rescuing an embryonic person are using their bodies to sustain the life of a very needy, vulnerable human person.

If it is immoral for an embryonic person to be gestated by someone other than the biological mother, what justifies the use of an incubator, which is essentially an artificial womb that gestates a child until it can live independent of a womb? An argument can definitely be made that it is preferable for a rescued embryonic person to be gestated by a living woman rather than by an incubator—certainly, a machine will eventually be invented that can keep an embryonic person alive from its earliest stages.

The language of *Donum vitae*, when it speaks of a right of a child to be "carried in the womb" and "brought up within marriage," can be misleading. For spouses to adopt an already born baby who is not genetically their own and to raise it within a marriage that is not the marriage of the biological parents of the child is *not* to violate any rights of the child. Rather, it is *repairing* the right of the child to be raised within marriage. The woman and her husband who rescue an embryonic person are honoring the right to life of the child as well as repairing its right to be raised within a marriage. Even a single woman who rescues a child honors its right to life, although she may not be able to provide a conventional family. She is not violating the rights of the child, but *offering* what she can.

Surrogacy

Some argue that *Donum vitae*'s condemnation of surrogacy rules out human embryo rescue, but I believe that the surrogacy condemned by *Donum vitae* is rightly understood to be *commercial* surrogacy, whereby a woman is *paid* to gestate (and sometimes conceive) a child.[4] The act of a woman who gestates and intends to raise as her own an abandoned embryonic person, for the purpose of rescuing the human embryo from indeterminate residence in a freezer or from a very premature death by thawing, resembles the act of a surrogate only in its matter and not at all in its intentionality, the primary determinant of morality. Such an act, much like the act of adopting born children, in fact, is a costly one financially, physically, and emotionally, not one for which she gets paid.

Cryopreservation

Some who maintain that human embryo rescue is wrong cite the statement in *Dignitas personae* that "cryopreservation is incompatible with the respect owed to human embryos." It gives these reasons: "It [cyropreservation] presupposes their production *in vitro*; it exposes them to the serious risk of death or physical harm, since a high percentage does not survive the process of freezing and thawing; it deprives them at least temporarily of maternal reception and gestation; it places them in a situation in which they are susceptible to further offense and manipulation."[5] Clearly, the condemnation being made here is of the cryopreservation that is a part of in vitro fertilization (IVF); it evidences disregard for human life, not the desire to save a human life. Moreover, simply to say cryopreservation is opposed to the respect owed to human persons does not mean it is intrinsically wrong; indeed, medical researchers are exploring the possibility of cryopreserving fully developed human bodies to help preserve cells until various treatments can be refined and, thereby, to prolong their lives. Finally, those who wish to rescue abandoned human embryos are not responsible for wrongs already done to them. They did not freeze the human embryos; rather, they want to rescue the tiny human persons imprisoned in freezers.

Complicity with Evil

Some argue that permitting the rescue of embryonic persons would be to cooperate with the evil of IVF. But those rescuing embryonic persons neither intend to create babies through IVF nor contribute anything to

---

4. CDF, *Donum vitae*, II.A.3.
5. CDF, *Dignitas personae* (September 8, 2008), n. 18.

the procedure. Indeed, it is not possible, in the sense the term *cooperate* has in moral theology, to cooperate with an evil that has *already* been performed, for cooperation means providing something that enables an action to take place. A more genuine concern is the possibility of being *complicit* with evil. Many have the reasonable fear that the practice of rescuing embryonic persons will facilitate the IVF industry by solving the problem of excess embryonic persons and, thereby, reducing the hesitancy of some people to approve of IVF. That is, the possibility that embryonic persons may be rescued mitigates, to some extent, the possibility that doing so involves complicity with the IVF industry. In my view, the good of enabling tiny living human persons to be born and have full lives is unlikely to be outweighed by the evil of reducing objections to IVF. The way to offset the problem of complicity is to continue to teach, speak, and legislate against IVF.[6]

Association with IVF

I think the debate about the morality of rescuing embryonic persons has been skewed from the start because of its link with IVF and various associated issues, such as surrogacy. Those associations have put the individuals defending the morality of rescuing abandoned embryonic persons on the defensive. Things might be different had the technique for transferring embryonic persons from one woman's uterus to another's been developed independent of IVF. For instance, consider the situation of a pregnant woman who has a rapidly growing cancer. Should she refuse treatment, almost certainly both she and her unborn child, not yet viable outside the womb, would die. Would not we find spectacular and morally acceptable the transference of her unborn child to the uterus of another woman, say, her sister, willing to gestate the child to birth? Many questions would arise about what reasons justify a transfer and to whom the transfer may be made, but our initial response to the procedure itself would, I believe, be quite enthusiastic. I do not think Francis Etheredge has met all the possible objections to his line of argument connecting the rights of a conceived child to the fact that God has permitted the conception of that child. I do, however,

---

6. Brandon Brown and Jason Eberl make extensive arguments against using the categories of cooperation, scandal, and complicity to object to embryo adoption in "Ethical Considerations in Defense of Embryo Adoption," in Brakman and Weaver, *Ethics of Embryo Adoption*, 103–118.

think he is right to insist that the human community has a responsibility to find ways of providing for the needs of embryonic persons whose rights have been severely violated in the manner of their coming to be.[7]

Discerning the Morality of Kinds of Actions

When no scriptural passage clearly speaks to the morality of an action, Catholic moral theology uses two primary ways to argue that a kind of action is immoral. A brief look at them here should help us understand the process of discerning the morality of the rescue of embryonic beings.

One way is to show that an action is intrinsically evil because it violates some moral principle based on human nature. As noted above, those who oppose the rescue of embryonic persons argue that a woman who gestates a frozen embryonic person is violating both the "reciprocal respect of their [the spouses'] right to become a father and a mother only through each other" and the right of the child "to be conceived, carried in the womb, brought into the world and brought up within marriage."[8] If either of those principles (or some other principle) demonstrates that adopting embryonic persons is intrinsically evil, it should never be done, no matter how good the consequences, even if millions of lives could be saved. Still, the fact that millions of lives can be saved through embryonic rescue puts the burden of proof on those who oppose it, even if, on the face of it, the procedure seems to violate some key principles.

The second way of evaluating the morality of a kind of action is to show that, even if the action is permissible in principle, the likelihood that it will result in even greater harms would make it imprudent, that is, immoral. For instance, it is not intrinsically immoral for a person under eighteen years of age to drink alcoholic beverages, but most people think there are good reasons for limiting the availability of alcoholic beverages to the young. Consideration needs to be given to the claim that permitting the rescue of frozen embryonic persons would lead to a number of serious harms or wrongs and perhaps should be forbidden on those grounds.

---

7. Francis Etheredge, "Frozen and Untouchable: A Double Injustice to the Embryo," *National Catholic Bioethics Quarterly* 16.1 (Spring 2016): 49–54, doi: 10.5840/ncbq20161616.
8. CDF, *Donum vitae*, II.A.1.

Since IVF has become a widely accepted and frequently used procedure to make babies—indeed, it is considered a routine procedure not only for couples struggling with infertility but also for same-sex couples—it is not remotely realistic to think we can close the lid on this Pandora's box. One way of dealing with the bad consequences that result from permitting the rescue of embryonic persons is to pass legislation that will forbid as many as possible of the bad consequences that might result. We also need to consider the very real possibility that promoting the rescue of frozen tiny human persons might help reduce the bad consequences of IVF and serve to support the fact that these are, in fact, human persons who should never have been made in a petri dish. And if that truth becomes widely recognized, it will become easier to achieve the prohibition of abortion.[9]

As the Church works to come to a conclusion about the morality of rescuing frozen embryonic persons, it would be reasonable to consult the *sensus fidelium*, the sense of the faithful.[10] The issue of rescuing frozen embryonic persons first came to my attention when, in 1996, England announced it was going to thaw and discard over three thousand embryonic persons who had been frozen for five years. The response of two hundred female members of a pro-life group in Italy, who offered to gestate the babies, seemed to be a marvelous spontaneous expression of the *sensus fidelium*.[11] I could imagine women standing up and shouting, "I have a uterus, give me that baby!" However they expressed their response, their immediate willingness to gestate the babies seemed a display of connaturality with the pro-life stance of the Church; it was the sense of the faithful that these abandoned tiny human persons needed to be loved and to be given life and that these women had the wherewithal to do that.

---

9. The Supreme Court of Alabama recently ruled that frozen embryos are children in *LePage v. Center for Reproductive Medicine*, SC-2022-0515 (Ala. 2024).
10. Janet E. Smith, "The *Sensus Fidelium* and *Humanae Vitae*," *Angelicum* 83.2 (2006) 271–297.
11. Francesco DeMartis, "Mass Pre-Embryo Adoption," *Cambridge Quarterly of Healthcare Ethics* 7.1 (January 1998): 101–103, doi:10.1017/S0963180 198701136.

Part 3: Defenses of Embryo Adoption

A Brief History of the Church's Approval of Organ Transplants

More than a decade ago, I researched how the Church discerned the morality of organ transplants.[12] What I learned there might be helpful in gaining clarity about the morality of the rescue of embryonic persons, since both it and organ transplants involve the use of body parts to help other persons. What we shall see is that the Church struggled to determine which principle or principles should guide the moral evaluation of organ transplants. Theologians argued that transplants are not morally permissible, since removal of an organ mutilates the body of the donor. Because organ transplants risk the health of the donor for the sake of the recipient and may lead to the death of some people of the sake of others, other theologians found the practice akin to the Nazi's killing Jews for the sake of Nazi Germany. Still others (most notably Pope Pius XII) thought the practice violates the principle of finality, which holds that each person's bodily parts are directed to the good of their owner and not to the good of other persons. Eventually, theologians (with the notable exception of Pius XII) found the proposed principles inapplicable and reached a consensus that the principle of charity supersedes the other principles.

The question of the morality of organ transplants did not arise until the pontificate of Pius XII, who was adamantly opposed to LOT. For the nearly two decades he served as pope (1939–1958), Pius XII spoke on the issue several times; he was very concerned to find the correct principle that should guide the determination of the morality of LOT. He never changed his thinking that LOT was intrinsically immoral, since in his view, it violates the principle of finality. His view has not stood, although it is not clear when it was decided that LOT is morally acceptable and is, indeed, a charitable and heroic act. The practice has never been explicitly and formally approved.[13] Even before Pius XII's death, Catholic hospitals started doing

---

12. Janet E. Smith, "Organ Transplants: A Study on Bioethics and the Ordinary Magisterium," in *The Ethics of Organ Transplantation*, ed. Steven J. Jensen (Washington, DC: Catholic University of America Press, 2011), 272–304. This article develops the historical narrative presented here.
13. Rev. John Gallagher, CSB, argues this point in "The Principle of Totality: Man's Stewardship of His Body," in *Moral Theology Today: Certitudes and Doubts*, ed. Donald McCarthy (St. Louis: Pope John Center, 1984), 233.

organ transplants. Subsequent popes spoke in favor of organ transplants, as though there had never been any condemnation of it.

In 1944, before Pius XII made any pronouncements on the issue, Rev. Bernard Cunningham wrote a dissertation on the subject of organ transplants, which played a key role in the eventual acceptance of LOT by theologians and physicians. Cunningham directed his arguments largely against the claim that the prohibition of mutilation establishes that organ transplantation is immoral.[14] He attempted to show that, in some important sense, our bodies are directed not only to our personal good but also to the good of others (an argument that also works against the principle of finality). Thus, just as we can cause some mutilation to our own bodies if our health requires it, we are permitted to endure some mutilation for the good of others.

Cunningham argued that, in a sense, we are all "one body," and thus we and our bodies are ordained to the good of others as well as to the good of ourselves; using our organs to help others is a logical fulfillment of our all being one body. Cunningham and several other moral theologians noted that a number of actions that compromise one's health for the sake of others were already considered moral, such as experimentation for medical purposes, blood transfusions, and skin grafts. That argument was met with the counterargument that those body parts are replenishable, whereas donated organs do not grow back. Still, those practices suggest that, in some respects, our bodies can be used for the benefit of others. (It might also have been noted that the reproductive organs of females are intrinsically ordered to the good of others!) Cunningham also noted that people are permitted to lay down their lives for others. Why should they not be permitted to generously donate organs to others? In the end, Cunningham and others appealed to the principle of charity, the principle of love for one's neighbor, as overriding the principle that we should not donate organs because to do so is to mutilate the body. There is no clear evidence that Pius XII took these arguments into account when developing his own position.

Before reviewing the reasons for Pius XII's condemnation of LOT, let us first address the misconception that it was based on his rejection of how Nazis employed the principle of totality to justify killing Jews for the sake of society. The principle of totality is used in bioethics to justify sacrificing the

---

14. Bert J. Cunningham, "The Morality of Organic Transplantation," PhD diss. (Catholic University of America, 1944).

good of a part for the sake of the whole. For instance, the principle justifies amputating a gangrenous limb to keep a person alive. Nazis sacrificed the good of Jews, a part of society, for the sake of the larger or whole community. Pius XII's opposition to using the principle of totality to justify killing Jews issued in an important distinction between an organic whole, such as a human body, where a part that exists for the sake of the whole can be sacrificed for the good of the whole, and a nonorganic whole, where the whole exists for the sake of the part, which cannot be sacrificed for the good of the whole. For example, the state exists for the sake of the individual, not the individual for the sake of the state.

Yet it was not the principle of totality, even as carefully defined, that guided Pius XII's thinking. Rather, he invoked the principle of finality, which holds that the organs God gave each one of us have as their *finality*, their *telos*, the well-being of each of us not the well-being of others. While we can sacrifice our lives for the sake of others, that sacrifice is properly understood not as a direct harm done to ourselves but as a consequence (or double effect) of our intending to save others. In Pius XII's view, organ donation involves our doing direct harm to ourselves for the sake of another. When he spoke on the issue of LOT in 1952 to a congress on histopathology, he invoked the principle of finality four times. He reiterated his position twice in 1953 and again in 1956.[15] The first successful kidney transplant between identical twins was performed in 1954, although it was not expected to become a common practice, since immunosuppressant drugs were not yet invented. Pius XII explicitly condemned the procedure among others in a talk on tissue transplantation delivered in 1956, two years before he died.

As mentioned, there is no evidence that Pius XII's judgment on the question of LOT—expressed in speeches, not in encyclicals—was formally overturned. That does not mean that organ transplants from living donors were not performed. On the contrary, US Catholic hospitals approved organ transplants in their ethical directives as early as 1948 and performed them in the 1960s, in spite of the fact that no magisterial document had been issued

---

15. These addresses can be found in *The Human Body*, selected and arranged by the Monks of Solesmes (Boston: St. Paul Editions, 1960): "Allocution to the First International Congress of Histopathology, September 13, 1952," 194–208; "Allocution to Delegates at the 26th Congress of Urology, October 8, 1953," 277–281; "Allocution to Military Surgeons, October 19, 1953," 281–283; and "Allocution to a Group of Eye Specialists, May 14, 1956," 373–384.

that approved the practice. Indeed, Pope St. Paul VI never mentioned organ transplants, and neither did Pope John Paul I, but their successors have greatly lauded LOT as being an act of charity, as though that had been the understanding all along. In 1984 Pope St. John Paul II gave the highest of praise to organ donors:

> I congratulate you on this initiative, which is an indication of your vitality and spirit that have impelled you to undertake this march. But above all I appreciate the purpose that has brought you together and mobilized: that is, to promote and encourage such a noble and meritorious act as that of donating one's blood or one's organ to those brothers and sisters who need it. This gesture is all the more praiseworthy inasmuch as it does not move you, in carrying it out, the desire for earthly interests or aims, but a generous impulse of heart, human and Christian solidarity: love of neighbour which forms the motive inspiring the Gospel message and which has indeed been defined as the new commandment (cf. Jn 13:34). In donating blood or an organ of your body, always have this human and religious perspective; may your gesture towards your brothers and sisters in need be made as an offering to the Lord, who identified himself with those who suffer because of illness, road accidents or accidents at work; may it be a gift made to the suffering Lord, who in his passion gave all of himself and shed his blood for the salvation of men. If you also put this supernatural intention, your humanitarian gesture, already so noble in itself, will rise and be transformed into a splendid witness of Christian faith and your merit will certainly not be lost."[16]

In 2005 John Paul II stated, "Since the time of my venerable predecessor, Pius XII, during whose pontificate the surgical practice of organ transplant

---

16. John Paul II, Address to the Participants in the Solidarity March Organized by the Leaders of the Volunteer Association of Italian Blood and Organ Donors (August 2, 1984), machine translated by Google. See Benedict XVI, Address to Participants at an International Congress Organized by the Pontifical Academy for Life (November 7, 2008); and Francis, Address to the Italian Association for the Donation of Organs, Tissues and Cells (AIDO) (April 13, 2019). In addition, the *Catechism* states that the practice is "in conformity with the moral law" (*Catechism of the Catholic Church*, 2nd ed. [Washington, DC: US Conference of Catholic Bishops / Libreria Editrice Vaticana, 2018 update], n. 2296).

began, the Church's Magisterium has continually made contributions in this field."[17]

Rescue of Embryonic Persons as an Act of Charity

Both donating organs and gestating an embryonic person who was made through IVF and abandoned are acts of charity whereby one puts one's own body parts in service of the needs of another. In both cases, there is risk involved for the donor and the woman gestating a baby, but the risks are undertaken for the well-being of another. Because of those self-sacrificial acts, other human beings are enabled to live and to bring all the gifts that they have to the world. Both procedures present challenges to bioethicists, since it was not immediately clear what principles should guide their evaluation, and at first glance, they seem to violate some established bioethical principles.

Practical Concerns with the Rescue of Embryonic Persons

As we have seen, even if the Church decides that the principle of charity permits the rescue of embryonic persons, that does not definitively settle the matter. This question arises: Even if an action is morally permissible in principle but leads, in some contexts, to many horrifically bad consequences, should it be permitted? Or, on the other hand, even if it has horrifically bad consequences on occasion, should it be denied as an option for those who would perform the action morally? It is worth observing that when the morality of LOT was being considered, the focus was on the transplantation of organs between identical twins, since immunosuppressant drugs had not yet been developed. There was no discussion of the many harms that could result should LOT become widely practiced: coercive practices in obtaining organs, the buying and selling of organs, the redefinition of death prompted by the supposed need to acquire more organs. Had they been considered, there may have been greater caution in promoting LOT.

On the other hand, is it just to outlaw or discourage a procedure that some may misuse but that could save the lives of others? Is it right to deny

---

17. John Paul II, Letter to the Pontifical Academy of Sciences (February 1, 2005), n. 2.

responsible and needy individuals access to a lifesaving procedure because of the possibility that evil people will profit from or misuse the same procedure? Analogously, some think that the way to combat gun violence in the United States is to forbid gun ownership. The argument is made that, although it is not intrinsically evil to own guns, so much gun violence occurs that we should give up our right to own guns.

Here are some possible problems with the rescue of embryonic persons, which could make this charitable act imprudent and, therefore, morally illicit:

As we observed earlier, permitting the rescuing of abandoned embryonic persons could lead to a greater acceptance of IVF, since it would address the problem of excess embryos. Does not that possibility compound the very problem that embryo rescue is designed to address?

Those who have excess embryonic persons may pressure relatives and friends to gestate their embryonic offspring for them.

Some women who do not want to or cannot gestate an abandoned embryonic person may hire other women to gestate their children. Homosexual couples may wish to hire a surrogate to gestate a child for them.

The need for surrogates will certainly lead to exploitation of the poor.

Should there be medical and social requirements for women who want to gestate an abandoned embryonic person, just as there are for those who wish to adopt already born children? For instance, if a woman has conditions that may result in a miscarriage or precariously early term delivery, is it fair to put the abandoned embryonic person at risk?

The decision on the morality of the rescue-adoption of an abandoned embryonic person will undoubtedly affect the response to and moral evaluation of other problematic situations. For instance, there are times when the transfer of an embryo or fetus from one woman to another may save the life of both the mother and the unborn child. Consider a pregnant woman with a lethal condition for which the recommended or only available treatment threatens the life of her unborn child. Would it not be an act of charity for another woman to gestate the unborn child, if it becomes possible to transfer an embryonic person from the womb of one woman to another?

All the above reflections address particular practical kinds of problems. There are, perhaps, greater, more theoretical concerns. Some argue that IVF, LOT, and allowing women to gestate another woman's child all contribute to the modern inability to understand that the body is an essential part of the person and to the modern tendency to think that the body is a mechanistic entity that we can mold to our own purposes—an understanding that has led to such barbarities as allowing and promoting transgender procedures and surgery. Those seem to me to be legitimate concerns. On the other hand, as mentioned earlier, women's willingness to place their bodies in service of gestating abandoned human persons is a witness to their valuable personhood. Great attention needs to be paid to a large number of cultural factors to determine the wisdom of allowing the rescue of abandoned, embryonic persons.

Promoting the Rescue of Embryonic Persons

There is no doubt that it will be difficult in our modern culture, which holds human life to be of such little value, to contain the harmful consequences that may arise from permitting the rescue of abandoned embryonic persons. Yet that many little frozen human persons, who would otherwise die in captivity, will mercifully live is certainly of inestimable value and makes it right to tolerate some bad consequences (although it is possible, in some social conditions, that the bad consequences would outweigh to good ones).[18]

We cannot underestimate the value of the witness to the humanity of the unborn that widespread rescue of embryonic persons would convey. We have an example of how the practice can lead to a more pro-life public policy in President George W. Bush's invitation of twenty-one individuals who were adopted as embryonic persons to a press conference announcing his decision to outlaw the harvesting of stem cells from living embryonic persons (a procedure that results in their death). He opened his remarks at the press conference with these words: "I have just met with 21 remarkable families. Each of them has answered the call to ensure that our society's most vulnerable members are protected and defended at every stage of life."[19] Surely many of those observing the press conference and learning of his decision had their respect for life deepened.

---

18. Weighing and balancing outcomes is a standard feature of prudent decision-making and not necessarily a sign that one subscribes to consequentialist ethics.
19. George W. Bush White House, "President Discusses Embryo Adoption and Ethical Stem Cell Research," news release, May 24, 2005, https://georgewbush-whitehouse.archives.gov/news/releases/2005/05/20050524-12.html.

Charities could be established to help those who want to rescue embryonic persons but do not have the financial means to do so. John Berkman and Kristen Carey have proposed a marvelous set of directives and procedures to be used by Catholic embryo adoption agencies that will separate the procedure from the IVF industry, ensure that adoptive parents are properly motivated, and fully respect the dignity of the embryonic person being rescued. A "comprehensive Catholic model of embryo adoption" should act "1) to serve the flourishing of human individuals (e.g., at a minimum the sanctity of human life and the option for the poor and marginalized), 2) to serve the common good ... of society, and 3) to avoid moral accommodation with the spirit and practices of those elements of the new 'reproductive technology' which neither serve the flourishing of individuals or the common good of our society."[20]

Berkman and Carey raise the possibility that the agency needs to challenge potential donors to examine whether they have a moral obligation to gestate as many as possible of the frozen embryonic persons they have had created. They also propose that the donors have an obligation to share, if not assume all, financial costs. They recognize that some donors will have no interest in going through with the donation if any burdens are put upon them and that making such just demands would be counterproductive to saving the lives of frozen embryonic persons in a world where there are more embryonic persons in need of rescue than there are rescuers. After all, in all matters, the good of the embryonic person should have primacy of place. Berkman and Carey also observe, "Ironically, it would seem that an important part of [the agency's] mission would be to advocate for public policies and individual decision-making that would put itself out of business."[21]

One practice (not considered by Berkman and Carey) that seems incompatible with the human dignity of the unborn child is that the agencies often ship the frozen unborn children to the adoptive couple. Shipping a baby by ground or even air mail seems to treat the frozen baby as a thing rather than a person. I think having at least one of the adoptive parents

---

20. John Berkman and Kristen N. Carey, "Ethical and Religious Directives for a Catholic Embryo Adoption Agency: A Thought Experiment," in Brakman and Weaver, *Ethics of Embryo Adoption*, 263.
21. Berkman and Carey, "Catholic Embryo Adoption Agency," 266.

travel to the place where the frozen baby is stored would be more in keeping with the dignity of the unborn child.

All in all, I think the rescuing of tiny human persons from living out their lives in a freezer or dying by being thawed is a good thing, indeed, a very good and merciful thing; it is generous and sacrificial and gives tremendous witness to the humanity of the smallest of human persons. That should help our culture in the fight against abortion, human embryo stem cell research, and a host of evils on the horizon, such as cloning.

Moreover, rather than increasing the use of IVF, the adoption of frozen human embryos may decrease it. Most infertile couples reasonably want to have their own biological children, and thus IVF is attractive to them. Some of these sadly do not know that IVF violates Church teaching on the moral ways of creating new human life. The presence of Catholic embryonic person adoption agencies may draw the attention of infertile Catholic couples, who can be taught the immorality of IVF and who will then consider rescuing a tiny human person imprisoned in a freezer. The Church has been woefully negligent in instructing Catholics and the larger society on the immorality of IVF; indeed, when I asked a bishop who has been vigorous in his defense of unborn children why the bishops do not speak out about IVF, he exclaimed, "Do we want people to think we are against helping infertile couples?" The presence of Catholic embryo adoption agencies may give bishops and priests confidence that they can speak out against IVF and, indeed, work against one of its worst consequences—the abandonment of embryonic persons.

The rescue of embryonic persons is also vastly superior to other proposed solutions. Researchers in China are developing artificial wombs that could gestate embryonic persons from conception in a petri dish to birth.[22] They would be accompanied by an AI robot that would monitor their development closely. Let me note that I am not opposed to artificial wombs in principle, and in fact, as stated previously, I view incubators as a form of artificial womb. Artificial wombs can rightly be considered a more highly developed incubator that can gestate babies from conception. Who knows, in the future such artificial wombs could help women who miscarry early.

---

22. Stephen Chen, "Chinese Scientists Create AI Nanny to Look after Embryos in Artificial Womb," *South China Morning Post*, January 31, 2022, https://www.scmp.com/news/china/science/article/3165325/chinese-scientists-create-ai-nanny-look-after-babies-artificial.

These women could conceive a child through an act of conjugal intercourse, and then, before a miscarriage is likely to happen, they could have their child placed in an artificial womb and gestated until birth.

One justification for alternative methods of gestation is that they may serve not only to rescue frozen embryonic persons but also to reduce the number of abortions; an abortion-minded woman could have her embryonic child transferred to an artificial womb or to a whole-body gestational donor. The benign uses of artificial wombs to rescue frozen human persons, unfortunately, are not the only ones being proposed, and perhaps they are not even the most probable ones. Artificial wombs could be used for such nefarious purposes as gestating little human persons to the stage of development when serious health conditions can be diagnosed, in order to kill those who do not measure up to the standard desired. Experiments could be done on the tiny human persons to yield important scientific information (and the little persons, if damaged, could be killed). Babies could be produced en masse to help populate areas suffering from underpopulation. They could be genetically manipulated to be in an IQ range that makes them suitable for menial jobs. Same-sex couples could have babies produced without having to hire a surrogate. Women who do not want their bodies disfigured by pregnancy might prefer to have their children gestated this way.

Another sci-fi-esque proposal is for people to donate their bodies to gestate little human persons in the eventuality that they are proclaimed to be in a persistent vegetative state or brain dead: "It seems plausible that some people would be prepared to consider donating their whole bodies for gestational purposes just as some people donate parts of their bodies for organ donation."[23] In this case, the process is called whole-body gestational donation. That such bizarre means of gestating babies are being proposed may be another reason for promoting embryonic person adoption, especially if facilitated in Catholic institutions. Furthermore, as I have stated earlier, if such bizarre methods are determined to be moral, they should not be preferred to the much more personal act of a woman's rescuing a tiny frozen

---

23. Anna Smajdor, "Whole Body Gestational Donation," *Theoretical Medicine and Bioethics* 44 (November 12, 2022): 113, doi: 10.1007/s11017-022-09599-8. I use the word *people* because Smajdor brings up the possibility that male bodies might be reconfigured to provide a uterus.

embryonic person.[24] It seems to be manifestly preferable, whenever possible, that embryonic persons be gestated by women who love and intend to raise them as their own.

It is somewhat unsettling that the Catholic Church has not made an official statement about the morality of embryonic person adoption, both because women have been adopting embryonic persons for over twenty-five years and also because there has been vigorous theological debate about the issue over that same period of time.[25] One hopes that this and other essays help those in positions of authority to settle this perplexing but ever-more urgent question.

---

24. I find it surprising that Pacholczyk, who opposes embryo adoption as a violation of the spousal relationship and of children, muses somewhat favorably about artificial wombs as a solution to abandoned frozen embryonic persons. See Pacholczyk, "On the Moral Objectionability of Human Embryo Adoption," 82.
25. See Editorial, "New Vatican Instruction Called Valuable 'Reference Point' on Bioethics," Catholic News Agency, December 16, 2008, https://www.catholicnewsagency.com/news/14629/new-vatican-instruction-called-valuable-reference-point-on-bioethics. *Dignitas personae* n. 19 speaks negatively about prenatal adoption, but the general consensus is that this judgment is in no way decisive. Indeed, Pacholczyk, who argues that embryo adoption is intrinsically evil, opines that *Dignitas personae* "did not speak the 'final word'" on the question, if only because the document does not offer clear guidance; rather, it raises challenging questions that some moral theologians believe they have answered.

17

Throw Open the Doors

Next Steps in Embryo Adoption

Christopher M. Reilly

Perhaps the defining moment of Christian action for the early Church was during Pentecost, when the shut-in apostles boldly flung open the doors and poured out into the crowds to preach the Good News. The apostles had been terrified and dejected, worried about the condemnation of those who doubted the radical teachings and invitation of the risen Christ that, at its core, calls us to an unwavering and unqualified love of God and our participation in God's infinite love for each neighbor. With the apostles, the fire of the Holy Spirit ultimately prevailed.

As prospective parents, teachers, and evangelists drawn to the extraordinarily charitable act of embryo adoption, we also pray that the Holy Spirit will inspire the unbounded charitable energy of Christian couples who desire to extend compassion and the fulfillment of purpose and justice owed to some of the most endangered and mistreated human beings—children of God who are literally frozen and held captive pending their demise, mistreatment in scientific experiments, and destruction. It is the adoptive couples who are at the center of the moral drama of embryo adoption and who are inappropriately discouraged by those who argue against the astonishing goodness of such an act of love. The focus of this chapter, then, is to examine next steps that may be taken to care for not only the embryonic children trapped in such a terrible state but also the prospective adoptive parents who find themselves in another terrible state: filled with the fire of the Holy Spirit to love, rescue, and raise these critically endangered and

PART 3: DEFENSES OF EMBRYO ADOPTION

maltreated persons, yet dismayed by the criticism or uncertainty of many in the Church, a lack of institutional and legal support, and gaps in crucial information for making wise decisions. This chapter, therefore, speaks to those who may engage and assist prospective adoptive parents—teachers in the Church, founders and managers of embryo adoption organizations, and researchers—as well as the political and legal advocates who want to end the scourge of in vitro fertilization (IVF) and cryopreservation or improve the legal framework for embryo adoptions. The chapter considers the following needs: (1) Church teaching, (2) Catholic embryo adoption organizations, (3) legal and political reform, and (4) associated research.

Next Steps for the Church

Clarification of Church teaching regarding the moral status of embryo adoption is greatly needed. Such a status has, unfortunately, become very difficult for Catholics to discern, given the divergence in explanations from instructions of the Congregation for the Doctrine of the Faith (CDF) and from Christian theology. Even trained moral theologians disagree over which moral principles and forms of reasoning are appropriate, sometimes going so far as to implicitly demote the virtues of mercy and compassion (not merely the emotional reactions associated with the virtues) to a marginal status. This is despite the centrality of such virtues to Christian action and their close relation to the theological virtue of charity.[1]

Debate and sincere discussion are enormously helpful to the Church in working through such moral questions. There are four very serious reasons, however, why Catholics need the Church's magisterium to issue a more timely and direct teaching that clarifies the moral goodness of embryo adoption. First, statements by the CDF are being variously—sometimes creatively—misinterpreted; those statements can be authoritatively clarified only by the magisterium. Second, public arguments that involvement in embryo adoption is a mortal sin confuse and discourage many of the most loving and charitably minded Christians from acting with confidence according to their conscientious deliberation. Such a lack of confidence in moral

---

1. Christopher M. Reilly, "Rescuing the Good Samaritan in Embryo Adoption and Beyond," *National Catholic Bioethics Quarterly* 20.3 (Autumn 2020): 487–498, doi: 10.5840/ncbq202020345.

reasoning may reverberate in other situations where Christians must weigh legalistic considerations that seem contrary to the goodness of charitable and merciful action toward other persons. Third, arguments for the grave immorality of embryo adoption as well as the portrayal of such a position as the proper interpretation of Church teaching place the Church itself in danger of a deeply consequential scandal that appears to pit the Church against the central roles of the virtues of charity, mercy, and compassion and the inviolable dignity of human life within Christian moral theology. In the face of opposition to embryo adoption, on what side of the road shall the Good Samaritan—Jesus's exemplar of the loving neighbor—walk? "The Good Samaritan, in fact, 'not only draws nearer to the man he finds half dead; he takes responsibility for him.'"[2] The fourth reason for clearing up the confusion of those opposed to embryo adoption is the importance, in bioethical arguments, of the moral difference between transfer of an embryo and the combined procedure of IVF and embryo transfer as well as surrogate motherhood. The moral issues associated with the second two actions do not apply reasonably to embryo transfer in itself, and this difference is at the core of moral evaluation of embryo adoption as well as clear understanding of the illicit nature of developing technologies—such as resolving ectopic pregnancies, utilizing artificial uteruses, and manipulating synthetic embryos—that may involve transfer of embryos or fetuses in some form.

The steps that the Church, including all Catholics, should take in regard to safeguarding and respecting human life are already outlined in detail in Church documents such as Pope St. John Paul II's encyclical *Evangelium vitae* and the CDF's instruction *Donum vitae*. Notably, Catholics must work to evangelize and advocate regarding an end to the practices of IVF and freezing live human zygotes and embryos (cryopreservation). It is morally absurd and publicly hypocritical to tolerate IVF, which is the very source of the problem of abandoned and frozen embryos, while defending the human dignity of already abandoned embryos and of natural procreation. The outcry against such violations in the practice of IVF has, unfortunately, been quite muted compared with concerns over such practices as

---

2. Congregation for the Doctrine of the Faith (CDF), *Samaritanus bonus* (July 14, 2020), I, citing Francis, Message for the Forty-Eighth World Communications Day (June 1, 2014).

abortion, contraception, and euthanasia. In an age when biotechnological advances will generate ever-more challenging moral questions, it is the proper concern of all Christians that our evangelization develop more energetically and effectively regarding every practice that imposes a technological domination over human life, procreation, and dignity. Embryo adoption is a loving response to the plight of the endangered embryonic person, but given the dire consequences of IVF and cryopreservation, it must also be part of a broader response to the excesses of a hyper-technological and utilitarian mindset prevalent in our culture. This does not mean, however, that serving the abandoned embryos should be a secondary effort subsumed under any political effort to ban the practice of IVF entirely; the practical and moral priority is defense of the life and dignity of the human being, through prohibition of cryopreservation and of the transfer of multiple embryos to an individual mother, rather than through compelling morally correct behavior. For organizations providing embryo adoption services, anti-IVF and anti-cryopreservation education and evangelization will require joyfully anticipating a day when their own services are no longer needed.[3]

Development and Management of Embryo Adoption Clinics

The facilitation of embryo adoption may occur in existing medical institutions or newly formed medical clinics or adoption-facilitating organizations, and the services provided by each organization will vary according to expertise and resources. For example, many organizations will not have the facilities needed to implement the actual transfer or care for (i.e., store and sustain) cryopreserved embryos that are not yet matched with adoptive couples. As the following outline of guidelines will demonstrate, however, there are numerous moral, practical, and pastoral considerations that are unlikely to be handled with the same moral reasoning and sensitivities outside a distinctly Catholic organization. Extensive cooperation with profit-oriented clinics, particularly those that also engage in IVF, can be morally

---

3. John Berkman and Kristen N. Carey, "Ethical and Religious Directives for a Catholic Embryo Adoption Agency: A Thought Experiment," in *The Ethics of Embryo Adoption and the Catholic Tradition: Moral Arguments, Economic Reality and Social Analysis*, ed. Sarah-Vaughan Brakman and Darlene Fozard Weaver (Cham, CE: Springer, 2007), 266.

illicit or generate scandal. For these reasons, it is far preferable that Catholics and Catholic hospitals establish embryo adoption clinics with participation and guidance from Church leaders as well as properly trained Catholic bioethicists. It is also preferable that the organizations and clinics take a comprehensive view of their responsibilities and services in caring for the embryonic persons, prospective and newly adoptive couples, biological parents and families of adopted embryos, and the public (through education and evangelization). The implementation of embryo adoption services is a complex and demanding ministry that requires vigilant adherence to proper guidelines and quality of care. The following section outlines considerations and suggestions for Catholic embryo adoption organizations, posing more questions than answers, in order to initiate a discussion among bioethicists, moral theologians, and nonprofit and medical leaders about best practices.

In 2007, John Berkman and Kristen Carey provided a somewhat similar and very helpful discussion of guidelines for prospective embryo adoption organizations, focusing largely on a description and critique of existing embryo adoption agencies' policies.[4] They indicated a desire to go beyond the abstract arguments and to address embryo adoption in practice. Unfortunately, there has been little progress in developing embryo adoption organizations with strong Catholic principles, and therefore, this chapter does not further describe existing adoption agencies but attempts a comprehensive review of the considerations to which innovators and new leaders will be oriented.

Most importantly, the leadership, staff, and clients should all clearly understand that the primary object of embryo adoption is saving the life of, caring for, and parenting a cryopreserved embryonic person that is abandoned or unwanted by its biological parents. The adoption services should, therefore, not be marketed as a convenient solution for infertile couples seeking to acquire and raise a child. If the sole object of the adoption is to fulfill the personal desires of the adoptive parents for a child, such as when a married couple is infertile or concerned about passing certain genetic health problems on to a biological child, there is the real danger of intentionally cooperating with the earlier formation of the child through IVF, technical domination of the creation of human life, and using the biological parents as

---

4. Berkman and Carey, "Catholic Embryo Adoption Agency," 251–273.

instrumentally convenient surrogates or donors. In other words, the object of the persons involved in embryo adoption has primary moral significance, even when the material nature and consequences of the act appears to be the same as in IVF. This is the main difference between embryo adoption and what has been termed *donor conception*. Adoption is oriented primarily to the needs of the adoptees, while donor conception focuses solely on the desires of the adults. The adoption organization will need to determine how to discuss such an object with prospective adoptive couples and whether it should be a consideration in screening clients. To date, Catholic bioethicists do not seem to have considered or offered guidance in this regard.

This is a very difficult teaching for many to accept and understand, because wanting to raise and love a child in a family is an admirable intention in itself. In *Dignitas personae*, however, the CDF states, "The proposal that these embryos could be put at the disposal of infertile couples as a *treatment for infertility* is not ethically acceptable for the same reasons which make artificial heterologous procreation illicit as well as any form of surrogate motherhood."[5] There are several clues to take note of here. First, the phrase "treatment for infertility" is identified in italics and is mentioned separately from "prenatal adoption," which is also identified in italics in the following paragraph; these are clearly intended to be understood as two different acts with different intentions and moral implications. Second, we are directed to the moral discussions of artificial heterologous procreation (such as IVF) and surrogate motherhood as guides for the moral reasoning applied to embryo transfer as a treatment for infertility. In both of those cases, the infertile couple directly utilizes a technology and the assistance of other persons to circumvent natural procreation (which, in this case, would be unlikely to result in a child without the extraordinary grace of God) to acquire a child. The emphasis is entirely on the desires of the couple, the treatment of the newly created child as an owned commodity, and an unfaithful method of achieving these purposes in the creation of the child. It is the very act of treating infertility that demeans the child. Similarly, when an infertile couple engages in the transfer of an embryo simply in order to resolve their infertility, their intention is to utilize the morally illicit method or context of creation (IVF) as a way to circumvent faithful reliance on God's grace in the creation of a child and a family. They are cooperating intentionally, immorally, and self-centeredly with the act of IVF—even

---

5. CDF, *Dignitas personae* (September 8, 2008), n. 19, emphasis original.

though it occurred previously—from the moment the genetic parents began the process. In the broader context, public and sustained demand by infertile couples for the acquisition of children generated from other couples has a structural similarity to the surrogacy industry, which encourages immoral methods for the creation of children for financial gain. (Note that such a market for the acquisition of children is far different from any widespread demand to adopt only existing, cryopreserved, and abandoned embryos; the latter demand is extinguished when the morally illicit abandonment of embryos ends.)

With embryo adoption that is primarily oriented to saving and respecting the life and dignity of an abandoned embryo, the only indignity to the child is initiated by the child's creation within the technical process of IVF (and by the child's cryopreservation and abandonment). The transfer of the child to the adoptive mother's womb is not an indignity, because it is a medical procedure that saves the life and promotes the welfare of the child (rather than a process intended solely to fulfill the acquisitive wishes of the adoptive parents). The adoption by the infertile (or fertile) couple is not an indignity to the child, because it is an act full of love and mercy for the existing, inherently dignified person who they are adopting. Neither the transfer nor the adoption is an indignity to God's role in procreation, because the couple is not seeking to circumvent natural procreation—not even by the fact that they may be unlikely to conceive through natural procreation—but extending a merciful welcome to a living, valued person. To be clear, if an infertile couple anticipates, enjoys, and treasures the opportunity to raise a child, it is a blessing not a sin. (Consider, as a parallel, the holy joy one experiences in a friendship of charity with God; the joy is not an indication of any transactional or acquisitive nature of the friendship, but is properly an effect of its inherent goodness.) As Berkman and Carey argue, "The desires to (a) aid an orphan and (b) find fulfillment in the raising of a child are perfectly compatible when rightly ordered.... In fact, it could very well be argued that a potential adoptive parent who has purely 'altruistic' motives, who foresees no personal fulfillment in raising a child, is precisely the kind of person who should not be raising a child."[6]

---

6. Berkman and Carey, "Catholic Embryo Adoption Agency," 259.

Part 3: Defenses of Embryo Adoption

Policies regarding Marital Status

This author recommends that, for Catholic organizations, the adoptive couples be a married woman and man, mutually consenting to their joint parenting of the child. While there may be a strong argument, given the moral weight of relieving the extreme danger and indignity experienced by the embryo, for the moral goodness of adopting endangered embryos in more varied parental and familial contexts or even volunteering to gestate and give birth to a child that will be subsequently adopted by another family, it does not seem prudent for a Catholic organization to provide those services; Catholics have a responsibility to uphold the dignity of marriage and avoid scandal.[7] This is not an issue that has been considered in the relevant bioethical and theological literature, but some precedent may be found in the efforts of Catholic adoption agencies (for born children) to maintain a strong moral identity and defense of the natural family, even in the face of legal mandates for adoption by single people and same-sex couples.

Policies for Obtaining Embryos

Policies for adoptee-embryo sourcing and selection will be perhaps the most morally significant and practically complex. Given the gravely immoral nature of IVF and cryopreservation of human embryos, Catholic embryo adoption organizations will need to balance a responsibility to avoid financial and ideological support for clinics that engage in IVF with the practical need to develop working relationships for obtaining the adoptees that will be transferred to adoptive couples. For example, while some compensation of cryopreservation facilities or IVF clinics is probably necessary, it should be kept to a minimum to avoid real and apparent support of their continued engagement in morally unacceptable practices; financial compensation of the biological parents should be avoided. One might doubt whether it is always immoral to give a payment to biological parents—essentially a ransom—for the extremely important and extraordinary purpose of saving the life and future of a human embryo. Such a practice, however, does

---

7. E. Christian Brugger argues for the goodness of serving as an emergency gestational mother in "In Defense of Transferring Heterologous Embryos," *National Catholic Bioethics Quarterly* 5.1 (Spring 2005), 95–112, doi: 10.5840/ncbq20055170.

not seem prudent in a context of otherwise willing donors of embryos, especially given the possibility (or at least appearance) that such payment practices will encourage and, therefore, cooperate with the acts of IVF and cryopreservation. Such payment for the embryos may also be illegal in the United States. In their policies, the source facilities should have clear guidelines for gathering and sharing important information about the health, origin, and any prior testing of the embryos as well as for ensuring required consent (and related documentation) from the biological parents and medical professionals or clinics involved. The embryo adoption organization will want to avoid, when possible, source facilities that sell human embryos or use them for the purpose of harmful experimentation. To avoid conflicts of interest and preserve moral integrity, the sources of adoptees should not be physicians, employees, or principals of the adoption organization.

Policies regarding Transfer

Policies about the embryo transfer itself will be necessary. For example, how many embryos may be transferred to the adoptive mother at one time, given that more embryos increase the odds of one or more successful implantations and births yet may create medical dangers for the mother and adoptees, lead to more births than the adoptive couple is prepared for, and often involve betting against the survival of some of the embryos? As proposed elsewhere, "an EA [embryo adoption] agency would typically only accept embryos into its care for which an adopting couple was pledged to gestate, or which the EA agency had very good reason to believe it would be able to place. For a Catholic embryo adoption agency would not wish to perpetuate the process of warehousing abandoned embryos. ... [It is also] morally important for the adopting couple to commit themselves to eventually implanting all of the embryos which they would have adopted."[8] The organization and adoptive couples might also consider giving preference to adoption of all embryonic progeny of the genetic parents, when feasible, so the adoptees may be raised in the same family.

There are many other ethical and practical decisions in the selection of adoptee embryos that can be improved by consulting with bioethicists, moral theologians, and persons with experience at other adoption organizations.

---

8. Berkman and Carey, "Catholic Embryo Adoption Agency," 264.

Part 3: Defenses of Embryo Adoption

Is it morally licit, for example, to select transferred embryos according to such criteria as their state of health, predicted future health, or perceived suitability for the adoptive family (such as race or gender), or does this enter into the prideful and controlling practice of eugenics, as when embryonic persons are selected for birth according to specific physical characteristics or mental capabilities? Is there even a good reason to utilize any available genetic testing results, such as concern about the need for medical intervention or special care, to make such decisions?[9] As Berkman and Carey indicate, "There are instances where certain forms of PGD [preimplantation genetic disagnosis] can be intended for the good of the embryo—to prepare medical treatments or gene therapy that could be done in utero or immediately upon birth—but this is rarely the intent in PGD."[10]

The organization will also need to decide, perhaps along with prospective adoptive couples, whether to transfer adoptee embryos formed with gametes from genetic parents other than the legal owners or parents of the embryos, thereby complicating the identity and extended familial relations of both the adoptee and the adoptive family. It will help in such decision-making to remember that the primary objective of embryo adoption is resolving the grave danger and harm done to the frozen embryo, and the primary objective in any adoption is to enhance the welfare of the adoptee. In ethical dilemmas where it is difficult to avoid scandal or significantly bad consequences, it seems prudent for Catholic embryo adoption organizations to take a conservative stance on diversifying their sourcing and selection policies, so long as the organizations are able to successfully save human embryos by matching them with appropriate adoptive couples.

Selecting and Testing Prospective Adoptive Parents

Prospective adoptive parents will need to be interviewed, screened, and medically tested. Screening of prospective parents should include careful assessment by trained employees, a home study, background checks, and evidence of appropriate parenthood education. Psychological assessments

---

9. For further consideration of genetic and other prenatal testing, see Christopher M. Reilly and Jonathan Scrafford, "Prenatal Testing and Diagnosis," in *Catholic Health Care Ethics: A Manual for Practitioners*, 3rd ed., ed. Edward J. Furton (Philadelphia: National Catholic Bioethics Center, 2020), 12.1–12.9.
10. Berkman and Carey, "Catholic Embryo Adoption Agency," 265.

and consideration of financial, insurance, and estate planning criteria may also be warranted.

Open or Closed Adoption Process

Policies will need to be set regarding the availability of and procedures for open or closed adoptions. Open adoptions involve sharing of information on an ongoing basis between the adoptive parents and the genetic parents. They also may involve contact between the adoptee and genetic parents, genetic siblings, and unrelated children of the genetic parents. Already by 2008, more than two-thirds of private domestic adoptions of born children in the United States included some ongoing contact with the birth parents, and the trend has been toward more open adoptions.[11] To what extent should the embryo adoption organization engage in "conditional relinquishment services" that enable the genetic parents of adoptee embryos to impose restrictions or preferences on the characteristics of prospective adoptive parents? Such options for setting conditions are certainly attractive to many genetic parents who tend to be reluctant about relinquishing control over their frozen embryos; liberal policies may, therefore, reduce the most important concern of genetic parents and enable more opportunities for adoption.[12] The organization must, however, protect the interests of the

---

11. Office of the Assistant Secretary for Planning and Evaluation, "National Survey of Adoptive Parents (NSAP)," US Department of Health and Human Services, accessed June 21, 2024, https://aspe.hhs.gov/national-survey-adoptive-parents-nsap.

12. For a review of multiple related studies, see Lucy Frith et al., "Conditional Embryo Relinquishment: Choosing to Relinquish Embryos for Family-Building through a Christian Embryo 'Adoption' Programme," *Human Reproduction* 26.12 (December 2011): 3327–3338, doi: 10.1093/humrep/der313. The authors state, "A predominant theme emerging from the data that influenced couples' disposition decisions was their feelings of responsibility for the future welfare of their embryos. This was reflected in their concern to find a 'good' home for their embryos—a view held by most participants, irrespective of their views of the embryos' status. . . . Further, most wanted to be involved in the process of selecting the families that would receive their embryos" (3334). Also worth noting is the following report: "A surprisingly large number of patients interested in donating embryos (42.2%), and of those who ultimately donated (48.0%), utilized donor eggs in embryo creation. These numbers are

Part 3: Defenses of Embryo Adoption

adoptees and prospective adoptive parents from overly restrictive or superfluous conditions on the opportunities for adoption and form potential future interference in family cohesion, privacy, and parental decision-making.

Counseling

The embryo adoption organization has a responsibility to both the adoptee and the adoptive parents to provide high quality, informative, and comprehensive counseling to prospective parents. Medical counseling will inform prospective parents of the nature and risks of the embryo transfer, including failure of the procedure and error in diagnosis and prediction of the health of the transferred embryos. Counseling is also warranted in regard to the interpretation, limitations, and morally appropriate use of genetic testing (e.g., avoiding eugenic intentions). Various psychological concerns may arise, and prospective parents should be prepared for the possibility of grief following a failed transfer and be apprised of resources for assistance in such an event. Prospective parents will need resources for parenting advice and counseling, including teaching and involving any other children in the process of adoption. A major consideration for parents is when and how to disclose the adoptee's origin and adoption status, with some indication by experts that early disclosure is preferable.[13] In a society where online networking and consumer genetic testing are widespread, parents will need to

---

much higher than the approximate 10% of IVF cycles which utilize donor egg within the practice. It is possible that these patients have a less genetically-centered definition, and experience, of family, which makes them more inclined both to use donor eggs and to donate embryos. It is also possible that donor egg recipients are more likely to have a desire to 'give back' and to donate embryos in order to help others achieve parenthood." Olivia Carpinello et al., "Just over One-Third of Patients Interested in Embryo Donation Complete Embryo Donation," *Fertility and Sterility* 114.3 suppl (September 2020): e102, doi: 10.1016/j.fertnstert.2020.08.309.

13. Nuffield Council on Bioethics, "Donor Conception: Ethical Aspects of Information Sharing," April 17, 2013, https://www.nuffieldbioethics.org/publications/donor-conception; and Elena Ilioi et al., "The Role of Age of Disclosure of Biological Origins in the Psychological Wellbeing of Adolescents Conceived by Reproductive Donation: A Longitudinal Study from Age 1 to Age 14," *Journal of Child Psychology and Psychiatry* 58.3 (March 2017): 315–324, doi: 10.1111/jcpp.12667.

be prepared for the possibility that disclosure and interaction with genetic relatives may occur outside their control.[14] Counselors must attend closely to the needs of the adoptive couple in relating to each other as they make mutually consenting and fulfilling decisions. The parents will also need information about the legal status and process of their adoption. Finally, Catholic organizations might engage in evangelization and greatly benefit prospective parents by offering (or providing referrals for) education in Catholic theology of the body and the gospel of life.

Other Policies and Protections

There are some particular issues that embryo adoption organizations will need to be prepared for, with attention to the welfare of the adoptee and prospective parents, error and disaster preparation, liability exposure, and so on. Policies should outline either the procedures or decision-making structures to be applied when unexpected events or legal considerations arise. The disposition of embryos who are in the care of the adoption organization yet, for various reasons, are not transferred is a very serious moral and practical concern.

In the current legal context in most jurisdictions, the legal protections and guidelines usually applied to the adoption of born children are not

---

14. European Society of Human Reproduction and Embryology (ESHRE) Working Group on Reproductive Donation, "Good Practice Recommendations for Information Provision for Those Involved in Reproductive Donation," *Human Reproduction Open* 2022.1 (February 2022): 1–26, doi: 10.1093/hropen/hoac001. "Direct-to-consumer genetic testing can: reveal the lack of a genetic link between the social parent and the offspring; reveal that a family member has donated gametes/embryos; or identify genetic relatives (a donor, siblings, family). Donor-conceived offspring and donors can connect through genetic information stored in these databases and offspring can be identified even before reaching the age set by national legislation. Even donors and donor-conceived offspring that are not registered on the ancestry databases themselves may be traced through relatives who use genetic testing for family tree research (Klotz, 2016), especially in combination with social media. Direct-to-consumer genetic testing can reveal matches, which may translate to a half-sibling, an aunt/uncle, a cousin, or a grandparent. By establishing contact with such genetic matches, they may be able to gain access to information about their donor or other same-donor offspring."

available for embryo adoption. Embryo adoption is most often considered to be a transfer of property, and embryo adoption organizations will need to carefully navigate such deficient legal frameworks with concern for protecting the adoptee and all adult parties from any indignities and harm. The adoption organization should, therefore, emphasize securing skilled and regular legal counsel as well as proactively assisting the adoptive parents. Location of services in jurisdictions with more favorable legal frameworks seems prudent until the demand and proliferation of embryo adoption services is ripe for expansion into other jurisdictions. This may mean, in turn, providing or referring for resources that assist prospective parents to travel longer distances in order to access the services.

Securing Resources

New embryo adoption organizations will have to plan carefully regarding the availability and need for resources. The provision of high-quality embryo adoption services, as discussed above, includes a much more comprehensive—and potentially expensive—array of services than just the medical procedure of embryo transfer and basic counseling. Organizations that have an institutional affiliation with larger entities, such as Catholic hospitals, may, therefore, have a strong advantage in providing the best care all around. Until the Church's magisterium clarifies in writing a favorable appraisal of embryo adoption, however, it may be difficult to secure sustained commitment from such institutions or from partner organizations. This reticence may also extend to populations of prospective financial supporters or investors. Significant work is needed, therefore, to identify, educate, and unify the potential supporters of embryo adoption in the current environment. This can be accomplished most effectively by tapping the resources of favorably minded organizations and Church leaders, welcoming potential supporters to discussions and planning for new embryo adoption organizations, and securing initial funds to hire fundraising staff and prospect research counsel. Given the investment required in identifying and cultivating financial support, collaboration between Catholic embryo adoption organizations or institutional consolidation will probably produce better results and more efficient use of resources than competition among individual organizations.

Embryo adoption organizations might appropriately plan on receiving income from fees charged to adoptive parents for services such as embryo thawing, embryo transfer, cycle coordination and documentation, and infectious disease screening and testing.[15] The adoptive parents may also pay for agency fees, home study fees, the genetic parent's related expenses, and medications. In their helpful article regarding the operation of embryo adoption agencies, Berkman and Carey have proposed that, in comparison to secular fertility clinics, "an EA agency should structure its fees so that the donating couple bears more of the costs of EA." Further, they state that "morally speaking, we argue the adopting couple are giving more of a gift to the relinquishing couple than vice versa. This becomes clear if we recognize that, at least in most cases, genetic parents have a grave responsibility to give their cryopreserved offspring an opportunity to live the human life cycle. Thus, a couple's relinquishing their embryos might be viewed as akin to an act of reparation to them."[16]

While obtaining fees from the donating couple seems to be an admirable goal, it is probably difficult to achieve in an environment where most genetic parents are already reluctant to relinquish control over embryos, and it may interfere with the goal of the adoption organization to save more lives. This author is also more than a little uncomfortable with communicating to the genetic parents about reparations, for there is much more to overcoming their engagement in a mortal sin than a physical act of atonement, and they should not be encouraged in any way to absolve themselves of their own responsibility to gestate, nurture, and raise their embryonic children (assuming they have the ability to parent and care for them). As awareness and advocacy of embryo adoption grows, we might expect a more-than-sustainable demand for these services, and existing medical centers, in particular, might see this as an opportunity for receiving positive net income that can support their ministries. Given the object of saving the lives of the adoptees, however, burdensome fees do not seem to be appropriate, neither do they

---

15. Minimum federal requirements for embryo donation in the United States can be found at US Food and Drug Administration, "Eligibility Determination for Donors of Human Cells, Tissues, and Cellular and Tissue-Based Products Guidance for Industry," August 2007, https://www.fda.gov/regulatory-information/search-fda-guidance-documents/eligibility-determination-donors-human-cells-tissues-and-cellular-and-tissue-based-products.
16. Berkman and Carey, "Catholic Embryo Adoption Agency," 269.

encourage a focus on prospective adoptive parents of any financial capacity who sincerely intend a pro-life object rather than (as a primary objective) eagerness to secure a preborn child to raise. Attention to raising charitable support is, therefore, crucial to the flourishing of such organizations.

The Legal Context and Reform

The third part of *Donum vitae* is concerned entirely with moral and civil law, and a subsection is titled "The Values and Moral Obligations that Civil Legislation Must Respect and Sanction in this Matter." In this subsection, the CDF states that "recourse to the conscience of each individual and to the self-regulation of researchers cannot be sufficient for ensuring respect for personal rights and public order." We should, therefore, give due consideration to legal reform that enables embryo adoption and protects the interests of the child and adoptive parents. As the CDF goes on to explain, "These human rights depend neither on single individuals nor on parents; nor do they represent a concession made by society and the State: they pertain to human nature and are inherent in the person by virtue of the creative act from which the person took his or her origin." Specific mention is made of the need to legally ban "techniques of artificial procreation" and also "embryo banks."[17]

The legal status and relevant laws or regulations concerning embryo adoption vary widely among jurisdictions throughout the world and among US states. In most cases, particularly in the United States, embryo adoption is treated under the law as the transfer of biological property. The property category within which human embryos are often placed is that of biological material rather than that of complete living organisms or animals. (Even livestock and animals that are subjects of scientific experiments have their own categories and legal rights regimes.) It is not surprising that such categorization as property without rights or dignity leads to deficient protection in the transfer of human embryos from genetic parents and fertility clinics to the adoptive parents. Property laws often do not address such crucial issues as the preservation or destruction of non-implanted embryos by the adoptive parents or embryo adoption organization and the precise nature of legal counsel and disclosures.

---

17. CDF, *Donum vitae* (February 22, 1987), III.

Adoption law, on the other hand, clearly attributes parental rights and responsibilities to the adoptive parents of born children. Custody issues are generally legislated and are supposed to be decided in favor of the best interests of the adoptee child above all else. Prospective parents are subject to legal requirements such as home studies, assessments, and (sometimes) post-adoption supervision. An adoption law regime is, therefore, greatly needed for embryo adoptions as well as for adoptions of born children. It will require significant efforts by pro-embryo, pro-life, and pro-adoption advocates to extend the adoption law regime to embryonic human persons.

Two European laws and two US state laws are worth noting. Germany's Embryo Protection Act of 1990 (revised and reinterpreted subsequently) places significant restrictions on IVF, selection and number of embryos for implantation, genetic testing, surrogacy arrangements, and so forth. Italy's Law 40/2004 bans IVF except for married couples, bans surrogacy, and restricts use of genetic testing. Louisiana has identified human embryos as juridical persons since 1986. Georgia Option of Adoption Act is unique in providing adoption-related protections and regulations for embryo transfers.[18] Finally, the legal assistance organization Americans United for Life has written detailed draft legislation for embryo adoption entitled Embryo Adoption Act and Custody of Embryonic Children Act.[19]

Research Needs

Researchers are developing a scientific and sociological literature (albeit with a secular orientation) regarding embryo and gamete donation as well as the experiences and practices of parents and children. Much more needs to be learned, however, about such concerns as disclosure of origin to adoptees, parenting of both adoptees and siblings, and future communication or interaction with biological parents and siblings. We lack accurate and comprehensive statistics about adoption prevalence, experiences, attitudes, and practices. Other topics of relevance to the success of embryo adoption

---

18. Elizabeth Bothamley Rex, "International Laws that Promote the Ethical Healthcare and Legal Protection of Human Embryos," Annual Summer Conference of the Center for Bioethics and Human Dignity, June 25, 2022.
19. See Americans United for Life, "Pro-Life Model Legislation and Guides," accessed June 10, 2024, https://aul.org/law-and-policy/.

include child psychology of adoptees, health risks for adoptive mothers, opportunities and related factors in identifying and sourcing adoptee embryos, societal impressions and effect, and best practices for evangelization or advocacy.

Next Steps toward Embryo Adoption

The presence of millions of frozen embryos and the continued enthusiasm of our contemporaries for the kind of treatment that, only a generation ago, was exclusively associated with Nazi experimentation—not to mention the operational and ideological hurdles of facilitating embryo adoption organizations—can be discouraging. As Pope St. John Paul II expressed, we can truly resolve the scourge of cryopreserved and destroyed embryos only by universal cessation of the practice of IVF. Christian hope, however, is founded in the revelation, teaching, and loving relationship of Christ, who, with the Holy Spirit, brings us to our fulfillment in the virtue of charity. Called, even destined, to love God and neighbor, our efforts to extend love to the very least of humanity will bear fruit in every single embryonic life that is saved and treasured. All we need to worry about is taking the next step.

Bibliography

Abad, Maria Rendón, Vicente Serra, Pilar Gámiz, José Maria de Los Santos, Josè Remohí, Alfredo T. Navarro, et al. "The Influence of Oxygen Concentration during Embryo Culture on Obstetric and Neonatal Outcomes: A Secondary Analysis of a Randomized Controlled Trial." *Human Reproduction* 35.9 (September 1, 2020): 2017–2025. DOI: 10.1093/humrep/deaa152.

Accad, Michel. "Heterologous Embryo Transfer: Magisterial Answers and Metaphysical Questions." *Linacre Quarterly* 81.1 (February 2014): 44. DOI: 10.1179/2050854913Y.0000000016.

Akin, Jimmy. *Teaching with Authority: How to Cut through Doctrinal Confusion & Understand What the Church Really Says*. El Cajon, CA: Catholic Answers Press, 2018.

Alabama Supreme Court. *See* Supreme Court of Alabama

Alexander, Irene. "The Error of Intentionalism," *National Catholic Bioethics Quarterly* 17.3 (Autumn 2017): 399–408. DOI: 10.5840/ncbq201717341.

———. "Embryo Adoption Part 2: Con (with Irene Alexander, PhD)." Hosted by Tom McGovern and Andrew Mullally. *Doctor, Doctor*. Podcase. Episode 299. YouTube. January 20, 2023. https://www.youtube.com/watch?v=q16J-piT8YQ. *See also* McCarthy, C. Ryan. "Embryo Adoption Part 1: Pro."

———, "Frozen Embryos, Unwanted Pregnancies, and Artificial Wombs: Which Options Are Morally Licit?" *Nova et Vetera* 19.4 (Fall 2021): 1111–1145.

———, "Is Artificial Impregnation Opposed to the Unity of Marriage? A New Look at the Question of Embryo Adoption." *Nova et Vetera* 16.1 (Winter 2018): 47–80.

———, "Redefining Direct and Indirect Abortions through 'the Perspective of the Acting Person': A Misreading of *Veritatis Splendor*." *Linacre Quarterly* 86.1 (February 2019): 28–46. DOI: 10.1177/0024363919838852.

Allen, John L., Jr. "Commitment to Truth is the Soul of Justice, Benedict XVI Says; Ali Agca and the Plot to Kill a Pope; Pope Meets with Neocatechumenal Way; Ethical Issues Facing Benedict XVI." The Word from Rome. *National Catholic Reporter* 5.19, January 13, 2006, https://nationalcatholicreporter.org/word/pfw011306.htm.

———. "Pope Benedict and Moral Theology." Lecture presented to the Society of Christian Ethics, Phoenix, Arizona, January 5, 2006.

Althaus, Catherine. "Can One 'Rescue' a Human Embryo? The Moral Object of the Acting Woman." In "Human Embryo Transfer," special issue, *National Catholic Bioethics Quarterly* 5.1 (Spring 2005): 113–141. DOI: 10.5840/ncbq20055171.

———. "Catherine Althaus Replies" [to David Wechter]. Colloquy. *National Catholic Bioethics Quarterly* 5.3 (Autumn 2005): 452. DOI: 10.5840/ncbq20055324.

———. "Establishing the Moral Object of Heterologous and Homologous Embryo Transfer." In *Contemporary Controversies in Catholic Bioethics*, edited by Jason T. Eberl, 169–187. New York: Springer, 2017. DOI: 10.1007/978-3-319-55766-3_13.

———. "Human Embryo Transfer and the Theology of the Body." In *Embryo Adoption and the Catholic Tradition: Moral Arguments, Economic Reality and Social Analysis*, edited by Sarah-Vaughan Brakman and Darlene Fozard Weaver, 43–67. Dordrecht, NL: Springer, 2007.

Alvare, Helen M. "Catholic Teaching and the Law concerning the New Reproductive Technologies." *Fordham Urban Law Journal* 30.1 (2002): 6, pp. 107–134. https://ir.lawnet.fordham.edu/ulj/vol30/iss1/6.

American College of Obstetricians and Gynecologists Committee on Practice Bulletins—Gynecology. "ACOG Practice Bulletin No. 200: Early Pregnancy Loss." *Obstetrics and Gynecology* 132.5 (November 2018): e197–e207. DOI: 10.1097/AOG.0000000000002899.

American College of Obstetricians and Gynecologists, Society for Maternal-Fetal Medicine, Torri D. Metz, Rana Snipe Berry, Ruth C. Fretts, Uma M. Reddy, et al. "Obstetric Care Consensus #10: Management of Stillbirth." *Journal of Obstetrics and Gynecology* 135.3 (March 2020): e110–e132. DOI: 10.1097/AOG.0000000000003719.

American Society for Reproductive Medicine Ethics Committee. "Compassionate Transfer: Patient Requests for Embryo Transfer for Nonreproductive Purposes." *Fertility and Sterility* 113.1 (January 2020): 62–65. DOI: 10.1016/j.fertnstert.2019.10.013.

———. "Defining Embryo Donation: An Ethics Committee Opinion." *Fertility and Sterility* 119.6 (June 2023): 944–947. DOI: 10.1016/j.fertnstert.2023.03.007.

Bibliography

———. "Posthumous Retrieval and Use of Gametes or Embryos: An Ethics Committee Opinion." *Fertility and Sterility* 110.1 (July 2018): 45–59. DOI: 10.1016/j.fertnstert.2018.04.002.
Americans United for Life. "Pro-Life Model Legislation and Guides." Accessed June 10, 2024. https://aul.org/law-and-policy/.
Amundsen, Darrel W. *Medicine, Society, and Faith in the Ancient and Medieval Worlds*. Baltimore: Johns Hopkins University Press, 1996.
Anderson, Matthew Lee. "#515: Embryo Adoption and Our Moral Imaginations: What Should America Do with Society's 'Surplus Embryos'?" *The Path Before Us, with Matthew Lee Anderson* (blog). December 8, 2023. https://matthewleeanderson.substack.com/p/515-embryo-adoption-and-our-moral.
Anderson, Whitney E. "Justice for the Orphan: The Ethics of 'Embryo Adoption.'" Master's thesis. University of St. Thomas, Minnesota, 2019.
Applegarth, Linda. "Embryo Donation: Counseling Donors and Recipients." In *Infertility Counseling: A Comprehensive Handbook for Clinicians*. Edited by Sharon N. Covington and Linda Hammer Burns, 356–369. Cambridge: Cambridge University Press, 2006.
Aquinas, Thomas, ed. *Catena aurea: Commentary on the Four Gospels Collected out of the Works of the Fathers*, English translation edited by John Henry Newman. Vol. 3, *St. Luke*. Translated by Thomas Dudley Ryder. Oxford: John Henry Parker, 1841; London: J. G. F. and J. Rivington, 1841.
———. *Commentary on the Nicomachean Ethics*. Translated by C. I. Litzinger. Chicago: Regnery, 1964. https://isidore.co/aquinas/english/Ethics.htm.
———. *Commentary on the Second Epistle to the Corinthians*, chap. 3, lect. 3. In John Cameron, *Novenas for the Church Year*, 94. Huntington, IN: Our Sunday Visitor, 2012.
———. *Commentum in quartum librum "Sententiarum" magistri Petri Lombardi*. Vol. 7/2. Parma: Peter Fiaccadori, 1858.
———. *Questiones de quolibet*. Edited by R. A. Gauthier. In *Opera omnia iussu Leonis XIII P. M. edita*. Vol. 25.2. Paris: Commissio Leonina, Éditions du Cerf, 1996.
———. *Scriptum super "Sententiis."* Transcribed by Robert Busa and Enrique Alarcón. Fundación Tomás de Aquino, Corpus Thomisticum. 2019. https://www.corpusthomisticum.org/iopera.html.
———. *Scriptum super "Sententiis,"* edited by Pierre Mandonnet and Maria Fabianus Moos. Paris: Lethielleux, 1929–1947.
———. *Summa contra Gentiles*. Translated by Laurence Shapcote. Green Bay: Aquinas Institute, 2018.
———. *Summa theologiae*. Collana reprint, 3rd ed. Turin: Edizione San Paolo, 1999.
———. *Summa theologiae*. Translated by Fathers of the English Dominican Province. 1920; New Advent, 2017. https://www.newadvent.org/summa.

___. *Summa theologiae*. Translated by Fathers of the English Dominican Province. Benziger, 1947; Thomistic Institute, 2017. https://aquinas101.thomistic institute.org/st-index.

___. *Summa theologiae*. Translated by Fathers of the English Dominican Province. New York: Benzinger, 1911–1925.

___. *Summa Theologiae: A Concise Translation*. Edited by Timothy McDermott. London: Methuen, 1991.

Arkes, Hadley. "May Embryos Be Adopted?" Opinion, Life Watch. *Crisis* 18.3 (March 2000): 12. https://crisismagazine.com/vault/life-watch-may-embryos-be-adopted.

Asci, Donald P. *The Conjugal Act as Personal Act: A Study of the Catholic Concept of the Conjugal Act in the Light of Christian Anthropology*. San Francisco: Ignatius Press, 2002.

Assaf, Andrea Kirk. "The Absurd Fate of Frozen Embryos: Interview with Law Professor Brian Scarnecchia." Zenit, February 25, 2010. https://zenit.org/2010/02/25/the-absurd-fate-of-frozen-embryos/.

Austriaco, Nicanor Pier Girorgio. *Biomedicine and Beatitude: An Introduction to Catholic Bioethics*. Washington, DC: Catholic University of America, 2011. See esp. "A Disputed Question: The Adoption of Abandoned Human Embryos," 109–110, and "The Use of 'Surplus' Human Embryos for Stem Cell Research," 237.

___. *Biomedicine and Beatitude: An Introduction to Catholic Bioethics*. 2nd ed. Washington, DC: Catholic University of America, 2021. See esp. "The Adoption of Abandoned Human Embryos," 138–141, "An Emerging Disputed Question: Use of an Artificial Womb," 141–143, and "The Use of 'Surplus' Human Embryos for Stem Cell Research," 345.

___. "Embryo Adoption and the Extended Inseparability Argument." *National Catholic Bioethics Quarterly* 21.1 (Spring 2021): 29–35. DOI: 10.5840/ncbq20212114.

___. "Embryo Adoption, Pregnancy, and the Conjugal Act." Colloquy. *National Catholic Bioethics Quarterly* 3.2 (Summer 2003): 239–241. DOI: 10.5840/ncbq20033250.

___. "On the Catholic Vision of Conjugal Love and the Morality of Embryo Transfer." In *Human Embryo Adoption*, edited by Thomas V. Berg and Edward J. Furton, 115–134. Philadelphia: National Catholic Bioethics Center, 2006.

Avila, Daniel. "The Present Standing of the Human Embryo in U.S. Law." *National Catholic Bioethics Quarterly* 1.2 (Summer 2001): 203–226. DOI: 10.5840/ncbq20011254.

Aznar, Justo, Miriam Martínez-Peris, and Pedro Navarro-Illana. "Moral Assessment of Frozen Human Embryo Adoption in the Light of the Magisterium of the Catholic Church." *Acta Bioéthica* 23.1 (June 2017): 137–149. DOI: 10.4067/S1726-569X2017000100137. *See also* Rodríguez Yunta, Eduardo.

Bibliography

———. "Valoración de la adopción de embriones humanos congelados desde el punto de vista de la filosofía moral, la ética laica y dos religiones monoteístas [Valuating Frozen Human Embryo Adoption from a Moral Philosophical Point of View, Lay Ethics and Two Monotheist Religions]." *Acta Bioéthica* 22.2 (November 2016): 187–194. DOI: 10.4067/S1726-569X2016000200005.

Bachiochi, Erika, ed. *Women, Sex and the Church*. Boston: Pauline Books and Media, see pages 204, 344, 2010.

Bagileo, Bridget. "Evaluating the Effectiveness of Arguments in the Embryo Adoption Debate." MA thesis, Catholic University of America, 2022. JSTOR, CU Theses—Open Access. https://www.jstor.org/stable/community.38761448.

Barahona, Mónica López. *See* López Barahona, Mónica.

Bauzon, Stéphane. "Catholic Reflections for an Updated *Donum Vitae Instruction*: A New Catholic Challenge in a Post-Christian Europe." *Christian Bioethics* 14.1 (April 2008): 42–57. DOI: 10.1093/cb/cbn001.

Bazelon, Emily. "Why Anonymous Sperm Donation Is Over, and Why That Matters." *New York Times*. December 3, 2023. https://www.nytimes.com/2023/12/03/magazine/anonymous-sperm-donation-genetic-testing.html/.

Benedict XVI. Address to Participants at an International Congress Organized by the Pontifical Academy for Life. November 7, 2008. https://www.vatican.va/content/benedict-xvi/en/speeches/2008/november/documents/hf_ben-xvi_spe_20081107_acdlife.html.

———. General audience, Vatican City, July 7, 2010. https://www.vatican.va/content/benedict-xvi/en/audiences/2010/documents/hf_ben-xvi_aud_20100707.html/.

———. *see also* Ratzinger.

Berg, Thomas V. Introduction to *Human Embryo Adoption: Biotechnology, Marriage, and the Right to Life*, edited by Thomas V. Berg and Edward J. Furton, 1–12. Philadelphia, PA: National Catholic Bioethics Center, 2006.

Berg, Thomas V., and Edward J. Furton. Afterword to *Human Embryo Adoption: Biotechnology, Marriage, and the Right to Life*, edited by Thomas V. Berg and Edward J. Furton, 327–332. Philadelphia, PA: National Catholic Bioethics Center, 2006.

———, eds. *Human Embryo Adoption: Biotechnology, Marriage, and the Right to Life*. Philadelphia, PA: National Catholic Bioethics Center, 2006. Co-published Thornwood, NY: Winchester Institute for Ethics and the Human Person, 2006.

Berkman, John. "Adopting Embryos in America: A Case Study and an Ethical Analysis." *Scottish Journal of Theology* 55.4 (November 2002): 438–460. DOI: 10.1017/S0036930602000455.

———. "Adopting Embryos." In *The Oxford Handbook of Religious Perspectives on Reproductive Ethics*, edited by Deana S. Davis, 261–283. Oxford: Oxford University Press, 2024.

———. "Gestating the Embryos of Others: Surrogacy? Adoption? Rescue?" *National Catholic Bioethics Quarterly* 3.2 (Summer 2003): 309–329. DOI: 10.5840/ncbq20033256.

———. "John Berkman Replies." Colloquy. *National Catholic Bioethics Quarterly* 4.1 (Spring 2004): 12–14. DOI: 10.5840/ncbq20044162.

———. "The Morality of Adopting Frozen Embryos in Light of *Donum Vitae*." *Studia Moralia* 40.1 (June 2002): 115–141.

———. "Response to Tonti-Filippini on 'Gestating the Embryos of Others.'" Colloquy. *National Catholic Bioethics Quarterly* 3.4 (Winter 2003): 660–664. DOI: 10.5840/ncbq2003341.

———. "Virtuous Parenting and Orphaned Embryos." In *Human Embryo Adoption: Biotechnology, Marriage, and the Right to Life*, edited by Thomas V. Berg and Edward J. Furton, 13–36. Philadelphia: National Catholic Bioethics Center, 2006.

Berkman, John, and Kristen N. Carey. "Ethical and Religious Directives for a Catholic Embryo Adoption Agency: A Thought Experiment." In *The Ethics of Embryo Adoption and the Catholic Tradition: Moral Arguments, Economic Reality and Social Analysis*, edited by Sarah-Vaughan Brakman and Darlene Fozard Weaver, 251–273. Dordrecht, NL: Springer, 2007.

Bianchi, Daniel. "The Adoption of Embryos in Malta: Acting in the Interest and Welfare of a Child in Embryonic Form?" *Medical Law Review* 19.3 (Summer 2011): 401–429. DOI: 10.1093/medlaw/fwr018.

Blackshaw, Bruce P. "Is Pregnancy Really a Good Samaritan Act?" *Christian Bioethics* 27.2 (August 2021): 158–168. DOI: 10.1093/cb/cbab004.

Blackshaw, Bruce P., and Nicholas Colgrove. "Frozen Embryos and the Obligation to Adopt." *Bioethics* 34.8 (October 2020): 857–861. DOI: 10.1111/bioe.12733. Response to Lovering, Rob. "A Moral Argument for Frozen Human Embryo Adoption."

Blackshaw, Bruce P., Nicholas Colgrove, and Daniel Rodger. "Inconsistency Arguments Still Do Not Matter." *Journal of Medical Ethics* 48.7 (July 2022): 485–487. DOI: 10.1136/medethics-2021-107644.

———. "Why Inconsistency Arguments Fail: A Response to Shaw." *New Bioethics* 28.2 (2022): 139–151. DOI: 10.1080/20502877.2022.2070960.

Bobier, Christopher. "A Practical Problem for Proponents of Heterologous Embryo Transfer." *National Catholic Bioethics Quarterly* 22.3 (Autumn 2022): 455–462. DOI: 10.5840/ncbq202222342.

Bonet Farriol, Enrique. "El debate teológico sobre el destino de los embriones humanos criopreservados." Extract from doctoral thesis, University of Navarra, Pamplona, Spain, 2006. *Excerpta e dissertationibus in sacra theologia* 49: 6.

Boswell, John. *The Kindness of Strangers: The Abandonment of Children in Western Europe from Late Antiquity to the Renaissance*. Chicago: University of Chicago Press, 1998.

Bibliography

Brakman, Sarah-Vaughan. "Paradigms, Practices and Politics: Ethics and the Language of Human Embryo Transfer/Donation/Rescue/Adoption." In *Pluralistic Casuistry: Moral Arguments, Economic Realities, and Political Theory*, edited by Mark J. Cherry and Ana S. Iltis, 191–210. New York: Spring, 2007. DOI: 10.1007/978-1-4020-6260-5_13.

———. "*Real* Mothers and Good Stewards: The Ethics of Embryo Adoption." In *The Ethics of Embryo Adoption and the Catholic Tradition: Moral Arguments, Economic Reality, and Social Analysis*, edited by Sarah-Vaughan Brakman and Darlene Fozard Weaver, 119–138. Dordrecht, NL, 2007.

———. "Who Is a Parent? The Philosophical Groundings of Parenthood and Moral Implications for Families." *The Family in America* 28.3 (2014): 349–367.

Brakman, Sarah-Vaughan, and Darlene Fozard Weaver. "Embryo Adoption before and after *Dignitas Personae*: Defending an Argument of Limited Permissibility." In *Contemporary Controversies in Catholic Bioethics*, edited by Jason T. Eberl, 147–167. Cham, CH: Springer, 2017. DOI: 10.1007/978-3-319-55766-3_12.

———, eds. *The Ethics of Embryo Adoption and the Catholic Tradition: Moral Arguments, Economic Reality, and Social Analysis*. New York: Springer, 2007.

———. "Introduction: The Ethics of Embryo Adoption and the Catholic Tradition." In *The Ethics of Embryo Adoption and the Catholic Tradition: Moral Arguments, Economic Reality, and Social Analysis*, edited by Sarah-Vaughan Brakman and Darlene Fozard Weaver, 3–23. Dordrecht, NL, 2007.

Brakman, Sarah-Vaughan, and Sally J. Scholz. "Adoption, ART, and a Reconception of the Maternal Body: Toward Embodied Maternity." In "Maternal Bodies," special issue, *Hypatia* 21.1 (Winter 2006): 54–73. DOI: 10.1111/j.1527-2001.2006.tb00964.x.

Breed, Glenn. "The Only Moral Option Is Embryo Adoption." *National Catholic Bioethics Quarterly* 14.3 (Autumn 2014): 441–447. DOI: 10.5840/ncbq20141436.

Brighouse, Harry, and Adam Swift. "The Goods of Parenting." In *Family-Making: Contemporary Ethical Challenges*, edited by Françoise Baylis and Carolyn McLeod, 11–28. New York: Oxford University Press, 2014.

Brown, Brandon, and Jason T. Eberl. "Ethical Considerations in Defense of Embryo Adoption." In *The Ethics of Embryo Adoption and the Catholic Tradition: Moral Arguments, Economic Reality, and Social Analysis*, edited by Sarah-Vaughan Brakman and Darlene Fozard Weaver, 103–118. Dordrecht, NL, 2007.

Brown, Francis, Samuel Rolles Driver, and Charles Augustus Briggs. *The Brown-Driver-Briggs Hebrew and English Lexicon: Coded with Strong's Concordance Numbers*. Biblesoft unabridged electronic database ed. Biblesoft, 2006. Available at Bible Hub. https://biblehub.com/hebrew/3045.htm.

Brown, James E. Letter to the editor. *Linacre Quarterly* 70.3 (August 2003): 181–182. DOI: 10.1080/20508549.2003.11877676.

Brown, Lauretta. "Frozen in Time: Catholic Ethicists Discuss the Fate of the Estimated 1 Million Human Embryos on Ice." *National Catholic Register*, January 17, 2023. https://www.ncregister.com/news/frozen-in-time-catholic-ethicists-discuss-the-fate-of-the-estimated-1-million-human-embryos-on-ice.

Browning, Don S. "Adoption and the Moral Significance of Kin Altrusim." In *The Morality of Adoption: Social-Psychological, Theological, and Legal Perspectives*, edited by Timothy P. Jackson, 52–77. Grand Rapids, MI: Eerdmans, 2005.

Brugger, E. Christian. "A Defense by Analogy of Heterologous Embryo Transfer." In *Human Embryo Adoption*, edited by Thomas V. Berg and Edward J. Furton, 197–228. Philadelphia: National Catholic Bioethics Center, 2006.

———. "In Defense of Transferring Heterologous Embryos." In "Human Embryo Transfer," special issue, *National Catholic Bioethics Quarterly* 5.1 (Spring 2005): 95–112. DOI: 10.5840/ncbq20055170.

———. "Rescuing Frozen Embryos: Is Adoption a Valid Moral Option?" Culture of Life Foundation, March 2010, http://culture-of-life.org/content/view/627/1/. (Website discontinued.) Reproduced at Life Issues, 2010, https://www.lifeissues.net/writers/bru/bru_10rescue_embryos.html.

———, ed. "Symposium on *Dignitas Personae*." Special issue. *National Catholic Bioethics Quarterly* 9.3 (Autumn 2009): 461–483. DOI: 10.5840/20099333. See esp. E. Christian Brugger, introduction, 461–465, and E. Christian Brugger, "Strengths and Weaknesses of *Dignitas Personae*," 481–483.

———. Review of *Catholic Bioethics and the Gift of Human Life*, by William E. May, 3rd ed. *National Catholic Bioethics Quarterly* 14.3 (Autumn 2014): 578–580, esp. 579. DOI: 10.5840/ncbq201414319.

Buchanan, Kelly. "New Law Library Report on the Legal Treatment of Embryos Created through IVF." *Law Library* (blog). Library of Congress. April 4, 2024. https://blogs.loc.gov/law/2024/04/new-law-library-report-on-the-legal-treatment-of-embryos-created-through-ivf/.

Bush, George W., White House. "President Discusses Embryo Adoption and Ethical Stem Cell Research." News release. May 24, 2005. https://georgewbush-whitehouse.archives.gov/news/releases/2005/05/text/20050524-12.html.

Buskmiller, Cara. "Cryopreserved Embryo Adoption: Not Now, Maybe Later." *National Catholic Bioethics Quarterly* 16.2 (Summer 2016): 225–231. DOI: 10.5840/ncbq201616220.

Cahill, Lisa Sowle. "Adoption: A Roman Catholic Perspective." In *The Morality of Adoption: Social-Psychological, Theological, and Legal Perspectives*, edited by Timothy P. Jackson, 148–171. Grand Rapids, MI: Eerdmans, 2005.

———. *Sex, Gender and Christian Ethics*. Cambridge: Cambridge University Press, 1996.

Cahn, Naomi. "Who Gets the Frozen Embryos?" *Forbes*. February 4, 2020. https://www.forbes.com/sites/naomicahn/2020/02/04/who-gets-the-frozen-embryos/?sh=684b54156cfd.

Bibliography

Campion, Bridget. "Parenthood Begins at Conception." Colloquy. *National Catholic Bioethics Quarterly* 3.3 (Autumn 2003): 441–442. DOI: 10.5840 /ncbq20033325.

Canon Law Society of America, ed. *Code of Canon Law: Latin-English Edition.* Washington, DC: CLSA, 1999.

Canosa, S., D. Cimadomo, A. Conforti, R. Maggiulli, A. Giancani, A. Tallarita, et al. "The Effect of Extended Cryo-Storage Following Vitrification on Embryo Competence: A Systematic Review and Meta-Analysis." *Journal of Assisted Reproduction and Genetics* 39.4 (April 2022): 873–882. DOI: 10.1007 /s10815-022-02405-3.

Carrasco de Paula, Ignacio. "The Respect Due to the Human Embryo: A Historical and Doctrinal Perspective." In *The Identity and Status of the Human Embryo: Proceedings of Third Assembly of the Pontifical Academy for Life*, edited by Juan de Dios Vial Correa and Elio Sgreccia, 48–73. Vatican City: Libreria Editrice Vaticana, 1998.

Carpinello, Olivia, B. Mitchell Bodily, Samad Jahandideh, Morine Cebert, Joshua C. Combs, Micah J. Hill, et al. "Just over One-Third of Patients Interested in Embryo Donation Complete Embryo Donation." *Fertility and Sterility* 114.3 suppl (September 2020): e102. DOI: 10.1016/j.fertnstert .2020.08.309.

Casanova, Carlos A. "The Underlying Assumptions of Germain Grisez's Critique of the Perverted Faculty Argument." *Espíritu* 69.159 (2020): 95–126.

Cataldo, Peter J. Letter to the editor in "Three Notes from Our Readers: Comments on Embryo Adoption." *Ethics & Medics* 26.11 (November 2001): 3–4. DOI: 10.5840/em2001261123.

Catechism of the Catholic Church, 2nd ed. Washington, DC: US Conference of Catholic Bishops / Libreria Editrice Vaticana, 2018 update.

Catholic Medical Association. "Embryo Adoption: A Debate." Transcript, Catholic Medical Association Annual Education Conference "Searching for the Truth: Medicine, Morality, and the Media," Denver, September 9, 2022. *See also* Golder, Barbara.

Catholic News Agency. "New Vatican Instruction Called Valuable 'Reference Point' on Bioethics." December 16, 2008. https://www.catholicnewsagency .com/news/14629/new-vatican-instruction-called-valuable-reference -point-on-bioethics

Catholic World News. "Christian Group Matches Frozen Embryos with Adoptive Parents." Catholic Culture (website). March 13, 2001. https://www .catholicculture.org/news/features/index.cfm?recnum=15050.

———. "White House Urged to Back 'Embryo Adoption.'" Catholic Culture (website). August 23, 2002. https://www.catholicculture.org /news/features/index.cfm?recnum=18796

Caulfield, Brian. "'Souls on Ice': With Frozen Embryo Technology, Life's Sanctity Is Lost." *National Catholic Register*, January 4, 1998.

———. "Where Do Frozen Embryos Belong?" *Human Life Review* 27.3 (Summer 2001): 7–13.

Cheely, Elizabeth Cason Crosby. "Embryo Adoption and the Law." In *The Ethics of Embryo Adoption and the Catholic Tradition: Moral Arguments, Economic Reality and Social Analysis*, edited by Sarah-Vaughn Brakman and Darlene Fozard Weaver, 275–306. Dordrecht, NL: Springer 2007.

Chen, Stephen. "Chinese Scientists Create AI Nanny to Look after Embryos in Artificial Womb." *South China Morning Post*. January 31, 2022. https://www.scmp.com/news/china/science/article/3165325/chinese-scientists-create-ai-nanny-look-after-babies-artificial.

Christensen, Jen, and Nadia Kounang. "Parents Welcome Twins from Embryos Frozen 30 Years Ago." CNN. November 21, 2022. https://www.cnn.com/2022/11/21/health/30-year-old-embryos-twins/index.html.

Clark, Cat. "To Become Father and Mother Only through Each Other." Colloquy. *National Catholic Bioethics Quarterly* 3.3 (Autumn 2003): 442–448. DOI: 10.5840/ncbq20033325.

Clark, Peter A. "Cryopreserved Embryos: A Catholic Alternative to Embryonic Stem Cell Research and Adoption." In *Embryonic Stem Cells: Basic Biology to Bioengineering*, edited by Michael S. Kallos, 33–46. London: IntechOpen, 2011.

Cohen, Eric. "Of Embryos and Empire: What the Embryo Debate Can Teach Us about American Civilization." *New Atlantis* 2 (Summer 2003). https://www.thenewatlantis.com/publications/of-embryos-and-empire.

Cole, Basil. Review of *Human Embryo Adoption: Biotechnology, Marriage, and the Right to Life*, edited by Thomas V. Berg and Edward J. Furton. *Thomist* 71.4 (October 2007): 657–660. DOI: 10.1353/tho.2007.0010.

Coleman, Kristin. "Defending Unborn Orphans: Embryo Adoption." *CedarEthics Online* 9.1 (Fall 2009): 5. https://digitalcommons.cedarville.edu/cedar_ethics_online/5/.

Colgrove, Nicholas. "Deadly Language Games: Theological Reflections on Emerging Reproductive Technologies." *Christian Bioethics* 30.2 (August 2024): 67–84. DOI: 10.1093/cb/cbae001.

Colgrove, Nicholas, Bruce P. Blackshaw, and Daniel Rodger, eds. *Agency, Pregnancy and Persons: Essays in Defense of Human Life*. New York: Routledge, 2023.

———. "Prolife Hypocrisy: Why Inconsistency Arguments Do Not Matter." *Journal of Medical Ethics* 47.12 (December 2021): e58. DOI: 10.1136/medethics-2020-106633.

Collins, Timothy P. "On Abandoned Embryos." *Linacre Quarterly* 75.1 (February 2008): 1–15. DOI: 10.1179/002436308803889747.

Congregation for the Doctrine of the Faith. *Dignitas personae*. September 8, 2008. https://www.vatican.va/roman_curia/congregations/cfaith/documents/rc_con_cfaith_doc_20081208_dignitas-personae_en.html.

Bibliography

———. *Doctrinal Commentary on the Concluding Formula of "Professio Fidei."* June 29, 1998. https://www.ewtn.com/catholicism/library/doctrinal-commentary-on-concluding-formula-of-professio-fidei-2038.
———. *Donum veritatis.* May 24, 1990. https://www.vatican.va/roman_curia/congregations/cfaith/documents/rc_con_cfaith_doc_19900524_theologian-vocation_en.html.
———. *Donum vitae.* February 22, 1987. https://www.vatican.va/roman_curia/congregations/cfaith/documents/rc_con_cfaith_doc_19870222_respect-for-human-life_en.html.
———. *Mysterium ecclesiae.* June 24, 1973. https://www.vatican.va/roman_curia/congregations/cfaith/documents/rc_con_cfaith_doc_19730705_mysterium-ecclesiae_en.html.
———. *Pastoralis actio.* October 20, 1980. https://www.vatican.va/roman_curia/congregations/cfaith/documents/rc_con_cfaith_doc_19801020_pastoralis_actio_en.html.
———. *Persona humana.* December 29, 1975. https://www.vatican.va/roman_curia/congregations/cfaith/documents/rc_con_cfaith_doc_19751229_persona-humana_en.html.
———. *Samaritanus bonus.* July 14, 2020. https://press.vatican.va/content/salastampa/en/bollettino/pubblico/2020/09/22/200922a.html.
———. *Proclaiming the Truth of Jesus Christ: Papers from the Vallombrosa Meeting.* Washington, DC: US Catholic Conference, 2000.
———. *Regarding the Instruction "Dignitas Personae."* December 12, 2008. https://www.vatican.va/roman_curia/congregations/cfaith/documents/rc_con_cfaith_doc_20081212_sintesi-dignitas-personae_en.html.
Connors, Ryan. "*Veritatis Splendor* at Thirty: Three Decades of Moral Teaching Founded on the Splendor of Truth." In "The Thirtieth Anniversary of *Veritatis Splendor*," edited by Romanus Cessario and Cajetan Cuddy, special issue, *National Catholic Bioethics Quarterly* 23.4 (Winter 2023): 655–668. DOI: 10.5840/ncbq202323452. See esp. pp. 659–661.
Connors, Stephanie Gray. *Conceived by Science: Thinking Carefully and Compassionately about Infertility and IVF.* Florida: Wongeese Publishing, 2021. See esp. appendix 1, "What to Do with Frozen Embryos?," 114–121.
———. Interview by Matt Fradd. YouTube. Posted as "The Most COMPLEX Pro-Life Issue??? w/ Stephanie Gray" by Matt Fradd on January 26, 2024. https://www.youtube.com/watch?v=mZNSD9pc_Zg.
Coolman, Holly Taylor. "Adoption and the Goods of Birth." *Journal of Moral Theology* 1.2 (2012): 96–114. https://jmt.scholasticahq.com/article/11244.
Cooperman, Alan. "Catholics Split on Embryo Issue." *Washington Post*, May 31, 2005. https://www.washingtonpost.com/archive/politics/2005/05/31/catholics-split-on-embryo-issue/0a8ad6d8-070c-4688-a385-d44d7f48f4ae/.

Corby, Paschal. "Estranged Fathers: The Alienation of Men in Heterologous Embryo Transfer." *National Catholic Bioethics Quarterly* 13.2 (Summer 2013): 287–297. DOI: 10.5840/ncbq201313250.

Corcoran, Gerald P. "Embryo Adoption." Colloquy. *National Catholic Bioethics Quarterly* 10.4 (Winter 2010): 644–646. DOI: 10.5840/ncbq20101041.

Cozzoli, Mauro. "The Human Embryo: Ethical and Normative Aspects." In *The Identity and Statute* [sic] *of the Human Embryo: Proceedings of the Third Assembly of the Pontifical Academy for Life (Vatican City, February 14–16, 1997)*, edited by Juan de Dios Vial Correa and Elio Sgreccia, 260–300. Vatican City: Libreria Editrice Vaticana, 1998. See esp. p. 295.

Crockin, Susan, and Lauren M. Nussbaum. "Embryo Donation: Legal Aspects." In *Third Party Reproduction: A Comprehensive Guide*, edited by James M. Goldfarb, 101–111. New York: Springer, 2013.

Cromer, Risa. *Conceiving Christian America: Embryo Adoption and Reproductive Politics*. New York: NYU Press, 2023.

Cromer, Risa. "Saving Embryos in Stem Cell Science and Embryo Adoption." *New Genetics & Society* 37.4 (2018): 362–386. DOI: 10.1080/14636778.2018.1546574.

Cunningham, Bert J. "The Morality of Organic Transplantation." PhD diss., Catholic University of America, 1944.

Cunningham, Mark W., Jr., and Babbette LaMarca. "Risk of Cardiovascular Disease, End-Stage Renal Disease, and Stroke in Postpartum Women and Their Fetuses after a Hypertensive Pregnancy." *American Journal of Physiology—Regulatory, Integrative, and Comparative Physiology* 315.3 (September 2018): R521–R528. DOI: 10.1152/ajpregu.00218.2017.

Davidson, JoAnn L. "A Birth Announcement." Colloquy. *National Catholic Bioethics Quarterly* 2.1 (Spring 2002): 9. DOI: 10.5840/ncbq20022171.

———. "A Successful Embryo Adoption." Case study. In "Respect for the Human Embryo," special issue, *National Catholic Bioethics Quarterly* 1.2 (Summer 2001): 229–233. DOI: 10.5840/ncbq20011255.

Davis, Dena S., ed. *The Oxford Handbook of Religious Perspectives on Reproductive Ethics*. New York: Oxford University Press, 2024.

Day, Angelique, Amy Dworsky, Kieran Fogarty, and Amy Damashek. "An Examination of Post-Secondary Retention and Graduation among Foster Care Youth Enrolled in a Four-Year University." *Children and Youth Services Review* 33.11 (2011): 2335–2341. DOI: 10/1016/j.childyouth.2011.08.004.

Delaquil, Edward. "Intention in Embryo Adoption." Colloquy. *National Catholic Bioethics Quarterly* 13.1 (Spring 2013): 17–18. DOI: 10.5840/ncbq201313165.

Bibliography

Dembitz, Lewis N., and Kaufmann Kohler. "Adoption." In *The Jewish Encyclopedia*, edited by Isodore Singer. Funk and Wagnalls, 1901–1906; Jewish Encyclopedia, 2002. https://www.jewishencyclopedia.com/articles/852-adoption.

DeMarco, Donald. "Technologized Parenthood and the Attenuation of Motherhood and Fatherhood." *Thought* (Fordham University): 63.4 (December 1988): 327–347. DOI: 10.5840/thought198863425.

———. "When Ethics Hits the Wall." *National Catholic Register*, February 13, 2009, https://www.ncregister.com/commentaries/when-ethics-hits-the-wall.

DeMartis, Francesco. "Mass Pre-Embryo Adoption." *Cambridge Quarterly of Healthcare Ethics* 7.1 (January 1998): 101–103. DOI:10.1017/S0963180198701136.

Denzinger, Heinrich, and Adolf Schönmetzer, eds. *Enchiridion symbolorum definitionum et declarationum de rebus fidei et morum*. 36th ed. Barcelona: Herder, 1976.

De Rosa, Francis M. "On Rescuing Frozen Embryos." *Linacre Quarterly* 69.3 (August 2002): 228–260. DOI: 10.1080/20508549.2002.11877649. *Compare* Geach, Mary C. Letter to the Editor.

———. "The Transfer of Abandoned Frozen Embryos: Identifying the Object of the Act." In "Human Embryo Transfer," special issue, *National Catholic Bioethics Quarterly* 5.1 (Spring 2005): 59–62. DOI: 10.5840/ncbq20055167.

De Vaux, Roland. *Ancient Israel: Its Life and Institutions*. London: Darton, Longman and Todd, 1961.

Devlin, Kayleen. "The World's First Artificial Womb for Humans." Video. BBC. October 15, 2019. https://www.bbc.com/news/av/health-50056405.

Devroey, P., M. Camus, E. Van Den Abbeel, L. Van Waesberghe, A. Wisanto, and A. C. Van Steirteghem. "Establishment of 22 Pregnancies after Oocyte and Embryo Donation." *British Journal of Obstetrics and Gynaecology* 96.8 (August 1989): 900–906. DOI: 10.1111/j.1471-0528.1989.tb03343.x.

Diamond, Sheila. "Theological Debate over Embryo Adoption: The Question Has Many Ramifications." *Ethics & Medics* 26.10 (October 2001): 3–4. DOI: 10.5840/em2001261021. Republished with minimal revision as "Theological Debate over Embryo Adoption." *Linacre Quarterly* 72.1 (February 2005): 70–73. DOI: 10.1080/20508549.2005.11877743.

Dicastery for Laity, Family and Life and Jérôme Lejeune Foundation. "Keys to Bioethics." Dicastery for Laity, Family and Life. Accessed October 19, 2023. https://laityinvolved.org/project/keys-to-bioethics/.

Doerflinger, Richard M. "On the Morality of Heterologous Embryo Transfer." Paper, The Westchester Institute Scholars Forum: On the Morality of Heterologous Embryo Transfer. Washington, DC, October 28–29, 2004.

———. Washington Insider. *National Catholic Bioethics Quarterly* 5.3 (Autumn 2005): 455–462. DOI: 10.5840/ncbq20055325. See esp. 457n10.

Donovan, Kevin. Interview by Catherin Hadro. *EWTN Pro-Life Weekly*. YouTube. Posted as "'Embryo Adoption' Debate" by EWTN on November 10, 2017. https://www.youtube.com/watch?v=Gkq0ZA8p8K8.

Drakopoulos, Panagiotis, Juan Garcia-Velasco, Ernesto Bosch, Christophe Blockeel, Michael de Vos, Samuel Santos-Ribeiro, et al. "ICSI Does Not Offer Any Benefit over Conventional IVF across Different Ovarian Response Categories in Non-Male Factor Infertility: A European Multicenter Analysis." *Journal of Assisted Reproduction and Genetics* 36.10 (August 2019): 2067–2076. DOI: 10.1007/s10815-019-01563-1.

Dworsky, Amy, and Mark E. Courtney. "Homelessness and the Transition from Foster Care to Adulthood." *Child Welfare* 88.4 (2009): 23–56.

Dworsky, Amy, Laura Napolitano, and Mark Courtney. "Homelessness during the Transition from Foster Care to Adulthood." *American Journal of Public Health* 103 suppl 2 (December 2013): S318–S323. DOI: 10.2105/AJPH.2013.301455.

Eberl, Jason T., ed. *Contemporary Controversies in Catholic Bioethics*. New York: Springer, 2017.

———. Review of *Human Embryo Adoption: Biotechnology, Marriage, and the Right to Life*, edited by Thomas V. Berg and Edward J. Furton. *Linacre Quarterly* 78.2 (May 2011): 232–234. DOI: 10.1179/002436311803888366.

———. "What *Dignitas Personae* Does Not Say." In "Responses to *Dignitas Personae*: Part I of II," special issue, *National Catholic Bioethics Quarterly* 10.1 (Spring 2010): 89–110. DOI: 10.5840/ncbq201010174. See esp. "Human Embryo Adoption," 93–97. Includes material from Brown, Brandon, and Jason T. Eberl. "Ethical Considerations in Defense of Embryo Adoption."

Ehrich, John. "Embryo Adoption." Colloquy. *National Catholic Bioethics Quarterly* 11.3 (Autumn 2011): 417. DOI: 10.5840/ncbq201111325.

———. "The Question of Human Embryo Adoption." Colloquy. *National Catholic Bioethics Quarterly* 11.2 (Summer 2011): 216. DOI: 10.5840/ncbq201111248.

Eijk, Willem Jacobus, Lambert M. Hendriks, and J. A. Raymakers, eds. *Manual of Catholic Medical Ethics: Responsible Healthcare from a Catholic Perspective*. English edition edited by John I. Fleming. Translated by M. Regina Van Den Berg and Janthony Raymakers. Brisbane, Australia: Connor Court Publishing, 2014. Original Dutch edition 2010.

Ellish, N. J., K. Saboda, J. O'Connor, P. C. Nasca, E. J. Stanek, and C. Boyle. "A Prospective Study of Early Pregnancy Loss." *Human Reproduction* 11.2 (February 1996): 406–412. DOI: 10.1093/humrep/11.2.406.

Elrod, Katie, and Paul Carpenter. "The Church's Best-Kept Secret: Church Teaching on Infertility Treatment." In *Women, Sex and the Church*, edited by Erika Bachiochi, 121–142. Boston: Pauline Books and Media, 2010.

Bibliography

Etheredge, Francis. *Conception: An Icon of the Beginning.* St. Louis, MO: En Route Books and Media, 2019.

———. "Embryo Adoption and Reciprocal Human Relationships." Colloquy. *National Catholic Bioethics Quarterly* 17.2 (Summer 2017): 196–198. DOI: 10.5840/ncbq201717219.

———. "Frozen and Untouchable: A Double Injustice to the Embryo." *National Catholic Bioethics Quarterly* 16.1 (Spring 2016): 49–54. DOI: 10.5840/ncbq20161616.

———. *Human Nature: Moral Norm.* St. Louis, MO: En Route Books and Media, 2023.

———. *The Human Person: A Bioethical Word.* St. Louis, MO: En Route Books and Media, 2017.

———. *Lord, Do You Mean Me? A Father-Catechist!* St. Louis, MO: En Route Books and Media, 2023.

———. *Mary and Bioethics: An Exploration.* St. Louis, MO: En Route Books and Media, 2020.

———. *The Prayerful Kiss.* St. Louis, MO: En Route Books and Media, 2019.

———. "A Reflection on the Language of the Body." *Communio* 24.2 (September 1997).

———. *Scripture: A Unique Word.* Newcastle upon Tyne, UK: Cambridge Scholars, 2014.

———. *Unfolding a Post-Roe World.* St. Louis, MO: En Route Books and Media, 2022

European Society of Human Reproduction and Embryology. "More Than 8 Million Babies Born from IVF since the World's First in 1978." *Science Daily.* July 3, 2018. https://www.sciencedaily.com/releases/2018/07/180703084127.htm.

European Society of Human Reproduction and Embryology Working Group on Reproductive Donation. "Good Practice Recommendations for Information Provision for Those Involved in Reproductive Donation." *Human Reproduction Open* 2022.1 (February 2022): 1–26. DOI: 10.1093/hropen/hoac001.

Euser, Saskia, Lenneke R. A. Alink, Anne Tharner, Marinus H. van Ijzendoorn, and Marian J. Bakermans-Kranenburg. "The Prevalence of Child Sexual Abuse in Out-of-Home Care: A Comparison between Abuse in Residential and in Foster Care." *Child Maltreatment* 18.4 (November 2013): 221–231. DOI: 10.1177/1077559513489848.

———. "The Prevalence of Child Sexual Abuse in Out-of-Home Care: Increased Risk for Children with a Mild Intellectual Disability." *Journal of Applied Research in Intellectual Disabilities* 29.1 (January 2016): 83–92. DOI: 10.1111/jar.12160.

Faggioni, Maurizio P. "The Question of Frozen Embryos." *L'Osservatore Romano* (English edition), May 29, 1996(?) or August 21, 1996.

Farris, Joshua, and S. Mark Hamilton. "Ransoming Embryos." Intersections. Center for Bioethics and Human Dignity, Trinity International University. January 18, 2019. https://www.cbhd.org/intersections/ransoming-embryos.

Faust, Katy. "A Children's Rights Perspective on Embryo Adoption." *Natural Family* 34.1 (2020): 2ff.

Feser, Edward. "In Defense of the Perverted Faculty Argument." In *Neo-Scholastic Essays*, 378–415. South Bend, IN: St. Augustine Press, 2015.

Finger, Reginald, and John Hissong. "Embryo Adoption: A Review of the Roman Catholic Conversation." Webinar. YouTube. Posted as "Embryo Adoption & Roman Catholicism" by Embryo Adoption Awareness Center on December 10, 2012. https://www.youtube.com/watch?v=8TM7ctCKeGk.

Finley, Kate. "Abortion, Adoption and Integrity." Chap. 8 in *Agency, Pregnancy and Persons*, edited by Nicholas Colgrove, Bruce P. Blackshaw, and Daniel Rodger. New York: Routledge, 2023.

Finnis, John. *Aquinas*. New York: Oxford University Press, 1998.

___. "Marriage: A Basic and Exigent Good." *Monist* 91.3–4 (July–October 2008): 392–393.

___. "Understanding *Dignitas Personae* on Embryo Adoption." In "Symposium on *Dignitas Personae*," special article, edited by E. Christian Brugger. *National Catholic Bioethics Quarterly* 9.3 (Autumn 2009): 474–477. DOI: 10.5840/20099333.

Finnis, John, Germain Grisez, and Joseph Boyle. "'Direct' and 'Indirect': A Reply to Critics of Our Action Theory." *Thomist* 65.1 (January 2001): 1–44. DOI: 10.1353/tho.2001.0014.

Fisher, John Steven, dir. *NaPro: A Quiet Revolution*. Blackfriars Media. YouTube. Posted by Dominican Friars on December 9, 2016. https://www.youtube.com/watch?v=6JT-m4-iEWE.

Fleming, Alex. "Striking a Balance between Embryo Transfer and the Goods of Marriage." *National Catholic Bioethics Quarterly* 17.3 (Autumn 2017): 461–473. DOI: 10.5840/ncbq201717346.

Francis, Address to the Italian Association for the Donation of Organs, Tissues and Cells (AIDO). April 13, 2019. https://www.vatican.va/content/francesco/en/speeches/2019/april/documents/papa-francesco_20190413_donazione-organi.html.

___. *Humana communitas*. January 6, 2019. https://www.vatican.va/content/francesco/en/letters/2019/documents/papa-francesco_20190106_lettera-accademia-vita.html.

___. *Laudato si'*. May 24, 2015. https://www.vatican.va/content/francesco/en/encyclicals/documents/papa-francesco_20150524_enciclica-laudato-si.html.

___. Message for the Forty-Eighth World Communications Day. June 1, 2014. https://www.vatican.va/content/francesco/en/events/event.dir.html/content

Bibliography

/vaticanevents/en/2014/1/24/papa-francesco_20140124_messaggio-comunicazioni-sociali.html

———. Message for the Thirty-Seventh World Youth Day. August 15, 2022. https://www.vatican.va/content/francesco/en/messages/youth/documents/papa-francesco_20220815_messaggio-giovani_2022.html.

Friedrich, Daniel. "A Duty to Adopt?" *Journal of Applied Philosophy* 30.1 (January 2013): 25–39. DOI: 10.1111/japp.12003.

Frith, Lucy, Eric Blyth, Marilyn S. Paul, and Roni Berger. "Conditional Embryo Relinquishment: Choosing to Relinquish Embryos for Family-Building through a Christian Embryo 'Adoption' Programme." *Human Reproduction* 26.12 (December 2011): 3327–3338. DOI: 10.1093/humrep/der313.

Furton, Edward J. "Embryo Adoption Reconsidered." In "Responses to *Dignitas Personae*: Part II of II." Special issue, *National Catholic Bioethics Quarterly* 10.2 (Summer 2010): 329–347. DOI: 10.5840/ncbq201010256.

———, ed. "Human Embryo Transfer." Special issue, *National Catholic Bioethics Quarterly* 5.1 (Spring 2005).

———. In This Issue. In "Responses to *Dignitas Personae*: Part I of II," special issue, *National Catholic Bioethics Quarterly* 10.1 (Spring 2010): 19–20. DOI: 10.5840/ncbq201010167.

———. In This Issue. In "Responses to *Dignitas Personae*: Part II of II," special issue, *National Catholic Bioethics Quarterly* 10.2 (Summer 2010): 227–228. DOI: 10.5840/ncbq201010248.

———. "On the Disposition of Frozen Embryos: An Approach to a Difficult Question." *Ethics & Medics* 26.9 (September 2001): 1–3. DOI: 10.5840/em200126918.

———, ed. "Responses to *Dignitas Personae*: Part I of II." Special issue, *National Catholic Bioethics Quarterly* 10.1 (Spring 2010).

———, ed. "Responses to *Dignitas Personae*: Part II of II." Special issue, *National Catholic Bioethics Quarterly* 10.2 (Summer 2010).

Furton, Edward J., and Louise A. Mitchell, eds. *What Is Man, O Lord? The Human Person in a Biotech Age: Proceedings of the Eighteenth Bishops' Workshop*. Boston: National Catholic Bioethics Center, 2002.

Gacek, Christopher M. "Conceiving Pregnancy: U.S. Medical Dictionaries and the Definitions of *Conception* and *Pregnancy*." *National Catholic Bioethics Quarterly* 9.3 (Autumn 2009): 543–557. DOI: 10.5840/20099336.

Gaines, Carla. "Embryo Adoption: An Opportunity for Life." *CedarEthics Online* 8.2 (Spring 2009): 1. https://digitalcommons.cedarville.edu/cedar_ethics_online/1/.

Gallagher, John. "The Principle of Totality: Man's Stewardship of His Body." In *Moral Theology Today: Certitudes and Doubts*, edited by Donald McCarthy, 217–242. St. Louis: Pope John Center, 1984.

Gallant, Kristen. "Twins Born from Embryos Frozen Nearly 30 Years Ago Break Record." WATE 6. November 21, 2022. https://www.wate.com/news/top-stories/twins-born-from-embryos-frozen-nearly-30-years-ago-break-record/.

Geach, Mary (Mrs. Mary Gormally). "Are There Any Circumstances in Which It Would Be Morally Admirable for a Woman to Seek to Have an Orphan Embryo Implanted in Her Womb?," part 1. In *Issues for a Catholic Bioethic*, edited by Luke Gormally, 341–346. London: Linacre Centre, 1999.

———. "The Female Act of Allowing an Intromission of an Impregnating Kind." In *Human Embryo Adoption*, edited by Thomas V. Berg and Edward J. Furton, 251–271. Philadelphia: National Catholic Bioethics Center, 2006.

———. Letter to the editor. *Linacre Quarterly* 70.1 (February 2003): 1. DOI: 10.1080/20508549.2003.11877658. Response to de Rosa, Frances M. "On Rescuing Frozen Embryos."

———. "Motherhood, IVF, and Sexual Ethics." In *Fertility and Gender: Issues in Reproductive and Sexual Ethics*," edited by Helen Watt, 169–183. Oxford: Anscombe Bioethics Centre, 2011.

———. "Reply to Finnis on Embryo Adoption." Colloquy. *National Catholic Bioethics Quarterly* 10.1 (Spring 2010): 9–11. DOI: 10.5840/ncbq201010166

———. "Rescuing Frozen Embryos." In *What Is Man, O Lord? The Human Person in a Biotech Age*, edited by Edward J. Furton and Louise A. Mitchell, 217–230. Boston: National Catholic Bioethics Center, 2002.

———. "Rescuing Frozen Embryos." Paper. The Westchester Institute Scholars Forum: On the Morality of Heterologous Embryo Transfer. Washington, DC, October 28–29, 2004.

Genovese, Eugene, and Elizabeth Fox-Genovese. *Fatal Self-Deception: Slaveholding Paternalism in the Old South*. New York: Cambridge University Press, 2011.

George, Robert P. Foreword to *Human Embryo Adoption: Biotechnology, Marriage, and the Right to Life*, edited by Thomas V. Berg and Edward J. Furton, xi–xiii. Philadelphia, PA: National Catholic Bioethics Center, 2006.

George, Robert P., and Christopher Tollefsen. *Embryo: A Defense of Human Life*. 2nd ed. Princeton, NJ: Witherspoon Institute, 2011. See esp. pp. 214–215.

Girgis, Sherif. "The Historic Christian Teaching against Contraception." *Public Discourse*. August 10, 2016. https://www.thepublicdiscourse.com/2016/08/17559/.

Glujovsky, Demián, Romina Pesce, Carlos Sueldo, Andrea Marta Quinteiro Retamar, Roger J. Hart, and Agustín Ciapponi. "Endometrial Preparation for Women Undergoing Embryo Transfer with Frozen Embryos or Embryos Derived from Donor Oocytes." *Cochrane Database of Systematic Reviews* 10.10 (October 28, 2020), CD006359. DOI: 10.1002/14651858.CD006359.pub3.

Bibliography

Goedeke, Sonja, and Deborah Payne. "Embryo Donation in New Zealand: A Pilot Study." *Human Reproduction* 24.9 (August 2009): 1939–1945. DOI: 10.1093/humrep/dep116.

Golder, Barbara. "Listening in Parables." Editorial (reflecting on a debate on the topic of "whether or not frozen embryos could be legitimately adopted, implanted, and brought to term by Catholic couples," held at the Catholic Medical Association Annual Education Conference in Denver, September 7, 2022). *Linacre Quarterly* 90.1 (March 2023): 5–7. DOI: 10.1177/00243639221146148. *See also* Catholic Medical Association.

Goldfarb, James M., ed. *Third Party Reproduction: A Comprehensive Guide*. New York: Springer, 2013.

Gormally, Luke, ed. *Issues for a Catholic Bioethic*. London: Linacre Center, 1999.

———. "The 'Various Problems' Presented by Embryo Adoption (n. 19)." In "Symposium on *Dignitas Personae*," special article, edited by E. Christian Brugger. *National Catholic Bioethics Quarterly* 9.3 (Autumn 2009): 470–474. DOI: 10.5840/20099333.

Gottlieb, Claes, Othon Lalos, and Frank Lindblad. "Disclosure of Donor Insemination to the Child: The Impact of Swedish Legislation on Couples' Attitudes." *Human Reproduction* 15.9 (September 2000): 2052–2056. DOI: 10.1093/humrep/15.9.2052.

Gouge, Michael. "Embryo Adoption Scenarios: Drawing Distinctions and Separating Cases." *National Catholic Bioethics Quarterly* 12.3 (Autumn 2012): 439–445. DOI: 10.5840/ncbq201212327.

Grabowski, John S., and Christopher Gross. "*Dignitas Personae* and the Adoption of Frozen Embryos: A New Chill Factor?" In "Responses to *Dignitas Personae*: Part II of II," special issue, *National Catholic Bioethics Quarterly* 10.2 (Summer 2010): 307–328. DOI: 10.5840/ncbq201010255.

Gregory, Eric. "A Protestant View: The Ethics of Embryo Adoption and the Catholic Tradition." In *The Ethics of Embryo Adoption and the Catholic Tradition: Moral Arguments, Economic Reality and Social Analysis*, edited by Sarah-Vaughn Brakman and Darlene Fozard Weaver, 199–218. Dordrecht, NL: Springer, 2007.

Griese, Orville N. "The Perils of 'Embryo Transfer': Problems with 'SET'—Ethical, Physiological, Legal." *Ethics & Medics* 9.11 (November 1984): 2–4. DOI: 10.5840/em198491122.

Grisez, Germain. "Should a Woman Try to Bear Her Dead Sister's Embryo?" In *The Way of the Lord Jesus*. Vol. 3, *Difficult Moral Questions*, 239–244. Quincy, IL: Franciscan Press, 1997.

———. *The Way of the Lord Jesus*. Vol. 2, *Living a Christian Life*. Chicago: Franciscan Press, 1993.

———. *The Way of the Lord Jesus*. Vol. 3, *Difficult Moral Questions*. Quincy, IL: Franciscan Press, 1997.

Grisez, Germain, Joseph Boyle, John Finnis, and William E. May. "'Every Marital Act Ought to Be Open to New Life': Toward a Clearer Understanding." *Thomist* 52.3 (July 1988): 365–426.

Grondin, Charles. "Ectopic Pregnancy and Double Effect." Catholic Answers. Accessed March 12, 2024. https://www.catholic.com/qa/ectopic-pregnancy-and-double-effect.

Gross, Christopher. "Artificial Wombs: Could They Deliver an Answer to the Problem of Frozen Embryos?" *Christian Bioethics* 30.2 (August 2024): 96–105. DOI: 10.1093/cb/cbae004.

Gullo, Giuseppe, Stamatios Petousis, Achilleas Papatheodorou, Yannis Panagiotidis, Chrysoula Margioula-Siarkou, Nikolaos Prapas, et al. "Closed vs. Open Oocyte Vitrification Methods Are Equally Effective for Blastocyst Embryo Transfers: Prospective Study from a Sibling Oocyte Donation Program." *Gynecologic and Obstetric Investigation* 85.2 (April 2020): 206–212. DOI: 10.1159/000506803.

Haas, John. "Bioethics in the New Millennium." *National Catholic Bioethics Quarterly* 1.1 (Spring 2001): 15–21. DOI: 10.5840/ncbq20011170.

Haas, John, and Tadeusz Pacholczyk. "Moral Contraindications to the Adoption of Abandoned, Frozen Human Embryos." *Linacre Quarterly* 90.2 (May 2023): 139–144. DOI: 10.1177/00243639231165252.

Heape, Walter. "Preliminary Note on the Transplantation and Growth of Mammalian Ova within a Uterine Foster-Mother." *Proceedings of the Royal Society of London* 48 (January 1891): 457–458. DOI: 10.1098/rspl.1890.0093.

Heymann, Devorah, Liat Vidal, Zeev Shoham, Elena Kostova, Marian Showell, and Yuval Or. "The Effect of Hyaluronic Acid in Embryo Transfer Media in Donor Oocyte Cycles and Autologous Oocyte Cycles: A Systematic Review and Meta-Analysis." *Human Reproduction* 37.7 (June 30, 2022): 1451–1469. DOI: 10.1093/humrep/deac097.

Hollowell, Anthony. "Virgin Suicide and Vital Conflicts." *National Catholic Bioethics Quarterly* 21.2 (Summer 2021): 87–102. DOI: 10.5840/ncbq202121227

Hordern, Joshua. "'A Knife into My Heart': Cries, Compassion and Ethical Life." *New Bioethics* 29.3 (September 27, 2022): 279–295. DOI: 10.1080/20502877.2022.2124604.

Horn, Trent. Interview by Matt Fradd. YouTube. Streamed as "Reviewing Trent's ABORTION Debate with @destiny on @whatever" by Matt Fradd on July 29, 2023. https://www.youtube.com/watch?v=dx1u_WqxuEA&t=1s. See esp. sec. "Human Embryo Adoption," 0:38:32–0:41:12.

Hornick, Matthew A., Ali Y. Mejaddam, Patrick E. McGovern, et al. "Technical Feasibility of Umbilical Cannulation in Midgestation Lambs Supported by EXTra-Uterine Environment for Neonatal Development (EXTEND). *Artificial Organs* 43.12 (December 2019): 1156–1161. DOI: 10.1111/aor.13524.

Hurst, Daniel J. "What You Should Know about Frozen Embryo Adoption." The Ethics and Religious Liberty Commission of the Southern Baptist Convention. January 19, 2018. https://erlc.com/resource/what-you-should-know-about-frozen-embryo-adoption/.
Hursthouse, Rosalind *Beginning Lives*. Oxford: Blackwell, 1987.
Ilioi, Elena, Lucy Blake, Vasanti Jadva, Gabriela Roman, and Susan Golombok. "The Role of Age of Disclosure of Biological Origins in the Psychological Wellbeing of Adolescents Conceived by Reproductive Donation: A Longitudinal Study from Age 1 to Age 14." *Journal of Child Psychology and Psychiatry* 58.3 (March 2017): 315–324. DOI: 10.1111 /jcpp.12667.
International Federation of Fertility Societies. "Chapter 8: Donation." In "IFF Surveillance 07," edited by H. Jones Jr. and J. Cohen, special issue, *Fertility and Sterility* 87.4 suppl 1 (April 2007): S28–S32. DOI: 10.1016/j.fertnstert.2007.01.092.
International Theological Commission. *The Hope of Salvation for Infants Who Die without Being Baptized*. January 19, 2007.
Iozzio, Mary Jo. "It Is Time to Support Embryo Adoption." *National Catholic Bioethics Quaterly* 2.4 (Winter 2002): 585–593. DOI: 10.5840/ncbq2002242.
Jackson, Timothy P., ed. *The Morality of Adoption: Social-Psychological, Theological, and Legal Perspectives*. Grand Rapids, MI: Eerdmans, 2005.
James, David N. "Ectogenesis: A Reply to Singer and Wells." *Bioethics* 1.1 (January 1987): 80–99. DOI: 10.1111/j.1467-8519.1987.tb00006.x.
Jamison, Tracy. "Embryo Adoption and the Design of Human Nature: The Analogy between Artificial Insemination and Artificial Impregnation." In "Responses to *Dignitas Personae*: Part I of II," special issue, *National Catholic Bioethics Quarterly* 10.1 (Spring 2010): 111–122. DOI: 10.5840/ncbq201010175.
Jarvis, Gavin E. "Early Embryo Mortality in Natural Human Reproduction: What the Data Say." *F1000 Research* 5 (November 25, 2016): 2765. DOI: 10.12688/f1000research.8937.2.
Jennie (no last name given). "Embryos on Ice: Jennie's Story." Interview by Kallie Fell. *Venus Rising*. Podcast. Season 4, episode 57. October 25, 2022. Center for Bioethics and Culture Network. https://cbc-network.org/2022/10/embryos-on-ice-jennies-story/.
Jensen, Steven J. "Causal Constraints on Intention: A Critique of Tollefsen on the Phoenix Case." *National Catholic Bioethics Quarterly* 14.2 (Summer 2014): 273–293. DOI: 10.5840/ncbq201414230.
Jérôme Lejeune Foundation. *See* Dicastery for Laity, Family and Life.
John Paul II. Address to the Meeting of the Adoptive Families Organized by the Missionaries of Charity. September 5, 2000. https://www.vatican.va/content/john-paul-ii/en/speeches/2000/jul-sep/documents/hf_jp-ii_spe_20000905_adozioni.html.

———. Address to the Participants in the Solidarity March Organized by the Leaders of the Volunteer Association of Italian Blood and Organ Donors. August 2, 1984. Machine translated by Google. https://www.vatican.va/content/john-paul-ii/it/speeches/1984/august/documents/hf_jp-ii_spe_19840802_donatori.html.

———. Address to the Participants in the Symposium on "*Evangelium Vitae* and Law" and the Eleventh International Colloquium on Roman and Canon Law. EWTN. May 24, 1996. https://www.ewtn.com/catholicism/library/i-appeal-to-worlds-scientific-authorities-halt-the-production-of-human-embryos-8784.

———. *Evangelium vitae*. March 15, 1995. https://www.vatican.va/content/john-paul-ii/en/encyclicals/documents/hf_jp-ii_enc_25031995_evangelium-vitae.html.

———. *Familiaris consortio*. November 22, 1981. https://www.vatican.va/content/john-paul-ii/en/apost_exhortations/documents/hf_jp-ii_exh_19811122_familiaris-consortio.html.

———. *Fides et ratio*. September 14, 1998. https://www.vatican.va/content/john-paul-ii/en/encyclicals/documents/hf_jp-ii_enc_14091998_fides-et-ratio.html.

———. General audience. Vatican City. September 16, 1998. https://www.vatican.va/content/john-paul-ii/en/audiences/1998/documents/hf_jp-ii_aud_16091998.html.

———. *Gratissimam sane*. February 2, 1994. https://www.vatican.va/content/john-paul-ii/en/letters/1994/documents/hf_jp-ii_let_02021994_families.html.

———. Letter to the Pontifical Academy of Sciences. February 1, 2005. https://www.vatican.va/content/john-paul-ii/en/messages/pont_messages/2005/documents/hf_jp-ii_mes_20050201_p-acad-sciences.html.

———. *Man and Woman He Created Them: A Theology of the Body*. Translated by Michael Waldstein. Boston: Pauline Books and Media, 2006.

———. *Mulieris dignitatem*. August 15, 1988. https://www.vatican.va/content/john-paul-ii/en/apost_letters/1988/documents/hf_jp-ii_apl_19880815_mulieris-dignitatem.html.

———. *Redemptoris custos*. August 15, 1989. https://www.vatican.va/content/john-paul-ii/en/apost_exhortations/documents/hf_jp-ii_exh_15081989_redemptoris-custos.html.

———. *The Theology of the Body: Human Love in the Divine Plan*. Boston: Pauline Books and Media, 1997.

———. *Original Unity of Man and Woman*. Boston: St. Paul Editions, 1981.

———. *Veritatis splendor*. August 6, 1993. https://www.vatican.va/content/john-paul-ii/en/encyclicals/documents/hf_jp-ii_enc_06081993_veritatis-splendor.html.

———. *The Way to Christ: Spiritual Exercises*. Translated by Leslie Wearne. San Francisco: Harper, 1994.

Jones, D. A. "The Human Embryo in the Christian Tradition: A Reconsideration." *Journal of Medical Ethics* 31.12 (December 2005): 710–714. DOI: 10.1136/jme.2004.011593.

Kaczor, Christopher. "Anthropological, Theological and Ethical Aspects of Human Life and Procreation (nn. 1–10)." In "Symposium on *Dignitas Personae*," special article, edited by E. Christian Brugger. *National Catholic Bioethics Quarterly* 9.3 (Autumn 2009): 464–467. DOI: 10.5840/20099333.

———. "The Artificial Womb and the End of Abortion." Chap. 10 in *Agency, Pregnancy and Persons*, edited by Nicholas Colgrove, Bruce P. Blackshaw, and Daniel Rodger. New York: Routledge, 2023.

———. "Artificial Wombs and Embryo Adoption." In *The Ethics of Embryo Adoption and the Catholic Tradition: Moral Arguments, Economic Reality and Social Analysis*, edited by Sarah-Vaughan Brakman and Darlene Fozard Weaver, 307–322. Dordrecht, NL: Springer, 2007.

———. "Could Artificial Wombs End the Abortion Debate?" *National Catholic Bioethics Quarterly* 5.2 (Summer 2005): 283–301. DOI: 10.5840/ncbq20055248.

———. *Defense of Dignity: Creating Life, Destroying Life, Protecting the Rights of Conscience*. Notre Dame, IN: University of Notre Dame Press, 2013. See esp. chap. 5, "Embryo Adoption and Artificial Wombs," and chap. 6, "The Ethics of Ectopic Pregnancy."

———. *The Edge of Life: Human Dignity and Contemporary Bioethics*. Dordrecht, NL: Springer, 2005. See esp. chap. 7, "Could Artificial Wombs End the Abortion Debate?"

———. Notes & Abstracts: Philosophy and Theology. *National Catholic Bioethics Quarterly* 7.2 (Summer 2007): 383–388, esp. "Licitness of Embryo Adoption," 386–388. DOI: 10.5840/ncbq20077264. Response to Steven Long, "An Argument for the Embryonic Intactness of Marriage."

———. Notes & Abstracts: Philosophy and Theology. *National Catholic Bioethics Quarterly* 9.1 (Spring 2009): 185–191, esp. 186. DOI: 10.5840/ncbq20099189.

———. Notes & Abstracts: Philosophy and Theology. *National Catholic Bioethics Quarterly* 14.4 (Winter 2014): 753–758, esp. 757–758. DOI: 10.5840/ncbq201414477.

———. Notes & Abstracts: Philosophy and Theology. *National Catholic Bioethics Quarterly* 21.1 (Spring 2021): 157–163. [Kaczor discusses artificial wombs.] DOI: 10.5840/ncbq202121114.

———. Review of *The Ethics of Pregnancy, Abortion, and Childbirth: Exploring Moral Choices in Childbearing*, by Helen Watt. *National Catholic Bioethics Quarterly* 17.2 (Summer 2017): 365–367, esp. 367. DOI: 10.5840/ncbq201717237.

Kalra, Suleena Kansal, and Thomas A. Molinaro. "The Association of In Vitro Fertilization and Perinatal Morbidity." *Seminars in Reproductive Medicine* 26.5 (September 2008): 423–435. DOI: 10.1055/s-0028-1087108.

Kant, Immanuel. *Groundwork of the Metaphysics of Morals*, edited by M. Gregor. Cambridge: Cambridge University Press, 1997.

Keenan, Jeffrey. "Development of the National Embryo Donation Center." In *The Ethics of Embryo Adoption and the Catholic Tradition: Moral Arguments, Economic Reality and Social Analysis*, edited by Sarah-Vaughn Brakman and Darlene Fozard Weaver, 221–230. Dordrecht, NL: Springer 2007.

Kellmeyer, Steve. "Embryo Adoption: A Form of In Vivo Organ Donation?" *National Catholic Bioethics Quarterly* 7.2 (Summer 2007): 263–270. DOI: 10.5840/ncbq20077255.

Kong, Fei, Yu Fu, Huifeng Shi, Rong Li, Yangyu Zhao, Yuanyuan Wang, et al. "Placental Abnormalities and Placenta-Related Complications following In-Vitro Fertilization: Based on National Hospitalized Data in China." *Frontiers in Endocrinology* 13 (June 30, 2022), 924070. DOI: 10.3389/fendo.2022.924070.

Krier, Jessie C., Tonika Duren Green, and Ashley Kruger. "Youths in Foster Care with Language Delays: Prevalence, Causes, and Interventions." *Psychology in the Schools* 55.5 (May 2018): 523–538. DOI: 10.1002/pits.22129.

Krivak, John A. "Heterologous Embryo Transfer as an Act of Adoption: A Moral Analysis based on a Catholic Theology of Adoption." PhD diss., Fordham University, 2015. ETD Collection for Fordham University (AAI3715378). ProQuest (3715378).

Landers, Ashley L., Saron M. Danes, Avery R. Campbell, and Sandy White Hawk. "Abuse after Abuse: The Recurrent Maltreatment of American Indian Children in Foster Care and Adoption." *Child Abuse and Neglect* 111 (January 2021), 104805. DOI: 10.1016/j.chiabu.2020.104805.

Lasnoski, Kent. "'Setting the Captives Free': Is There Precedent for Embryo Adoption in Scripture and Medieval Christian Tradition?" Posted by Charles Camosy. *Catholic Moral Theology* (blog), January 28, 2013. https://catholicmoraltheology.com/setting-the-captives-free-is-there-precedent-for-embryo-adoption-in-scripture-and-medieval-christian-tradition/.

———. "Setting the Captives Free: Precedent for Embryo Adoption in Scripture and the Catholic Tradition." *Josephinum Journal of Moral Theology* 20.1 (2013): 88–112.

———. "The Moral Basis for the Adoption of Abandoned, Frozen Human Embryos." *Linacre Quarterly* 90.2 (May 2023): 135–138. DOI: 10.1177/00243639231165245.

Latkovic, Mark S. "The Dignity of the Person: An Overview and Commentary on *Dignitas Personae*." In "Responses to *Dignitas Personae*: Part II of II," special issue, *National Catholic Bioethics Quarterly* 10.2 (Summer 2010): 283–305. DOI: 10.5840/ncbq201010254. See esp. pp. 293–296.

Lauritzen, Paul. "From Rescuing Frozen Embryos to Respecting the Limits of Nature: Reframing the Embryo Adoption Debate." In *The Ethics of Embryo Adoption and the Catholic Tradition: Moral Arguments, Economic Reality and Social Analysis*, edited by Sarah-Vaughn Brakman and Darlene Fozard Weaver, 161–174. Dordrecht, NL: Springer 2007.

Lee, Henry C., Jeffrey B. Gould, W. John Boscardin, Yasser Y. El-Sayed, and Yair J. Blumenfeld. "Trends in Cesarean Delivery for Twin Births in the United States: 1995–2008." *Obstetrics and Gynecology* 118.5 (November 2011): 1095–1101. DOI: 10.1097/AOG.0b013e3182318651.

Leies, John A. *Handbook on Critical Life Issues*. Revised 3rd ed. Philadelphia: National Catholic Bioethics Center, 2016. See esp. pp. 100–101.

Leies, John A., Donald G. McCarthy, and Edward J. Bayer. *Handbook on Critical Life Issues*. 2nd ed. Edited by Louise A. Mitchell. Brighton, MA: National Catholic Bioethics Center, 2004. See esp. pp. 104–105.

———. *Handbook on Critical Life Issues*. 3rd ed. Philadelphia: National Catholic Bioethics Center, 2010.

Lejeune, Jérôme. *The Concentration Can: When Does Human Life Begin? An Eminent Geneticist Testifies*. San Francisco: Ignatius Press, 1992.

Lensen, Sarah, Diana Osavlyuk, Sarah Armstrong, Caroline Stadelmann, Aurélie Hennes, Emma Napier, et al. "A Randomized Trial of Endometrial Scratching before In Vitro Fertilization." *New England Journal of Medicine* 380.4 (January 24, 2019): 325–334. DOI: 10.1056/NEJMoa1808737.

Leslie, Laurel K., Jeanne N. Gordon, Katina Lambros, Kamila Premji, John Peoples, and Kristin Gist. "Addressing the Developmental and Mental Health Needs of Young Children in Foster Care." *Journal of Developmental and Behavioral Pediatrics* 26.2 (April 2005): 140–151. DOI: 10.1097/00004703-200504000-00011.

Lester, Caroline. "Embryo 'Adoption' Is Growing but It's Getting Tangled in the Abortion Debate." *New York Times*, February 17, 2019. https://www.nytimes.com/2019/02/17/health/embryo-adoption-donated-snowflake.html.

Letterie, Gerard. "In Re: The Disposition of Frozen Embryos: 2022." *Fertility and Sterility* 117.3 (March 2022): 479. DOI: 10.1016/j.fertnstert.2022.01.001.

Letter to the Editor. *Linacre Quarterly* 76.4 (November 2009): 363–366. DOI: 10.1179/002436309803889007.

Letter to the Editor. *Linacre Quarterly* 78.4 (November 2011): 375–380. DOI: 10.1080/002436311803888212.

Liao, S. Matthew. "The Right of Children to Be Loved." *Journal of Political Philosophy* 14.4 (November 2006): 420–440. DOI: 10.1111/j.1467-9760.2006.00262.x.

———. *The Right to Be Loved.* New York: Oxford University Press, 2015.
LifeSite News. "Top Catholic Ethicists Duel over Frozen Embryo Adoption." August 2, 2011. https://www.lifesitenews.com/news/top-catholic-ethicists-duel-over-frozen-embryo-adoption/.
Lomax, Geoffrey P., and Alan O. Trounson. "Correcting Misperceptions about Cryopreserved Embryos and Stem Cell Research." *Nature Biotechnology* 31.4 (April 5, 2013): 288–290. DOI: 10.1038/nbt.2541.
Long, Steven A. "An Argument for the Embryonic Intactness of Marriage." *Thomist* 70.2 (April 2006): 267–288. DOI: 10.1353/tho.2006.0019.
———. "A Brief Disquisition regarding the Nature of the Object of the Moral Act according to St. Thomas Aquinas." *Thomist* 67.1 (January 2003): 45–71. DOI: 10.1353/tho.2003.0037.
Lopes, Ana S., Veerle Frederickx, Gunther Van Kerkhoven, Rudi Campo, Patrick Puttemans, and Stephan Gordts. "Re-Expansion and Cell Survival of Human Blastocysts following Vitrification and Warming Using Two Vitrification Systems." *Journal of Assisted Reproduction and Genetics* 32.1 (January 2015): 83–90. DOI: 10.1007/s10815-014-0373-2.
López Barahona, Mónica, Ramón Lucas Lucas, and Slavador Antuñano Alea. "The Moral Licitness of Adopting Frozen Embryos, with Answers to Objections." In *Human Embryo Adoption: Biotechnology, Marriage, and the Right to Life*, edited by Thomas V. Berg and Edward J. Furton, 273–295. Philadelphia: National Catholic Bioethics Center, 2006.
Lovering, Rob. "A Moral Argument for Frozen Human Embryo Adoption." *Bioethics* 34.3 (March 2020): 242–251. DOI: 10.1111/bioe.12671.
Lubov, Deborah Castellano. "Pope Francis: Church a 'Field Hospital for Vulnerable.'" Vatican News. May 14, 2022. https://www.vaticannews.va/en/pope/news/2022-05/pope-francis-audience-village-of-francis.html.
Lyerly, Anne Drapkin, Karen Steinhauser, Corrine Voils, Emily Namey, Carolyn Alexander, Brandon Bankowski, et al. "Fertility Patients' Views about Frozen Embryo Disposition: Results of a Multi-Institutional U.S. Survey." *Fertility and Sterility* 93.2 (February 2010): 499–509. DOI: 10.1016/j.fertnstert.2008.10.015.
Lysaught, M. Therese. "Embryo Adoption?" *Human Life Review* 29.4 (Fall 2003): 94–98.
———. "Embryo Adoption? The Dilemmas of Fertility." *Commonweal* 130, September 26, 2003, 15–19.
MacCallum, Fiona, and Sarah Keeley. "Embryo Donation Families: A Follow-Up in Middle Childhood." *Journal of Family Psychology* 22.6 (December 2008): 799–808, doi: 10.1037/a0013197.
MacCallum, Fiona, and Susan Golombok. "Embryo Donation Families: Mothers' Decisions regarding Disclosure of Donor Conception." *Human Reproduction* 22.11 (November 2007): 2888–2895. DOI: 10.1093/humrep/dem272.

Bibliography

MacCallum, Fiona, Susan Golombok, and Peter Brinsden. "Parenting and Child Development in Families with a Child Conceived through Embryo Donation." *Journal of Family Psychology* 21.2 (June 2007): 278–287. DOI: 10.1037/0893-3200.21.2.278.

MacKinnon, Grace. "Can Frozen Embryos Be Saved?" *Catholic Answers Magazine*, January 1, 2002. https://www.catholic.com/magazine/print-edition/can-frozen-embryos-be-saved.

―――. "Theologians Argue Frozen Embryos' Fate." *Catholic Medical Quarterly*, November 2001: 4. www.cmq.org.uk/CMQ/2001/frozen_embryos.htm. Reprinted from *HLI Reports* 19.8 (August 2001).

Machin, Laura. "A Hierarchy of Needs? Embryo Donation, In Vitro Fertilisation and the Provision of Infertility Counselling." *Patient Education and Counseling* 85.2 (November 2011): 264–268. DOI: 10.1016/j.pec.2010.09.014.

Maertens-Pizzo, Colten P. "Artificial Wombs Replace One Violence with Another." *Ethics & Medics* 45.11 (November 2020): 1–2. DOI: 10.5840/em2020451119.

Maheshwari, Abha, Shilpi Pandey, Edwin Amalraj Raja, Ashalatha Shetty, Mark Hamilton, and Siladitya Bhattacharya. "Is Frozen Embryo Transfer Better for Mothers and Babies? Can Cumulative Meta-Analysis Provide a Definitive Answer?" *Human Reproduction Update* 24.1 (January–February 2018): 35–58. DOI: 10.1093/humupd/dmx031.

Mahowald, Mary B. "Embryo *Adoption*? An Egalitarian Perspective." In *The Ethics of Embryo Adoption and the Catholic Tradition: Moral Arguments, Economic Reality and Social Analysis*, edited by Sarah-Vaughn Brakman and Darlene Fozard Weaver, 175–198. Dordrecht, NL: Springer 2007.

Malone, Jay R. "Ethics of Cryopreserved Embryo Adoption: Defrosting *Dignitas Personae*." *Health Care Ethics USA* 27.4 (Fall 2019): 2–14.

Mao, Yuling, Ni Tang, Yanfen Luo, Ping Yin, and Lei Li. "Effects of Vitrified Cryopreservation Duration on IVF and Neonatal Outcomes." *Journal of Ovarian Research* 15.1 (September 8, 2022): 101. DOI: 10.1186/s13048-022-01035-8.

Marquis, Don. "Why Abortion Is Immoral." *Journal of Philosophy* 86.4 (April 1989): 183–202. DOI: 10.2307/2026961.

Marshall, Alfred. *The Interlinear NRSV-NIV Parallel New Testament in Greek and English*. Grand Rapids, MI: Zondervan, 1994.

Matheson, Jonathan. "Moral Caution and the Epistemology of Disagreement." *Journal of Social Philosophy* 47.2 (Summer 2016): 125–126. DOI: 10.1111/josp.12145.

May, William E. *Catholic Bioethics and the Gift of Human Life*. Huntington, IN: Our Sunday Visitor, 2000. See esp. chap. 3, part 5, "'Rescuing' Frozen Embryos," 94–108, 115–118.

———. *Catholic Bioethics and the Gift of Human Life*. 2nd ed. Huntington, IN: Our Sunday Visitor, 2008. See esp. chap. 3, part 5, "'Rescuing' Frozen Embryos," 95–112, 119–125.

———. *Catholic Bioethics and the Gift of Human Life*. 3rd ed. Huntington, IN: Our Sunday Visitor, 2013. See esp. chap. 3, part 6, "'Rescuing' Frozen Embryos," 113, 120.

———. Colloquy. *National Catholic Bioethics Quarterly* 10.4 (Winter 2010): 646–647. DOI: 10.5840/ncbq20101041.

———. "Dr. May Responds." Colloquy. *National Catholic Bioethics Quarterly* 11.2 (Summer 2011): 216–217. DOI: 10.5840/ncbq201111248.

———. "Embryo Adoption and Conscience." Colloquy. *National Catholic Bioethics Quarterly* 11.4 (Winter 2011): 619–620. DOI: 10.5840/ncbq20111141.

———. "The Embryo Adoption Debate: Gormally vs. Finnis." Culture of Life Foundation. October 9, 2009. http://culture-of-life.org/content/view/596/110/. (Website discontinued.)

———. Letter to the editor in "Three Notes from Our Readers: Comments on Embryo Adoption." *Ethics & Medics* 26.11 (November 2001): 4. DOI: 10.5840/em2001261123.

———. "On 'Rescuing' Frozen Embryos: Why the Decision to Do So Is Moral." In "Human Embryo Transfer," special issue, *National Catholic Bioethics Quarterly* 5.1 (Spring 2005): 51–57. DOI: 10.5840/ncbq20055166. This is a revised version of the presentation at the Westchester Institute Scholars Forum and was later revised as "The Object of the Acting Woman in Embryo Rescue."

———. Presentation. The Westchester Institute Scholars Forum: On the Morality of Heterologous Embryo Transfer. Washington, DC, October 28–29, 2004. This was later revised and published as "On 'Rescuing' Frozen Embryos."

———. "Rescuing Frozen Embryos." Chap. 3, part 5, in *Catholic Bioethics and the Gift of Human Life*, 94–118. Huntington, IN: Our Sunday Visitor, 2000.

———. "Rescuing Frozen Embryos." Chap. 3, part 5, in *Catholic Bioethics and the Gift of Human Life*, 2nd ed., 95–125. Huntington, IN: Our Sunday Visitor, 2008.

———. "The Embryo Rescue Debate." Colloquy. *National Catholic Bioethics Quarterly* 4.1 (Spring 2004): 9–10. DOI: 10.5840/ncbq20044162.

———. "The Morality of 'Rescuing' Frozen Embryos." In *What Is Man, O Lord? The Human Person in a Biotech Age: Proceedings of the Eighteenth Bishops' Workshop*, edited by Edward J. Furton and Louise A. Mitchell, 201–215. Boston: National Catholic Bioethics Center, 2002.

———. "The Object of the Acting Woman in Embryo Rescue." In *Human Embryo Adoption: Biotechnology, Marriage, and the Right to Life*, edited by Thomas V. Berg and Edward J. Furton, 135–163. Philadelphia: National Catholic Bioethics Center, 2006. This is a revised version of "On 'Rescuing' Frozen Embryos" and was later revised as chap. 3, part 5, "'Rescuing' Frozen Embryos," of *Catholic Bioethics and the Gift of Human Life*, 2nd ed.

Bibliography

Mayer, Ryan C. "Is Embryo Adoption a Form of Surrogacy?" *National Catholic Bioethics Quarterly* 11.2 (Summer 2011): 249–266. DOI: 10.5840/ncbq201111252.

McCarthy, C. Ryan. "Embryo Adoption." Interview by Tom McGovern [?]. *Doctor, Doctor*. Podcast. Episode 27. July 20, 2019. Soundcloud. https://soundcloud.com/user-546435917/dd-27-embryo-adoption (Podcast not available.)

———. "Embryo Adoption Part 1: Pro (with Fr. Ryan McCarthy)." Hosted by Tom McGovern and Andrew Mullally. *Doctor, Doctor*. Podcast. Episode 298. YouTube. January 13, 2023. https://www.youtube.com/watch?v=R5io-MlxaWk. *See also* Alexander, Irene. "Embryo Adoption Part 2: Con."

———. *What To Do with the Least of Our Brothers? Finding Moral Solutions to the Problem of Endangered Embryos*. Charlotte, NC: Saint Benedict Press, 2015.

McGovern, Celeste. "Brave New Womb: Embryos' Dilemma." *National Catholic Register*, May 25, 2003.

McTavish, James. "Suffering, Death, and Eternal Life." *Linacre Quarterly* 83.2 (May 2016): 139. DOI: 10.1080/00243639.2016.1166338.

Meaney, Joseph. "The Question of Embryo Adoption." The Moral Mind. National Catholic Bioethics Center. March 18, 2025. https://www.ncbcenter.org/messsages-from-presidents/ethicsofembryoadoption.

Meilaender, Gilbert C. *Not by Nature But by Grace: Forming Families through Adoption*. Catholic Ideas for a Secular World. Notre Dame, Indiana: University of Notre Dame Press, 2016. See esp. chap. 5, "Adopting Embryos."

Menart, Teresa. "Is Adoption the Best Solution to the Plight of Frozen Embryos?" Colloquy. *National Catholic Bioethics Quarterly* 1.3 (Autumn 2001): 293–294. DOI: 10.5840/ncbq20011325.

Miller, Kevin E. Review of *The Edge of Life: Human Dignity and Contemporary Bioethics*, by Christopher Kaczor. *National Catholic Bioethics Quarterly* 8.3 (Autumn 2008): 589–592. DOI: 10.5840/ncbq20088347. See esp. 592.

Miller, Monica Migliorino. "Adopting Embryos: Here's Why Not—A Rejoinder in the Bioethical Debate." *National Catholic Register*, May 15, 2009. https://www.ncregister.com/commentaries/adopting-embryos-here-s-why-not.

———. "Extremely Insightful." *National Catholic Register* [?], March 15 [2009?].

Mirus, Jeff. "On Melting Snowflakes and Saving Babies: The State of the Question." Catholic Culture. September 5, 2013. https://www.catholicculture.org/commentary/on-melting-snowflakes-and-saving-babies-state-question/?repos=6&subrepos=0&searchid=2494423.

[Moraczewski, Albert S.?]. "Human Embryo Transplantation: Who Will Decide—Lawyers or M.D.'s." *Ethics & Medics* 4.2 (February 1979): 2. DOI: 10.5840/em1979426.

Moschella, Melissa. "Gestation Does Not Necessarily Imply Parenthood: Implications for the Morality of Embryo Adoption and Embryo Rescue." *American*

Catholic Philosophical Quarterly 92.1 (Winter 2018): 21–48. DOI: 10.5840/acpq20171130137.

———. "Sexual Ethics, Human Nature, and the 'New' and 'Old' Natural Law Theories." *National Catholic Bioethics Quarterly* 19.2 (Summer 2019): 251–278. DOI: 10.5840/ncbq201919218.

———. "Sexual Ethics, Practical Reason, and the Magisterium: A Response to Irene Alexander." *National Catholic Bioethics Quarterly* 22.1 (Spring 2022): 99–127. DOI: 10.5840/ncbq20222219.

Mullen, David J. Letter to the editor in "Three Notes from Our Readers: Comments on Embryo Adoption." *Ethics & Medics* 26.11 (November 2001): 4. DOI: 10.5840/em2001261123.

Mumusoglu, Sezcan, Mehtap Polat, Irem Yarali Ozbek, Gurkan Bozdag, Evangelos G. Papanikolaou, Sandro C. Esteves, et al. "Preparation of the Endometrium for Frozen Embryo Transfer: A Systematic Review." *Frontiers in Endocrinology* 12 (July 9, 2021)L 688237. DOI: 10.3389/fendo.2021.688237.

Murphy, Timothy F. "Dignity, Marriage and Embryo Adoption: A Look at *Dignitas Personae*." *Reproductive Biomedicine Online* 23.7 (December 2011): 860–868. DOI: 10.1016/j.rbmo.2011.06.001.

Napier, Stephen. "Moral Justification and Human Acts: A Reply to Christopher Oleson." *Linacre Quarterly* 76.2 (May 2009): 150–162. DOI: 10.1179/002436309803889214.

National Conference of Catholic Bishops Committee on Doctrine. *The Teaching Ministry of the Diocesan Bishop: A Pastoral Reflection*. Washington, DC: NCCB, 1992.

National Embryo Adoption Center. "About." Accessed February 29, 2024. https://www.embryodonation.org/about.

Nehrbass, Daniel. "What If We Are Catholic … Can We Still Pursue Embryo Adoption?" Nightlight Christian Adoptions. March 18, 2022. https://nightlight.org/2022/03/what-if-we-are-catholic-can-we-still-do-embryo-adoption/.

NeJaime, Douglas. "Who Is a Parent?" American Bar Association, May 10, 2021. https://www.americanbar.org/groups/family_law/publications/family-advocate/2021/spring/who-a-parent/.

Nelson, Margaret K., Rosanna Hertz, and Wendy Kramer. "Gamete Donor Anonymity and Limits on Numbers of Offspring: The Views of Three Stakeholders." *Journal of Law and Bioscience* 3.1 (April 2016): 39–67. DOI: 10.1093/jlb/lsv045.

Nelson, Thomas K. "Personal Relatedness and Embryo Adoption." Colloquy. *National Catholic Bioethics Quarterly* 14.4 (Winter 2014): 601–602. DOI: 10.5840/ncbq201414463.

Bibliography

———. "Personhood and Embryo Adoption." *Linacre Quarterly* 79.3 (August 2012): 261–274. DOI: 10.1179/002436312804872767.

———. "Reply to Brother Breed on Embryo Adoption." Colloquy. *National Catholic Bioethics Quarterly* 15.3 (Autumn 2015): 422–423. DOI: 10.5840/ncbq201515341.

Nichols, Arland K. Colloquy. *National Catholic Bioethics Quarterly* 11.4 (Winter 2011): 620–622. DOI: 10.5840/ncbq20111141.

———. *Handbook on Critical Life Issues*. 4th ed. Broomall, PA: National Catholic Bioethics Center, 2024. See esp. "Prenatal Adoption," 225–228, 237.

Nightline Christian Adoptions. "The Beginning of Embryo Adoption." Accessed March 22, 2024, https://nightlight.org/testimonial/the-beginning-of-embryo-adoption/.

Nolt, John. "How Harmful Are the Average American's Greenhouse Gas Emissions?" *Ethics, Policy and the Environment* 14.1 (May 2011): 3–10. DOI: 10.1080/21550085.2011.561584.

Nuffield Council on Bioethics. "Donor Conception: Ethical Aspects of Information Sharing." April 17, 2013. https://www.nuffieldbioethics.org/publications/donor-conception.

O'Connell, Gerald, "Death of the 'Ice Babies.'" *Tablet* (UK), August 10, 1996.

O'Donovan, Oliver. *Begotten or Made?* New York: Oxford University Press, 1984.

Oesterle, John. *Logic: The Art of Defining and Reasoning*, 2nd ed. Upper Saddle River, NJ: Prentice Hall, 1963.

Okby, Rania, Avi Harlev, Kira Nahum Sacks, Ruslan Sergienko, and Eyal Sheiner. "Preeclampsia Acts Differently in In Vitro Fertilization versus Spontaneous Twins." *Archives of Gynecology and Obstetrics* 297.3 (March 2018): 653–658. DOI: 10.1007/s00404-017-4635-y.

Oleson, Christopher. "*Dignitas Personae* and the Question of Heterologous Embryo Transfer." *Linacre Quarterly* 76.2 (May 2009): 133–149. DOI: 10.1179/002436309803889250.

———. "The Immorality of Heterologous Embryo Transfer." Paper. The Westchester Institute Scholars Forum: On the Morality of Heterologous Embryo Transfer. Washington, DC, October 28–29, 2004.

———. "More Thoughts on *Dignitas Personae* and Embryo Rescue: A Reply to Stephen Napier." *Linacre Quarterly* 76.3 (August 2009): 250–264. DOI: 10.1179/002436309803889151.

———. "The Nuptial Womb: On the Moral Significance of Being with Child." In *Human Embryo Adoption: Biotechnology, Marriage and the Right to Life*, edited by Thomas V. Berg and Edward J. Furton, 165–196. Philadelphia: National Catholic Bioethics Center, 2006.

Onder, Robert F. "Practical and Moral Caveats on Heterologous Embryo Transfer." In "Human Embryo Transfer," special issue, *National Catholic Bioethics Quarterly* 5.1 (Spring 2005): 75–94. DOI: 10.5840/ncbq20055169.

O'Rourke, Kevin D. "Catholic Principles and In Vitro Fertilization." *National Catholic Bioethics Quarterly* 10.4 (Winter 2010): 709–722, esp. 720. DOI: 10.5840/ncbq20101048.

Overall, Christine. *Why Have Children? The Ethical Debate.* Cambridge, MA: MIT Press, 2012.

Pacholczyk, Tadeusz. "Examining Some Objections to Heterologous Transfer of 'Abandoned' Embryos." Presentation. The Westchester Institute Scholars Forum: On the Morality of Heterologous Embryo Transfer. Washington, DC, October 28–29, 2004.

———. "Frozen Embryo Adoptions Are Morally Objectionable." In *The Catholic Citizen: Debating the Issues of Justice*, edited by Kenneth D. Whitehead, 84–101. South Bend, IN: St. Augustine Press, 2004.

———. "Germany and Italy Have Done It—Shouldn't We?" Making Sense of Bioethics 42. December 2008. https://www.ncbcenter.org/making-sense-of-bioethics-cms/column-042-germany-and-italy-have-done-it-shouldnt-we.

———. "On the Moral Objectionability of Human Embryo Adoption." In *The Ethics of Embryo Adoption and the Catholic Tradition: Moral Arguments, Economic Reality and Social Analysis*, edited by Sarah-Vaughn Brakman and Darlene Fozard Weaver, 69–83. Dordrecht, NL: Springer 2007.

———. "Orphans in Liquid Nitrogen." Making Sense of Bioethics 137. November 2016. https://www.ncbcenter.org/making-sense-of-bioethics-cms/column-137-orphans-in-liquid-nitrogen.

———. "What Should We Do with the Frozen Embryos?" Making Sense of Bioethics 48. June 2009. https://www.ncbcenter.org/making-sense-of-bioethics-cms/column-048-what-should-we-do-with-the-frozen-embryos.

———. "Some Moral Contraindications to Embryo Adoption." In *Human Embryo Adoption: Biotechnology, Marriage, and the Right to Life*, edited by Thomas V. Berg and Edward J. Furton, 37–53. Philadelphia: National Catholic Bioethics Center, 2006.

Partridge, Emily A., Marcus G. Davey, Matthew A. Hornick, et al. "An Extra-Uterine System to Physiologically Support the Extreme Premature Lamb." *Nature Communications* 8 (2017): 15112. DOI: 10.1038/ncomms15112.

Partridge, Emily A., Marcus G. Davey, Matthew A. Hornick, and Alan W. Flake. "An EXTrauterine Environment for Neonatal Development: EXTENDING Fetal Physiology beyond the Womb." *Seminars in Fetal and Neonatal Medicine* 22.6 (December 2017): 404–409. DOI: 10.1016/j.siny.2017.04.006.

Patel, Bonnie G., and Brooke V. Rossi. "Embryo Donation: Medical Aspects." In *Third Party Reproduction: A Comprehensive Guide*, edited by James M. Goldfarb, 95–100. New York: Springer, 2014.

Bibliography

Patterson, Colin. "Embryo Adoption: Some Further Considerations." *Linacre Quarterly* 82.1 (February 2015): 34–38. DOI:10.1179/2050854914Y0000000029.

Paul VI. *Humanae vitae*. July 25, 1968. https://www.vatican.va/content/paul-vi/en/encyclicals/documents/hf_p-vi_enc_25071968_humanae-vitae.html.

Pinches, Charles. *Theology and Action: After Theory in Christian Ethics*. Grand Rapids, MI: Eerdmans, 2002.

Pincus, G., and E.V. Enzmann. "Can Mammalian Eggs Undergo Normal Development In Vitro?" *Biological Sciences* 20.2 (February 1934): 121–122. DOI: 10.1073/pnas.20.2.121.

Pius XII. "Allocution to a Group of Eye Specialists, May 14, 1956." In *The Human Body*, selected and arranged by the Monks of Solesmes, 373–384. Boston: St. Paul Editions, 1960.

———. "Allocution to Delegates at the 26th Congress of Urology, October 8, 1953." In *The Human Body*, selected and arranged by the Monks of Solesmes. Boston: St. Paul Editions, 1960, 277–281.

———. "Allocution to Military Surgeons, October 19, 1953." In *The Human Body*, selected and arranged by the Monks of Solesmes, 281–283. Boston: St. Paul Editions, 1960.

———. "Allocution to the First International Congress of Histopathology, September 13, 1952." In *The Human Body*, selected and arranged by the Monks of Solesmes, 194–208. Boston: St. Paul Editions, 1960.

———. "Allocution to the Second World Congress on Fertility and Sterility. May 19, 1956." In *The Human Body*, selected and arranged by the Monks of Solesmes, 384–394. Boston: St. Paul Editions, 1960.

Pomană, Cristina-Diana, Prabhu Chandra Mishra, Elvira Brătilă, and Diana Mihai. "The Fate of Frozen Embryos: Their Destruction, Adoption or Donation?" *Ginecologia.ro* 9.32 (2021): 17ff.

Pontifical Academy for Life Tenth General Assembly. *Final Communique on "The Dignity of Human Procreation and Reproductive Technologies. Anthropological and Ethical Aspects."* February 2004. https://www.vatican.va/roman_curia/pontifical_academies/acdlife/documents/rc_pont-acd_life_doc_20040316_x-gen-assembly-final_en.html.

Pontifical Council for Justice and Peace. *Compendium of the Social Doctrine of the Church*. Rome: Libreria Editrice Vaticana, 2004.

Post, Stephen G. "Adoption: A Protestant Agapic Perspective." In *The Morality of Adoption: Social-Psychological, Theological, and Legal Perspectives*, edited by Timothy P. Jackson, 172–187. Grand Rapids, MI: Eerdmans, 2005.

Pruss, Alexander R. "I Was Once a Fetus: That Is Why Abortion Is Wrong." In *Persons, Moral Worth, and Embryos: A Critical Analysis of Pro-Choice Arguments*, edited by Stephen Napier, 19–42. New York: Springer, 2011.

Pugeda, Teofilo Giovan S., III. "An Overview of the Embryo Adoption Debate." *Philippiniana Sacra* 57.173 (May–August 2022): 187–214.

___. "Embryo Reception and Maternal Identity." *Linacre Quarterly* 90.3 (August 2023): DOI: 10.1177/00243639231184026.
Quigley, Muireann. "A Right to Reproduce?" *Bioethics* 24.8 (October 2010): 403–411. DOI: 10.1111/j.1467-8519.2008.00722.x.
Ramirez, Nicholas. "Homologous Embryo Transfer: An Issue for Certain Arguments against Embryo Rescue and Embryo Adoption." Colloquy. *National Catholic Bioethics Quarterly* 24.3 (Autumn 2024): 407–410. DOI: 10.5840/ncbq202424332.
___. "Heterologous Embryo Transfer: A Thomistic Approach." *National Catholic Bioethics Quarterly* 24.3 (Autumn 2024): 437–446. DOI: 10.5840/ncbq202424335.
Ratzinger, Joseph. *Daughter Zion: Meditations on the Church's Marian Belief.* Translated by John M. McDermott. San Francisco: Ignatius Press, 1983.
___. *See also* Benedict XVI.
Rebovich, Kelsey. "The Infant Incubator in Europe (1860–1890)." *Embryo Project Encyclopedia*. Arizona State University. November 2, 2017, https://keep.lib.asu.edu/items/173300.
Reiber, David T. "The Morality of Artificial Womb Technology." *National Catholic Bioethics Quarterly* 10.3 (Autumn 2010): 515–527. DOI: 10.5840/ncbq201010332.
Reilly, Christopher M. "Embryo Adoption: A Radically Counter-Cultural Act of Mercy." *Dignitas* 27.1–4 (Spring–Winter 2020): 28–32.
___. "Rescuing the Good Samaritan in Embryo Adoption and Beyond." *National Catholic Bioethics Quarterly* 20.3 (Autumn 2020): 487–498. DOI: 10.5840/ncbq202020345.
Reilly, Christopher M., and Jonathan Scrafford. "Prenatal Testing and Diagnosis." In *Catholic Health Care Ethics: A Manual for Practitioners*, 3rd ed., edited by Edward J. Furton, 12.1–12.9. Philadelphia: National Catholic Bioethics Center, 2020.
Repenshek, Mark F. "Therapeutic Access to the Embryo: Can Therapeutic IVF Be Justified?" *National Catholic Bioethics Quarterly* 11.4 (Winter 2011): 735–756. DOI: 10.5840/ncbq201111410.
Rex, Elizabeth B. "Bioethics: IVF and the Controversy of Embryo Adoption." Interview by Rafael Gonzalez. YouTube. Posted by My Catholic Two Cents on July 22, 2024. https://www.youtube.com/watch?v=JDMSZkMdzvA.
___. "Dr. Elizabeth Rex, The Morality of Embryo Adoption—What Is the Catholic Church's Position." Interview by Dave Maroney and Joan Maroney and online seminar. YouTube. Posted by Divine Mercy for America on November 4, 2022. https://www.youtube.com/watch?v=08DGJMPSZdg.
___. "Embryo Adoption and Conscience." Colloquy. *National Catholic Bioethics Quarterly* 11.4 (Winter 2011): 622–623. DOI: 10.5840/ncbq20111141.

Bibliography

———. "Embryo Adoption and the Bodily Relationship of Biological Mother and Child." Colloquy. *National Catholic Bioethics Quarterly* 15.2 (Summer 2015): 208–209. DOI: 10.5840/ncbq201515224.

———. "Impregnation versus Implantation in the Embryo Adoption Debate." Colloquy. *National Catholic Bioethics Quarterly* 17.3 (Autumn 2017): 381–386. DOI: 10.5840/ncbq201717339.

———. "International Laws that Promote the Ethical Healthcare and Legal Protection of Human Embryos." Annual Summer Conference of the Center for Bioethics and Human Dignity. June 25, 2022.

———. "IVF, Embryo Transfer, and Embryo Adoption: A Response to Repenshek and Delaquil." *National Catholic Bioethics Quarterly* 14.2 (Summer 2014): 227–234. DOI: 10.5840/ncbq201414226.

———. "The Magisterial Liceity of Embryo Transfer: A Response to Charles Robertson." *National Catholic Bioethics Quarterly* 15.4 (Winter 2015): 701–722. DOI: 10.5840/ncbq201515471.

Rex, Elizabeth B., and Charles Robertson. *A Handbook on the Moral Arguments in the Embryo Adoption Debate: What Does the Catholic Church Teach? A Three-Year Scholarly Debate in the Pages of the "National Catholic Bioethics Quarterly," [and] A Webinar Debate Hosted by the Institute for Theological Encounter with Science & Technology*. St. Louis, MO: En Route Books and Media, 2024. This book is a transcript of Rex and Robertson, "The Moral Arguments in the Embryo Adoption Debate," and a reprint of Rex, "IVF, Embryo Transfer, and Embryo Adoption"; Robertson, "A Thomistic Analysis"; Rex, "The Magisterial Liceity"; Robertson, "Navigating an Impasse"; and Rex, "Impregnation versus Implantation."

———. "The Moral Arguments in the Embryo Adoption Debate." Webinar Debate. Hosted by the Institute for Theological Encounter with Science and Technology. May 8, 2021. YouTube. Posted as "WCAT TV Presents … ITEST Welcomes Dr. Charles Robertson and Dr. Elizabeth Rex on Embryo Adoption" by WCAT TV on May, 9, 2021. https://www.youtube.com/watch?v=FLPC PI9heTk. *See also* "ITEST Webinar: The Moral Arguments in the Embryo Adoption Debate." Institute for Theological Encounter with Science and Technology. May 8, 2021. https://faithscience.org/embryo-adoption/.

Roberts, Elizabeth F. S. "Abandonment and Accumulation: Embryonic Futures in the United States and Ecuador." *Medical Anthropology Quarterly* (new series) 25.2 (June 2011): 232–253.

Robertson, Charles. "A Thomistic Analysis of Embryo Adoption." *National Catholic Bioethics Quarterly* 14.4 (Winter 2014): 673–695. DOI: 10.5840/ncbq201414470.

———. "Embryo Adoption and the Incarnation." Colloquy. *National Catholics Bioethics Quarterly* 17.3 (Autumn 2017): 381–386. DOI: 10.5840/ncbq201717339.

———. "The Ethics of Embryo Adoption and Embryo Rescue: A Thomistic Approach." PhD diss., University of St. Thomas (Houston), 2017.

———. "Generation, Gestation, and Birth: An Important Element in the Embryo Adoption Debate." *Linacre Quarterly* 85.1 (February 2018): 35–48. DOI: 10.1177/0024363918756388.

———. "Is Marriage a Basic Good?" *Proceedings of the American Catholic Philosophical Association* 90 (2016): 163–173. DOI: 10.5840/acpaproc20182871.

———. "Lawrence Dewan, Legal Obligation, and the New Natural Law." *Thomist* 83.3 (July 2019): 437–459. DOI: 10.1353/tho.2019.0027.

———. "Navigating an Impasse in the Embryo Adoption Debate: A Response to Elizabeth Rex." *National Catholic Bioethics Quarterly* 16.3 (Autumn 2016): 409–417. DOI: 10.5840/ncbq201616339.

Robertson, John A. "Ethical and Legal Issues in Human Embryo Donation." *Fertility and Sterility* 64.5 (November 1995): 885–894. DOI: 10.1016/s0015-0282(16)57897-2.

Rodger, Daniel, and Bruce P. Blackshaw. "Detached from Humanity: Artificial Gestation and the Chrisitian Dilemma." *Christian Bioethics* 30.2 (August 2024): 85–95. DOI: 10.1093/cb/cbae002.

Rodríguez Yunta, Eduardo. "Commentario a: Moral Assessment of Frozen Human Embryo Adoption in the Light of the Magisterium of the Catholic Church." *Acta Bioéthica* 23.1 (June 2017): 150–151. DOI: 10.4067/s1726-569x2017000100150. See also Aznar, Justo, Miriam Martínez-Peris, and Pedro Navarro-Illana, "Moral Assessment."

Romanis, Elizabeth Choe. "Artificial Womb Technology and the Frontiers of Human Reproduction: Conceptual Differences and Potential Impications." *Journal of Medical Ethics* 44.11 (November 2018): 751–755. DOI: 10.1136/medethics-2018-104910.

Rowland, Tracey. "St Joseph the Man, the Knight, the Prince, the Saint." *Catholic Weekly*. August 14, 2022. https://www.catholicweekly.com.au/st-joseph-the-man-the-knight-the-prince-the-saint/.

Rulli, Tina. "Preferring a Genetically-Related Child." In "New Developments in Family Ethics," edited by Monika Betzler and Jörg Löschke, special issue, *Journal of Moral Philosophy* 13.6 (November 2016): 669–698.

———. "The Unique Value of Adoption." In *Family-Making: Contemporary Ethical Challenges*, edited by Françoise Baylis and Carolyn McLeod, 109–130. New York: Oxford University Press, 2014.

Ryan, Peter F. "New Problems concerning Procreation." In "Symposium on *Dignitas Personae*," special article, edited by E. Christian Brugger. *National Catholic Bioethics Quarterly* 9.3 (Autumn 2009): 467–470. DOI: 10.5840/20099333.

Bibliography

———. "Our Moral Obligation to the Abandoned Embryo." In *Human Embryo Adoption: Biotechnology, Marriage, and the Right to Life*, edited by Thomas V. Berg and Edward J. Furton, 297–325. Philadelphia: National Catholic Bioethics Center, 2006.

Salas Valdivia, César, Gabriela Carpio Valderrama, Angélica Alejandra Bernedo Moscoso, Analucía Torres Flor, and Miriam Berríos Garaycochea. "Adopción embrionaria: estado de la cuestión ético-jurídica en el Perú." *Persona y Bioética* 26.2 (2022): e2627. DOI: 10.5294/pebi.2022.26.2.7.

Sampaio de Oliviera, Janaína, and Valéria Silva Galdino Cardim. "ADOÇÃO DOS EMBRIÕES EXCEDENTÁRIOS E SUAS IMPLICAÇÕES À LUZ DO ORDENAMENTO JURÍDICO BRASILEIRO [Adoption of Excedentary Embryos and Their Implications in the Light of the Brazilian Legal Order." *Argumenta Journal Law* 39 (2023): 57–82. DOI: 10.35356/argumenta.v0i39.2240.

Saunders, William L. "Embryo Adoption Appears to Be Morally Licit." In *The Catholic Citizen: Debating the Issues of Justice. Proceedings from the 26th Annual Conference of the Fellowship of Catholic Scholars, September 26–28, 2003, Arlington Virginia*, edited by Kenneth D. Whitehead, 75–83. South Bend, IN: St. Augustine's Press, 2004.

———. *The Whole Truth about Stem Cell Research*. Washington, DC: Family Research Council, 2001.

Saward, John. *Redeemer in the Womb: Jesus Living in Mary*. San Francisco: Ignatius Press, 1993.

Schudt, Karl. "What Is Chosen in the Act of Embryo Adoption?" In "Human Embryo Transfer," special issue, *National Catholic Bioethics Quarterly* 5.1 (Spring 2005): 63–71. DOI: 10.54840/ncbq20055168.

Sciupac, Elizabeth Podrebarac, Anna Schiller, and Kelsey Beveridge. "U.S. Teens Take after Their Parents Religiously, Attend Services Together and Enjoy Family Rituals." Pew Research Center. September 10, 2020. https://www.pewresearch.org/religion/2020/09/10/u-s-teens-take-after-their-parents-religiously-attend-services-together-and-enjoy-family-rituals/.

Scorcone, Suzanne. "Update on Reproductive Technologies." In *The Interaction of Catholic Bioethics and Secular Society: Proceedings of the Eleventh Bishops' Workshop, Dallas, Texas*, edited by Russell E. Smith, 93–113. Braintree, MA: Pope John Center, 1992. See esp. p. 98.

Scarnecchia, D. Brian. *Bioethics, Law, and Human Life Issues: A Catholic Perspective on Marriage, Family, Contraception, Abortion, Reproductive Technology, and Death and Dying*. Lanham, MD: Scarecrow, 2010. See esp. pp. 158, 163–164, 178, 179–195.

———. Interview by Andrea Kirk Assaf. *See* Assaf, Andrea Kirk.
Secretariat of Pro-Life Activities. *Questions and Answers: The Instruction "Dignitas Personae: On Certain Bioethical Questions."* Washington, DC: US Conference of Catholic Bishops, December 9, 2008. https://dioceseofraleigh.org/sites/default/files/2019-01/Q-and-A_on_Dignitas_Personae.pdf.
——— [?]. "*Dignitas Personae* (Instruction on Certain Bioethical Questions)—Excerpts." In "Diocesan Natural Family Planning Ministry," special issue, *USCCB Forum* [*NFP Forum?*] 20.1–2 (Winter–Spring 2009): 1–4. https://www.usccb.org/resources/Winter-spring2009.pdf. See esp. pp. 3–4, question 5.
Shaw, Joshua. "Why Inconsistency Arguments Matter." *New Bioethics* 28.1 (2022): 40–53. DOI: 10.1080/20502877.2021.2007643.
Shpall, Sam. "Parental Love and Procreation." *Philosophical Quarterly* 73.1 (January 2023): 206–226. DOI: 10.1093/pq/pqac017.
Sibai, Baha M., John Hauth, Steve Caritis, Marshall D. Lindheimer, Cora MacPherson, Mark Klebanoff, et al. "Hypertensive Disorders in Twin versus Singleton Gestations." *American Journal of Obstetrics and Gynecology* 182.4 (April 2000): 938–942. DOI: 10.1016/s0002-9378(00)70350-4.
Simkulet, William. "The Inconsistency Argument: Why Apparent Pro-Life Inconsistency Undermines Opposition to Induced Abortion." *Journal of Medical Ethics* 48.7 (July 2022): 461–465. DOI: 10.1136/medethics-2020-107207.
Smajdor, Anna. "In Defense of Ectogenesis." *Cambridge Quarterly of Healthcare Ethics* 21.1 (January 2012): 90–103. DOI: 10.1017/S0963180111000521.
———. "Whole Body Gestational Donation." *Theoretical Medicine and Bioethics* 44 (November 12, 2022): 113. DOI: 10.1007/s11017-022-09599-8.
Smith, Janet. "Adopting Embryos: Why Not?" *National Catholic Register*. March 27, 2009. https://www.ncregister.com/commentaries/adopting-embryos-why-not.
———. *"Humanae Vitae": A Generation Later*. Washington, DC: Catholic University of America Press, 1991.
———. "Organ Transplants: A Study on Bioethics and the Ordinary Magisterium." In *The Ethics of Organ Transplantation*, edited by Steven J. Jensen, 2011, 272–304. Washington, DC: Catholic University of America Press.
———. "The *Sensus Fidelium* and *Humanae Vitae*." *Angelicum* 83.2 (2006): 271–297.
Smith, Janet E., and Christopher Kaczor. *Life Issues, Medical Choices: Questions and Answers for Catholics*. Cincinnati, OH: Servant Books, 2007. See esp. "Is It Morally Permissible to 'Adopt' a Frozen Embryo?," chap. 3, question 21, pp. 68–69.
Smith, William B. "Rescue the Frozen?" *Homiletic and Pastoral Review* 96.1 (October 1995): 72–74.
———. "Response" [to Surtees]. *Homiletic and Pastoral Review* 96.11–12 (August–September 1996): 16–17. *See* Surtees, Geoffrey, and William Smith.

Bibliography

Snow, David, Alan Cattapan, and Françoise Baylis. "Contesting Estimates of Cryopreserved Embryos in the United States." *Nature Biotechnology* 33.9 (September 2015): 909. DOI: 10.1038/nbt.3342.

"'Snowflake Babies': Exploring the Church's Teaching." *EWTN Pro-Life Weekly*. YouTube. Posted by EWTN on March 16, 2018. https://youtu.be/qCDo6t wcaHQ?feature=shared.

Snowflakes Embryo Adoption Program. *See* Nightlight Christian Adoptions.

___. "Embryo Adoption-Donation." Nightlight Christian Adoptions. Accessed February 29, 2024. https://nightlight.org/snowflakes-embryo-adoption -donation/.

Söderström-Anttila, Viveca, Tuija Foudila, Ulla-Riitta Ripatti, and Rita Siegberg. "Embryo Donation: Outcome and Attitudes among Embryo Donors and Recipients." *Human Reproduction* 16.6 (June 2001): 1120–1128. DOI: 10.1093/humrep/16.6.1120.

Song, Jianjuan, Tingting Liao, Kaiyou Fu, and Jian Xu. "ICSI Does Not Improve Live Birth Rates but Yields Higher Cancellation Rates Than Conventional IVF in Unexplained Infertility." *Frontiers in Medicine* 7 (February 10, 2021), 614118. DOI: 10.3389/fmed.2020.614118.

Stairs, Jocelyn, Tina Y. J. Hsieh, and Daniel L. Rolnik. "In Vitro Fertilization and Adverse Pregnancy Outcomes in the Elective Single Embryo Transfer Era." *American Journal of Perinatology*. E-pub December 26, 2022. DOI: 10.1055 /a-1979-8250.

Stanmeyer, John. "An Embryo Adoptive Father's Perspective." In *The Ethics of Embryo Adoption and the Catholic Tradition: Moral Arguments, Economic Reality and Social Analysis*, edited by Sarah-Vaughn Brakman and Darlene Fozard Weaver, 231–236. Dordrecht, NL: Springer 2007.

Stanmeyer, Suzanne. "An Embryo Adoptive Mother's Perspective." In *The Ethics of Embryo Adoption and the Catholic Tradition: Moral Arguments, Economic Reality and Social Analysis*, edited by Sarah-Vaughn Brakman and Darlene Fozard Weaver, 237–249. Dordrecht, NL: Springer 2007.

Stempsey, William E. "Heterologous Embryo Transfer: Metaphor and Morality." In *The Ethics of Embryo Adoption and the Catholic Tradition: Moral Arguments, Economic Reality and Social Analysis*, edited by Sarah-Vaughan Brakman and Darlene Fozard Weaver, 25–41. Dordrecht, NL: Springer, 2007.

St. Hilaire, Anselm L. "Pregnancy, Marriage, and the Parents of Jesus." Colloquy. *National Catholic Bioethics Quarterly* 3.3 (Autumn 2003): 441. DOI: 10.5840/ncbq20033325.

Strege, John. *A Snowflake Named Hannah: Ethics, Faith, and the First Adoption of a Frozen Embryo*. Grand Rapids, MI: Kregel Publications, 2020.

Sullivan, Ezra. Interview by Prudence Robertson. *EWTN Pro-Life Weekly*. YouTube. Posted as "A Catholic Solution to IVF: Baptize Embryonic Children?" by EWTN on March 1, 2024. https://www.youtube.com/watch?v=tvNK2q-bAk28.

Sullivan, Francis A. *Magisterium: Teaching Authority in the Catholic Church*. Eugene, OR: Wipf and Stock, 2002.

Supreme Court of Alabama. *LePage v. Center for Reproductive Medicine*. SC-2022-0515 (Ala. 2024).

Surtees, Geoffrey, and William Smith. "Adoption of a Frozen Embryo" and "Response." *Homiletic and Pastoral Review* 96.11–12 (August–September[?] 1996): 7–17.

Tarabrin, Roman. "Case Study of the Moral Dilemma: Orthodox Christianity vs. New Reproductive Technologies." In "37th Annual Conferenc of the European Association of Centres of Medical Ethics (EACME): Smart Ethics. Trends to the Future, September 9–11, Cluj-Napoca, Romania," special issue, *Studia Universitatis Babeș-Bolyai Bioethica* 66 special issue (September 2021): 172–173. DOI: 10.24193/subbbioethica.2021.spiss.118.

Tennessee Code §36-2-401.

Terho, A. M., S. Pelkonen, S. Opdahl, L. B. Romundstad, C. Bergh, U. B. Wennerholm, et al. "High Birth Weight and Large-for-Gestational Age in Singletons Born after Frozen Compared to Fresh Embryo Transfer, by Gestational Week: A Nordic Register Study from the CoNARTaS Group." *Human Reproduction* 36.4 (March 18, 2021): 1083–1092. DOI: 10.1093/humrep/deaa304.

Theobald, Rachel, Sioban SenGupta, and Joyce Harper. "The Status of Preimplantation Genetic Testing in the UK and USA." *Human Reproduction* 35.4 (April 28, 2020): 986–998. DOI: 10.1093/humrep/deaa034.

Tollefsen, Christopher. "Aquinas's Four Orders, Normativity, and Human Nature." *Journal of Value Inquiry* 52.3 (August 2018): 243–256. DOI: 10.1007/s10790-018-9657-6.

———. "Could Human Embryo Transfer Be Intrinsically Immoral?" In *The Ethics of Embryo Adoption and the Catholic Tradition: Moral Arguments, Economic Reality and Social Analysis*, edited by Sarah-Vaughan Brakman and Darlene Fozard Weaver, 85–102. Dordrecht, NL: Springer, 2007.

———. "Divine, Human, and Embryo Adoption: Some Criticisms of *Dignitas Personae*." In "Responses to *Dignitas Personae*: Part I of II," special issue, *National Catholic Bioethics Quarterly* 10.1 (Spring 2010): 75–85. DOI: 10.5840/ncbq201010173.

———. "In Vitro Fertilization Should Not Be an Option for a Woman." In *Contemporary Debates in Bioethics*, edited by Arthur Caplan and Robert Arp, 451–459. Hoboken, NJ: Wiley, 2014.

———. "Is a Purely First Person Account of Human Action Defensible?" *Ethical Theory and Moral Practice* 9.4 (August 2006): 441–460.

———. "Response to Robert Koons and Matthew O'Brien's 'Objects of Intention: A Hylomorphic Critique of the New Natural Law Theory.'" *American

Bibliography

    Catholic Philosophical Quarterly 87.4 (Fall 2013): 751–778. DOI: 10.5840/acpq201387455.

———. Review of *Fertility and Gender: Issues in Reproductive and Sexual Ethics*, edited by Helen Watt. *Catholic Social Science Review* 17 (2012): 301–304. DOI: 10.5840/cssr20121725.

Tonti-Filippini, Nicholas. *About Bioethics*. 5 volumes. Ballarat and Brisbane, Australia: Connor Court, 2012–2017.

———. "Frozen Embryo 'Rescue.'" Letter to the editor. *Linacre Quarterly* 64.1 (February 1997): 3–4. DOI: 10.1080/20508549.1999.11878370.

———. "Nicholas Tonti-Filippini Replies." Colloquy. *National Catholic Bioethics Quarterly* 3.3 (Autumn 2003): 448–452. DOI: 10.5840/ncbq20033325.

———. "Nicholas Tonti-Filippini Replies." Colloquy. *National Catholic Bioethics Quarterly* 4.1 (Spring 2004): 11–12. DOI: 10.5840/ncbq20044162.

———. "The Embryo Rescue Debate: Impregnating Women, Ectogenesis, and Restoration from Suspended Animation." In *Human Embryo Adoption: Biotechnology, Marriage, and the Right to Life*, edited by Thomas V. Berg and Edward J. Furton, 69–114. Philadelphia: National Catholic Bioethics Center, 2006. This is a lightly edited reprint of "The Embryo Rescue Debate," *National Catholic Bioethics Quarterly* 3.1.

———. "The Embryo Rescue Debate: Impregnating Women, Ectogenesis, and Restoration from Suspended Animation." *National Catholic Bioethics Quarterly* 3.1 (Spring 2003): 111–137. DOI: 10.5840/ncbq20033181. This article was lightly edited and reprinted as "The Embryo Rescue Debate" in *Human Embryo Adoption*.

Tossati, Marco, "Chiesa divisa sugli embrioni." *La stampa*, July 22 (or 27?), 1966.

Treff, Nathan R., and Diego Marin. "The 'Mosaic' Embryo: Misconceptions and Misinterpretations in Preimplantation Genetic Testing for Aneuploidy." *Fertility and Sterility* 116.5 (November 2021): 1205–1211. DOI: 10.1016/j.fertnstert.2021.06.027.

Trevett, Thomas, and Anthony Johnson. "Monochorionic Twin Pregnancies." *Clinics in Perinatology* 32.2 (June 2005): 475–494. DOI: 10.1016/j.clp.2005.02.007.

Tully, Patrick A. "Cryopreserved Embryos and *Dignitas Personae*: Another Option?" *Kennedy Institute of Ethics Journal* 22.4 (December 2012): 367–389. DOI: 10.1353/ken.2012.a495159.

Turner, Joseph V., and Lucas A. McLindon. "Bioethical and Moral Perspectives in Human Reproductive Medicine." *Linacre Quarterly* 85.4 (November 2018): 385–398. DOI: 10.1177/0024363918816697.

United States Conference of Catholic Bishops. "*Dignitas Personae*, Vatican Instruction on Bioethics, Welcomed for Guidance on Issues of Procreation, Medical Research." News release. December 12, 2008. Archived at the Internet

Archive. https://web.archive.org/web/20090124205434/http://www.usccb.org/comm/archives/2008/08-196.shtml.

———. "Life-Giving Love in an Age of Technology." November 17, 2009. https://www.usccb.org/beliefs-and-teachings/what-we-believe/love-and-sexuality/life-giving-love-in-an-age-of-technology.

United States Conference of Catholic Bishops Natural Family Planning Program. "Unitive and Procreative Nature of Intercourse." United State Conference of Catholic Bishops. Accessed November 6, 2023. https://www.usccb.org/issues-and-action/marriage-and-family/natural-family-planning/catholic-teaching/upload/Unitive-and-Proc-Nature-of-Interc.pdf.

University of Navarre. *The Navarre Bible: Pentateuch*. Edited by José María Casciaro, Gonzalo Aranda, Santiago Ausín, et al. Translated by Michael Adams. English ed. edited by James Gavigan, Brian McCarthy, and Thomas McGovern. Dublin: Four Courts Press, 1999.

US Department of Health and Human Services Office of the Assistant Secretary for Planning and Evaluation. "National Survey of Adoptive Parents (NSAP)." Accessed June 21, 2024. https://aspe.hhs.gov/national-survey-adoptive-parents-nsap.

US Food and Drug Administration. "Eligibility Determination for Donors of Human Cells, Tissues, and Cellular and Tissue-Based Products Guidance for Industry." August 2007. https://www.fda.gov/regulatory-information/search-fda-guidance-documents/eligibility-determination-donors-human-cells-tissues-and-cellular-and-tissue-based-products.

———. Revisions to Exceptions Applicable to Certain Human Cells, Tissues, and Cellular and Tissue-Based Products. 81 Fed. Reg. 40512. August 22, 2016.

Vacca, Michael Arthur. "Equivalence of the Moral Objects in Embryo Adoption and Heterologous IVF." *National Catholic Bioethics Quarterly* 22.3 (Autumn 2022): 437–446. DOI: 10.5840/ncbq202222340.

Valera, Mária Ángeles, Carmela Albert, Julián Marcos, Zaloa Larreategui, Lorena Bori, and Marcos Meseguer. "A Propensity Score-Based, Comparative Study Assessing Humid and Dry Time-Lapse Incubation, with Single-Step Medium, on Embryo Development and Clinical Outcomes." *Human Reproduction* 37.9 (August 25, 2022): 1980–1993. DOI: 10.1093/humrep/deac165.

Van Ijzendoorn, Marinus H., Everline M. Euser, Peter Prinzie, Femmie Juffer, Marian J. Bakermans-Kranenburg. "Elevated Risk of Child Maltreatment in Families with Stepparents but Not with Adoptive Parents." *Child Maltreatment* 14.4 (November 2009): 375. DOI:10.1177/1077559509342125.

Van Ljzendoorn, Marinus H., and Femmie Juffer. "The Emanuel Miller Memorial Lecture 2006: Adoption as Intervention. Meta-Analytic Evidence for

Bibliography

Massive Catch-Up and Plasticity in Physical, Socio-Emotional, and Cognitive Development." *Journal of Child Psychology and Psychiatry* 47.12 (December 2006): 1228–1245. DOI: 10.1111/j.1469-7610.2006.01675.x.

Vatican Council II. *Dei verbum*. November 18, 1965. https://www.vatican.va/archive/hist_councils/ii_vatican_council/documents/vat-ii_const_19651118_dei-verbum_en.html.

———. *Gaudium et spes*. December 7, 1965. https://www.vatican.va/archive/hist_councils/ii_vatican_council/documents/vat-ii_const_19651207_gaudium-et-spes_en.html.

———. *Lumen gentium*. November 21, 1964. https://www.vatican.va/archive/hist_councils/ii_vatican_council/documents/vat-ii_const_19641121_lumen-gentium_en.html.

Vatican News. "Pope: May We Hear the Voice of the Unborn through Science." May 21, 2023. https://www.vaticannews.va/en/pope/news/2023-05/pope-may-we-hear-the-voice-of-the-unborn-through-science.html.

Verrier, Nancy Newton. *The Primal Wound*. Baltimore: Gateway Press, 1993.

Vial Correa, Juan de Dios, and Elio Sgreccia, eds. *The Identity and Statute* [sic] *of the Human Embryo: Proceedings of the Third Assembly of the Pontifical Academy for Life (Vatican City, February 14–16, 1997)*. Vatican City: Libreria Editrice Vaticana, 1998.

Villar, J., L. Say, A. M. Gulmezoglu, M. Merialdi, M. D. Lindheimer, A. P. Betran, et al. "Eclampsia and Preeclampsia: A Worldwide Health Problem for 2000 Years." In *Preeclampsia*, edited by H. Critchley, A. MacLean, L. Poston, and J. Walker, 57–72. London: Royal College of Obstetricians and Gynaecologists Press, 2003.

Violette, Caroline J., Rachel S. Mandelbaum, Shinya Matsuzaki, Joseph G. Ouzounian, Richard J. Paulson, and Koji Matsuo. "Assessment of Abnormal Placentation in Pregnancies Conceived with Assisted Reproductive Technology." *International Journal of Gynecology and Obstetrics* 163.2 (November 2023): 555–562. DOI: 10.1002/ijgo.14850.

Virzera, Diane L. "Unthawing Frozen Embryos: The Legal & Ethical Conundrum of Embryo Adoption." *Human Life Review* 35.1/2 (2009): 85ff.

Vohr, Betty R. "Neurodevelopmental Outcomes of Premature Infants with Intraventricular Hemorrhage across A Lifespan." *Seminars in Perinatology* 46.5 (August 2022), 151594. DOI: 10.1016/j.semperi.2022.151594.

Von Balthasar, Hans Urs. *Mary for Today*. Translated by Robert Nowell. Slough, UK: St. Paul Publications, 1987.

Warmflash, David. "Why Don't We Have Artificial Wombs for Premature Infants?" Up Worthy Science. March 2, 2018. https://upworthyscience.com/dont-artificial-wombs-premature-infants/particle-13.

Waters, Brent. "Adoption, Parentage, and Procreative Stewardship." In *The Morality of Adoption: Social-Psychological, Theological, and Legal Perspectives*, edited by Timothy P. Jackson, 32–51. Grand Rapids, MI: Eerdmans, 2005.

Watt, Helen. "A Brief Defense of Frozen Embryo Adoption." In "Respect for the Human Embryo," special issue, *National Catholic Bioethics Quarterly* 1.2 (Summer 2001): 151–154. DOI: 10.5840/ncbq20011250.

———. "Are There Any Circumstances in Which It Would Be Morally Admirable for a Woman to Seek to Have an Orphan Embryo Implanted in Her Womb?," part 2. In *Issues for a Catholic Bioethic*, edited by Luke Gormally. London: Linacre Centre, 1999, 347–352.

———. "Becoming Pregnant or Becoming a Mother? Embryo Transfer with and without a Prior Maternal Relationship." In *Human Embryo Adoption: Biotechnology, Marriage, and the Right to Life*, edited by Thomas V. Berg and Edward J. Furton, 55–67. Philadelphia: National Catholic Bioethics Center, 2006.

———. "Beyond Double Effect: Side Effects and Bodily Harm." In *Human Values: New Essays on Ethics and Natural Law*, edited by David S. Oderberg and Timothy D. Chappell, 236–251. Houndmills, UK: Palgrave Macmillan, 2004.

———. *The Ethics of Pregnancy, Abortion and Childbirth: Exploring Moral Choices in Childbearing*. New York: Routledge, 2016. See esp. "Accepting Donor Embryos ('Embryo Adoption')," pp. 112–114.

———, ed. *Fertility and Gender: Issues in Reproductive and Sexual Ethics*. Oxford: Anscombe Bioethics Centre, 2011.

———. Letter to the editor in "What To Do With Spare Embryos." Letters to the editor. *Lancet* 347.9013 (May 25, 1996): 1488–1489. DOI: 10.1016/S0140-6736(96)91726-2.

———. "The Origin of Persons." In *The Identity and Status of the Human Embryo: Proceedings of Third Assembly of the Pontifical Academy for Life*, edited by Juan de Dios Vial Correa and Elio Sgreccia, 342–364. Vatican City: Libreria Editrice Vaticana, 1998.

———. "Parenthood and New Reproductive Technologies: Anthropological Considerations." In *The Dignity of Human Procreation and Reproductive Technologies: Anthropological and Ethical Aspects*, edited by Juan de Dios Vial Correa and Elio Sgreccia. Vatican City: Libreria Editrice Vaticana, 2005.

Weaver, Darlene Ford. "Embryo Adoption: Expanding the Terms of the Debate. In *Applied Ethics in a World Church*, edited by Linda Hogan, 199–207. New York: Orbis, 2008.

———. "Embryo Adoption Theologically Considered: Bodies, Adoption, and the Common Good." In *The Ethics of Embryo Adoption and the Catholic Tradition: Moral Arguments, Economic Reality and Social Analysis*, edited by

Sarah-Vaughn Brakman and Darlene Fozard Weaver, 141–159. Dordrecht, NL: Springer 2007.

———. "Water Is Thicker Than Blood: Adoptive Families and Catholic Tradition." *Concilium* 2 (2016): 98–110.

Wechter, David. "Response to Catherine Althaus on Heterologous Embryo Transfer." Colloquy. *National Catholic Bioethics Quarterly* 5.3 (Autumn 2005): 451–452. DOI: 10.5840/ncbq20055324. Corrected reprint of misprinted Colloquy in Summer 2005.

Weiss, Joanna. "How 'Snowflake Babies' Could Change IVF Politics." *Politico*, October 6, 2024. https://politico.com/news/magazine/2024/10/06/adopting-discarded-embryos-ivf-crisis-00169174.

West, Christopher. *Theology of the Body Explained: A Commentary on John Paul II's Man and Woman He Created Them*, rev. ed. Boston: Pauline Books and Media, 2007.

West, Ryan. "Anger and the Virtues: A Critical Study in Virtue Individuation." *Canadian Journal of Philosophy* 46.6 (June 24, 2016): 883–884. DOI: 10.1080/00455091.2016.1199232.

Whitehead, Kenneth D., ed. *The Catholic Citizen: Debating the Issues of Justice. Proceedings from the 26th Annual Conference of the Fellowship of Catholic Scholars, September 26–28, 2003, Arlington Virginia*. South Bend, IN: St. Augustine's Press, 2004.

Widdows, Heather, and Fiona MacCallum. "Disparities in Parenting Criteria: An Exploration of the Issues, Focusing on Adoption and Embryo Donation." *Journal of Medical Ethics* 28.3 (June 2002): 139–142. DOI: 10.1136/jme.28.3.139.

Wilding, Martin Graham, Clemente Capobianco, Nadia Montanaro, Genc Kabili, Loredana Di Matteo, Enrico Fusco, et al. "Human Cleavage-Stage Embryo Vitrification Is Comparable to Slow-Rate Cryopreservation in Cycles of Assisted Reproduction." *Journal of Assisted Reproduction and Genetics* 27.9–10 (September 2010): 549–554. DOI: 10.1007/s10815-010-9452-1.

Williams, Thomas D. "Can Embryos Be Adopted?" Interview by Zenit. Catholic Online. June 5, 2005. https://www.catholic.org/featured/headline.php?ID=2236.

———. "Heterologous Embryo Transfer and the Meaning of 'Becoming a Mother.'" In *Human Embryo Adoption: Biotechnology, Marriage, and the Right to Life*, edited by Thomas V. Berg and Edward J. Furton, 229–249. Philadelphia: National Catholic Bioethics Center, 2006.

———. "The Least of My Brethren: The Ethics of Heterologous Embryo Transfer." *Human Life Review* 31.3 (Summer 2005): 87–98.

Wilson, Aaron. "What Christians Should Know about Embryo Adoption." The Gospel Coalition. February 16, 2017. https://www.thegospelcoalition.org/article/what-christians-should-know-about-embryo-adoption/.

___. "Why My Wife and I Choose to Adopt Embryos." Lifeway Research (website). April 16, 2018. https://research.lifeway.com/2018/04/16/why-my-wife-and-i-chose-to-adopt-embryos/.

Wooden, Cindy. "Adopting Embryos Raises Moral Questions, Vatican Officials Say." Catholic News Service. December 12, 2008. Archived at the Internet Archive. https://web.archive.org/web/20110112204018/http://www.catholicnews.com/data/stories/cns/0806229.htm.

World Health Organization. "WHO COVID-19 Dashboard." Accessed January 22, 2023. https://covid19.who.int/.

World Population Review. "Sperm Donation Laws by Country 2024." Accessed February 28, 2024. https://worldpopulationreview.com/country-rankings/sperm-donation-laws-by-country.

Xiao, Yaling, Xue Wang, Ting Gui, Tao Tao, and Wei Xiong. "Transfer of A Poor-Quality along with A Good-Quality Embryo on In Vitro Fertilization / Intracytoplasmic Sperm Injection-Embryo Transfer Clinical Outcomes: A Systematic Review and Meta-Analysis." *Fertility and Sterility* 118.6 (December 2022): 1066–1079. DOI: 10.1016/j.fertnstert.2022.08.848.

Yanaihara, Atsushi, Takeshi Yorimitsu, Hiroshi Motoyama, Motohiro Ohara, and Toshihiro Kawamura. "Clinical Outcome of Frozen Blastocyst Transfer; Single vs. Double Transfer." *Journal of Assisted Reproduction and Genetics* 25.11–12 (November–December 2008): 531–534. DOI: 10.1007/s10815-008-9275-5.

Young, C. M. "The Ethics of Frozen Embryo Transfer: A Moral Study of 'Embryo Adoption.'" Doctoral Thesis in Philosophy. Rome, 2004.

Zhang, Yali. "A Comparison of Preterm Birth Rate and Growth from Birth to 18 Years Old between In Vitro Fertilization and Spontaneous Conception of Twins." *Twin Research and Human Genetics* 24.4 (August 2021): 228–233. DOI: 10.1017/thg.2021.33.

Zhu, Tian. "In Vitro Fertilization." *Embryo Project Encyclopedia*. Arizona State University. July 22, 2009. https://embryo.asu.edu/pages/vitro-fertilization.

Ziadeh, Saed M. "The Outcome of Triplet versus Twin Pregnancies." *Gynecologic and Obstetric Investigation* 50.2 (August 2000): 96–99. DOI: 10.1159/000010290.

Zimon, Alison E., Donal S. Shepard, Jeffrey Prottas, Kristin L. Rooney, Jeanie Ungerleider, and Yara A. Halasa-Rappel, et al. "Embryo Donation: Survey of *In-Vitro* Fertilization (IVF) Patients and Randomized Trial of Complimentary Counseling." *PLoS One* 14.8 (August 15, 2019), e0221149. DOI: 10.1371/journal.pone.0221149.

Bibliography

Zwicker, Jill Glennis, and Susan Richardson Harris. "Quality of Life of Formerly Preterm and Very Low Birth Weight Infants from Preschool Age to Adulthood: A Systematic Review." *Pediatrics* 121.2 (February 2008): e366–e376. DOI: 10.1542/peds.2007-0169.

Index

abortion, 63, 75, 77, 126, 154–155, 166, 168, 182, 190, 192, 268, 289–299, 315

Accad, Michel, 72, 188

act of admission *See* feminine act of admission

Adam and Eve, 242–246, 257, 260

admission *See* feminine act of admission

adoption as a spiritual status and social practice. *See also* children's rights to love and life; embryo adoption: adultery and, 233–234; biblical history of adoption and, 220; Catholic identity and, 221–223; counter objections and, 238; defective marital acts and, 233–235; definition of HET and, 229; definition of marital act and, 234–235; definition of prenatal adoption and, 230–232; dignity and, 220; *Donum vitae* and, 233; EA is not intrinsically wrong and, 230–232; Francis and, 220; impasse on status of EA and, 227–230; implications for Christian parents and, 223–224; Jesus and, 220, 221–222; justifying prenatal adoption and, 225–227; lack of focus on meanings of adoption and, 219; moral significance of kinship and, 224–225; natural law and, 219, 235–237; neither natural nor conventional and, 235–237; overview of, 219–221, 239–240; Paul and, 222; prenatal orphans and, 220–221; primacy of adoption and, 222–223; procreative infidelity and, 229, 232–238; rescue of embryos and, 228–231; self-identity and, 222–223; subordination of kinship and, 221–223; theology of the family and, 221–223

adultery, 126, 147, 229, 232–234, 301

Akin, Jimmy, xi–xii, 25

Alexander, Irene, xiii, 151, 202n15, 206n22, 215–217

Althaus, Catherine, 176, 187–188

Andrew, James, 203n17

Annunciation: Adam and Eve and, 242–246, 257, 260; answer to three objections and, 259–260; Aquinas and, 257, 262; Baptism and, 242; child-as-gift and, 252–253; definition of human conception and, 262–263; differences between Incarnation and EA and, 253–254; *Dignitas personae* and, 246–247; divine adoption and, 251; EA compared and contrasted with, 106–107, 250–255; feminine act of admission and, 105–107; Francis and, 241–242, 257; *Gaudium et spes* and, 249; grace and, 250; image of God and, 246–247; Immaculate Conception and, 241–242, 249; impasse on status of EA and, 241; Incarnation of Christ and, 242, 249–255; Jesus and, 242, 249–263; John Paul II and, 244, 255; Joseph as guardian of the Redeemer and, 254–255; love of God and, 251; Marian relationship and, 255–263; natural law and, 247; overview of, 241–244; parenthood as gift from God and, 253–254; parents as equal to Mary and Joseph and, 252–253; personhood and, 241–243, 253, 256–257; priority of the action of God in conception and, 245–246; psychological and spiritual suffering of Mary and, 247–248; salvation history context and, 242–243, 253; self-gift and, person as, 253; theological commentary on, 249–250; Trinity and, 244–249; verb *to know*, 244–249; virginity and, 244–245; will of God and, 252

Aquinas, Thomas, St.: Annunciation and, 257, 262; becoming a parent and, 93, 96–98; children's rights to love and life and, 75; definition of adoption and, 93; differing orders of reason and, 207n23; ensoulment and, 262; happiness as not found in created things and, 75; natural law and, 103, 158, 179–185, 190; next steps if EA is illicit and, 158; procreative dimension of marital union and, 179–185, 190; *Summa contra Gentiles*, 181–184; Trinity and, 95; wrongness of fornication and, 196

artificial wombs, 34, 47–49, 156, 217–218, 279–283, 301, 314–315

attitude of dominion, 203–205

Augustine of Hippo, 75

Austriaco, Nicanor Pier Giorgio, iv, 53, 82, 156, 176, 214, 227

Baptism, 77–78, 167n27, 191, 223, 242, 250

becoming a parent. *See also* children's rights to love and life; parenthood; protecting the dignity of the child: Aquinas and, 93, 96–98; criteria for a successful defense of extended inseparability and, 100–104; divine adoption and, 89–92, 95–98; *Donum vitae* and, 81–88, 100–103; EA makes spouses parents through each other and, 86–91; ET does not make a woman to be a mother and, 91–99; ET is wrong for making a woman a mother apart from her spouse and, 83–84; *Evangelium vitae* and, 88; extended inseparability and, 82, 84, 92, 100–104; God's role in, 89–99; HET and, 85, 89; infidelity and, 83–84; Jesus and, 91–92; John Paul II and, 88; legal generation and, 94, 96, 99; marital bond and, 83; as moral category, 88–89; moral equivalence of natural and adoptive parenthood and, 85–86; motherhood categories and, 92–94; natural generation and, 94–99; objections to arguments based on, 85–86; overview of, 81–82; permanent commitment and, 87; personhood and, 89; principle based on, 81–82; procreation terminating at conception and, 85–86; real and rational relations and, 97–98; relevance and application of the parenthood principle and, 99–100; rescue of embryos and, 100–102; "term from which"

and, 94–98; "term to which" and, 94–96; traditional adoption and, 85–88; Trinity and, 95; virtuous parenthood and, 87
Berkman, John, xiii, 87, 219, 305, 313, 321–323, 326, 331
Biblical history of adoption, 32–33
bioethics (Catholic), 5, 155, 157, 162, 166–167, 193, 321–322
Bobier, Christopher, xiii, 63
Boleyn, Anne, 201
Brakman, Sarah-Vaughan, x, 58, 87–88, 212n35
Brave New World (Huxley), 38
Brighouse, Harry, 64
Brown, Louise, 38, 270, 274
Brugger, E. Christian, 85, 187
Bush, George W., 304
Buskmiller, Cara, xi, 3
Carey, Kristen, 313, 321–323, 326, 331
Catholic bioethics, 5, 155, 157, 162, 166–167, 193, 321–322
Catholic Church. *See also* Congregation for the Doctrine of the Faith (CDF); John Paul II; magisterium: artificial procreation condemned by, 275; *Catechism of the Catholic Church*, 35, 71–72, 76–77, 266, 273–274, 278, 283; conjugal act and procreation and, 59; cryopreservation as intrinsically evil and, 280; EA teachings of, ix–x; history of adoption in, 220; identity of Catholics and, 221–223; impasse on status of EA and, 24, 73, 125; IVF stance of, 41; postnatal adoption supported by, 220, 278; rescue of embryos and, 265; sexual ethics of, 54–55, 59–60, 115–118, 173–174, 197–198; as thinking in centuries, ix
Caulfeld, Brian, 129

CDF. *See* Congregation for the Doctrine of the Faith
chastity, xii, 105, 109–111, 144
children's rights to love and life. *See also* protecting the dignity of the child: Aquinas and, 75; arguments in support of adoption obligation and, 65–69; benefits to children of adoption and, 68–69; benefits to parents of children and, 64–65; *Catechism of the Catholic Church* and, 71–72, 76–77; considerations in favor of traditional adoption and, 69–80; consumerism and climate change and, 73–74; death's harms and, 75–76; differing opinions on EA and, 70–73; *Dignitas personae* and, 71; EA distinguished from traditional adoption and, 70; *Evangelium vitae* and, 77; flourishing life and, 64–65; God's role in, 75–78; harm imprint and, 73–74; harmfulness of embryonic death and, 74–80; harms of foster care and, 65–67; *Instruction on Children's Baptism* and, 77; Jesus and, 76–79; John Paul II and, 67, 69, 77; *Laudato si'* and, 74; love present within adoptions and, 67; moral ambiguity and, 70–73; moral preferability of traditional adoption and, 69–80; overview of, 63–64; parental rights and, 64–67; prima facie duty to help those in need and, 66–67; prioritization of traditional adoption and, 80; pro tanto obligation to adopt foster children and, 65; religious formation, parental role in, 79; right to become a parent and, 65; right to procreate distinguished from right to parent and, 65; unbaptized infants and, 77–78

Christ. *See* Jesus Christ
Christian Nightlight Adoptions, 19n6
Christian parenting, 223–224
Christianity and Christians. *See* Catholic Church; Jesus Church. *See* Catholic Church
Code of Canon Law (Canon Law Society of America), 28
Cohen, Eric, 127–128
Commentary on the Sentences (Aquinas), 93
conception *See also* in vitro fertilization: definition of, 262–263; donor conception and, 314; Immaculate Conception, 241–242, 249; Jesus and, 241–242, 249; priority of the action of God in, 245–246; procreation terminating at, 85–86
Congregation for the Doctrine of the Faith (CDF). *See also Dignitas personae; Donum vitae*: artificial wombs and, 282; authority of documents issued by, 29; criteria for authority of teachings and, 41; definition of dissent and, 31; finality of the sexual act and, 60n11; infallibility and, 28–29; magisterium and, 28–31, 282; natural moral law and, 28; next steps in EA and, 318–319; noninfallible teachings and, 30; surrogate motherhood and, 37
consequentialism, 153–154
contraception, 110, 174, 182, 198–201, 274–275, 320
counseling for EA, 14, 21, 328, 330
COVID-19, 3
crisis embryo transfer (CET), 34, 36–38
cryopreservation, 23, 34, 39, 42, 126, 135, 156–160, 164, 213, 267, 279–283, 302, 319–320
Cunningham, Bernard, 307
deposit of faith, 26

destruction of embryos, 6, 24, 25, 39–40, 43, 45, 117, 126, 157, 164–165, 184, 300, 317, 332
Devroey, Paul, 17
Dignitas personae (CDF): aims of, x; Annunciation and, 246–247; children's rights to love and life and, 71; as closest to definitive statement on liceity of embryo adoption, ii; *Donum vitae* and, ii, 43; impasse on status of EA and, 42–49; introduction of, 46–47; magisterium and, 25, 29, 41–47, 267–268, 293–294; next steps in EA and, 322; overview of, x–xi; papal approval of, 29; protecting the dignity of the child and, 206–207; publication of, x; resolving duty of existent embryos and, 42–49; respect for embryos and, 42; scholarship on, x–xi; Theology of the Body and, 117, 267–268, 293–294; writing of, x–xi
dignity, 37–39, 48, 81–82, 126, 157, 165–166, 220, 313–314. *See also* protecting the dignity of the child
divine adoption, 89–92, 95–98, 251
divine revelation, 27, 35
dogma, x, 27, 30
domination of technology, 156, 159, 207
Donum vitae (CDF): adoption as a spiritual status and social practice and, 233; artificial wombs and, 48; becoming a parent and, 81–88, 100–103; *Dignitas personae* and, x, 43; magisterium and, 29, 36–37, 40, 43, 266–268, 275–279, 293–295; moral contraindications to EA and, 140–144, 148; next steps if EA is illicit and, 152, 156–157, 165; next steps in EA and, 319–320, 322; papal approval of, 29; protecting

382

Index

the dignity of the child, 195–201, 204, 206, 211–214, 217–218; rescue of embryonic persons and, 298, 301–302; Theology of the Body and, 266–268, 275–279, 293–295
duty to existent embryos, 42–49. *See also* destruction of embryos; next steps if EA is illicit; next steps in EA; rescue of embryos
Edwards, Robert, 38
embryo adoption (EA). *See also* medical aspects of EA: aims and motivation for current volume on, x–xi; Catholic Church's teaching on, ix–x; chapter summaries of current volume on, iii–vi; *Dignitas personae* and, x; ET's relation to, 8–13, 38, 293–296; IVF as basis of, ix; legal status of, xii; limbo of ethical status of, ix; overview of, ix–xiv; personhood and, xi; pressure to find definitive answer on, ix–x; selection of chapters for current volume on, xi; structure of current volume on, xi–xiv; Supreme Court and, xi
embryo destruction, 6, 24, 25, 39–40, 43, 45, 117, 126, 157, 164–165, 184, 300, 317, 332
Embryo Protection Act (1990, Germany), 333
embryo rescue. *See* rescue of embryos
embryo transfer (ET). *See also* crisis embryo transfer; heterologous embryo transfer; voluntary embryo transfer: becoming a parent and, 83–84, 91–99; definition and procedure of, 8–13; EA's relation to, 8–13, 38, 293–294; forms of, 126–127; liceity of, 293–296; magisterium and, 38; medical aspects of EA and, 8–13; morality of EA and, 293–296; as not making a woman to be a mother and, 91–99; organ transplants and, 102; as wrong for making a woman a mother apart from her spouse and, 83–84
embryos in storage. *See* destruction of embryos; duty to existent embryos; impasse on status of EA; next steps if EA is illicit; next steps in EA; rescue of embryos
Enzmann, Ernst, 38
ET. *See* embryo transfer
Etheredge, Francis, v, 241, 303
Ethics of Embryo Adoption and the Catholic Tradition (Vaughan-Brakman and Fozard Weaver), x
Evangelium vitae (John Paul II), 77, 88, 168–169, 294, 319
existent embryos. *See* destruction of embryos; impasse on status of EA; next steps if EA is illicit; next steps in EA; rescue of embryos
experimentation, 39–40, 157
extended inseparability: becoming a parent and, 82, 84, 92, 100–104; criteria for a successful defense of, 100–104; generative faculty objections and, 54–57; impasse on status of EA and, 54, 60; implications of, 61; procreative dimension of marital union and, 177–178; protecting the dignity of the child and, 214–215; responses to, 57–61
extraordinary and ordinary care distinction, 161–163
FDA (US Food and Drug Administration), 18, 21–22
feminine act of admission: chastity and, 105, 110–111; defective marriage acts and, 108; definition of impregnation and, 107; EA compared and contrasted with Annunciation and, 106–107; ecclesiastical authority

and, 113; feminine aspect of reproductive integrity and, 111; how a woman should get pregnant and, 111–112; Joseph and, 106; magisterium and, 113; male marriage act contrasted with female act and, 109–110; Mary's act at the Annunciation and, 105–106, 111–112; natural generation and, 108; nature of the female marriage act and, 109–110; objections to EA and, 108–109; overview of, 105, 114; replies to defences of EA and, 112–114; reproductive integrity and, 105, 110–114; rescue of embryos and, 107, 112; why just adoption and, 107–108

Finley, Kate, 63

Fisichella, Rino, 46–47

foster care, 65–67, 69–70, 73, 79–80

Francis, Pope: adoption as a spiritual status and social practice and, 220; Annunciation and, 241–242, 257; Church as field hospital and, 220; consumerism and climate change and, 74; dignity and, 269; *Laudato si'*, 74; listening to the voice of the embryo and, 268; Mary and, 257; personhood and, 242

future of frozen embryos. *See* destruction of embryos; duty to existent embryos; next steps if EA is illicit; next steps in EA; rescue of embryos

Gabriel, 105

Gaudium et spes (Second Vatican Council), 118, 132, 249

Geach, Mary (Mrs. Mary Gormally), iv, 105, 176–178, 233–237

generative faculty objections: Catholic sexual ethics and, 54–55, 59–60; devaluation of adoption objection and, 58; extended inseparability and, 54–57; flawed reasoning objection and, 59; great good of EA objection and, 57–58; impasse on status of EA and, 60–61; implications of the extended inseparability argument and, 61; licit and illicit pregnancies and, 53–55; marriage bond and, 54; naturalistic fallacy and, 59; overview of, 53–54; pregnancy as proxy for sex and, 54–55; procreation-conjugal act link objection and, 59; responses to extended inseparability argument and, 57–61; teleological ordering of sex and, 55–56, 59–60

gestational intimacy, 185–186, 190–191

gift of the self, 118–124, 185, 192, 253, 256

Girgis, Sherif, 198

God: becoming a parent role of, 89–99; children's rights to love and life role of, 75–78; image of, 144, 147–148, 246–247; laws and mercy of, 147–148; love of, 78, 251, 277, 317; magisterium's relation to, 26, 29, 33, 35, 44; parenthood as gift from, 253–254; priority of action in conception of, 245–246; will of, 77, 249–252, 257, 260

Gormally, Mary, iv, 105. *See* Geach, Mary

Grabowski, John, 88, 211n35

Grisez, Germain, 89, 154–155, 223–224

Gross, Christopher, 88, 211n35

Haas, John, 166–167

harmfulness of embryonic death, 74–80

Heape, Walter, 38

HEG (heterologous external gestation), 217–218

Henry VIII, 201

hermeneutic of the gift, 118–124

heterologous embryo transfer (HET): becoming a parent and, 85, 89; definition of, 229; dignity and, 196–197, 210–214; humanizing the terminology and, 298–300; as intrinsically wrong, 85; as not involving failure to respect dignity, 196–197, 210–214; protecting the dignity of the child and, 196–197, 210–217; rescue of embryos and, 298–300

heterologous external gestation (HEG), 217–218

Horn, Trent, ix

Human Embryo Adoption (NCBC), x

Humanae vitae (Paul VI), 55n3, 122n14, 269–277

Hume, David, 59

Hursthouse, Rosalind, 64

Immaculate Conception, 241–242, 249

impasse on status of EA: adoption as a spiritual status and social practice and, 227–230; Annunciation and, 241; Catholic Church and, 24, 73, 125; *Dignitas personae* and, 42–49; extended inseparability and, 54, 60; generative faculty objections and, 60–61; next steps in EA and, 318–320, 330; rescue of embryonic persons and, 316

in vitro fertilization (IVF): associations with, 303–304, 314; as basis of EA, ix; Catholic Church's stance on, 41; development of, 38; first birth conceived through, i, 38; instrumentalization necessarily involved in, 206; John Paul II and, 39–47; magisterium as not yet making infallible pronouncements about, 38, 41, 74; medical aspects of EA and, 5, 8; moral contraindications to EA and, 126–128, 131, 143–145, 149–150; prevalence of, ix–x, 38; protecting the dignity of the child and, 206; rescue of embryos and, 303–304, 314; standard protocols of, 203–205

infidelity, 83–84, 229, 232

inseparability. *See* extended inseparability

Instruction on Children's Baptism (CDF), 77

International Theological Commission, 77

IVF. *See* in vitro fertilization (IVF)

Jacob, 32

Jesus Christ: ability to teach authoritatively in name of, 25–26; adoption as a spiritual status and social practice and, 220, 221–222; Annunciation and, 106, 242, 249–263; Apostles and, 25–26; becoming a parent and, 91–92; children's rights to love and life and, 76–79; conception and, 241–242, 249; divinity of, 92; Incarnation of, 242, 249–255; magisterium and, 25–26; Mary and, 255–263

John Paul II. *See also* Theology of the Body and magisterium; Theology of the Body arguments: adoption as a concrete way of equal love, 67–69; Annunciation and, 244, 255; authority of teachings of, 41; becoming a parent and, 88; children's rights to love and life and, 67, 69, 77; election of, 274; embryo production and, 39–47; *Evangelium vitae*, 77, 88, 168–169, 294, 319; hermeneutic of the gift and, 118–124; IVF and, 39–47; legal status of embryos and, 40–41; magisterium and, 39–47; *Man and Woman*

385

He Created Them, 118–119, 271; moral contraindications to EA and, 133; next steps if EA is illicit and, 153–154, 166–169; next steps in EA and, 319; organ transplants and, 309–310; procreative dimension of marital union and, 176, 185, 186, 188; resolving duty of existent embryos and, 42–49; *Veritatis splendor,* 153–154, 166–168
Joseph, 105, 106, 254–255
Juvenal, 166
Keenan, Jeffrey, xi, 17
kinship, moral significance of, 221–225
Lasnoski, Kent, ix, xii, 115
Laudato si' (Pope Francis), 74
law, natural. *See* natural law
legal generation, 94, 96, 99
legal status of embryos, xi, 17–18, 20, 23–24
Levin, Yuval, 128
Liao, S. Matthew, 68–69
Long, Stephen, 176, 179, 182
Lovering, Rob, 72
magisterium. *See also* Theology of the Body and magisterium: adoption in general and, 35; adrogation and, 32–33; ancient Israelite society and, 32–33; artificial wombs and, 48; authority and teachings of, 25–31, 35; bishops' relation to, 26, 29; CDF's relation to, 28–31; crisis embryo transfer (CET) and, 34, 36–38; definition of adoption and, 31–32; deposit of faith and, 26; destruction of embryos and, 39–40; *Dignitas personae* and, 25, 29, 41–47, 267–268, 293–294; dissent and, 31; divine revelation and, 27, 35; dogma and, 27; *Donum vitae* and, 29, 36–37, 40, 43, 266–268, 275–279, 293–295; ET and, 38; experimentation and, 39–40; feminine act of admission and, 113; forms of prenatal adoption and, 34–35; God's relation to, 26, 29, 33, 35, 44; history of adoption and, 31–33; infallibility and, charism of, 27–30; IVF and, 38, 41, 74; Jesus and, 25–26; John Paul II and, 39–47; legal status of embryos and, 40–41; levels of authority in, 28–29; modern forms of adoption and, 33; moral contraindications to EA and, 132–136; motives for adoption and, 32; natural law and, 27–28; nature of adoption and, 31–35; NCBC and, 48; New Testament views on adoption and, 33; next steps in EA and, 318–319; Old Testament views on adoption and, 32–33; overview of, 25–31; Pope's relation to, 29; posthumous adoption and, 32–33; primary object of infallibility and, 27; property transfer and, EA as, 33–34; *res fidei et morum* as primary subject matter of, 26–27; resolving duty of existent embryos and, 42–49; responses of the faithful to authoritative teachings of, 30; Roman Empire and, 32; second object of infallibility and, 27; surrogate motherhood and, 36; US bishops and, 47; voluntary embryo transfer (VET) and, 34, 38–39; with extrauterine gestation (WEG) and, 34, 47–49; without embryo transfer (WET) and, 34–36
Man and Woman He Created Them (John Paul II), 118–119, 271
marital bond, 83, 140, 301
Marquis, Don, 75
marital acts, 108, 129, 137, 233–235. *See also* adoption as a spiritual

status and social practice; procreative dimension of marital union

Mary. *See also* Annunciation: act at the Annunciation of, 105–106, 111–112; feminine act of admission and, 105–106, 111–112; Jesus and, 255–263; Marian Relationship to Christ and, 255–263; parents as equal to Joseph and, 252–253; psychological and spiritual suffering of, 247–248

Matheson, Jonathan, 73

May, William, 187

medical aspects of EA: act itself and, 8–10; antigen exposure and, 11; ART patients and, 7–8; circumstances of freezing and, 5–8; commonality of single-embryo transfer and, 5; consequences and, 10–15; counseling for EA and, 14; definition of EA and, 4, 15–16; disclosing EA status of children and, 14–15; donors considered as parents by children and, 13; embryo discard and, 6; ET and, 8–13; fertilization as prior to EA and, 8–9; framework of fertilization and gestation and, 15–16; gynecology and, 8–10; hypertensive disorders and, 13; infertility and, 7; IVF and, 5, 8; live birth potential and, 6; miscarriages and, 11; number of embryos in cryostorage and, 3; obstetrical consequences and, 10–13; overview of, 3–4; preference for EA children and, 14; procedure itself and, 8–10; psychiatry and, 13–15; rates of pregnancy and, 10–13; reasons for EA and, 7; reasons for embryo storage and, 3–4; screenings and tests and, 8, 14; steps in process of EA and, 8–10; terminology and, 4–5; twins and, 11–13; underemphasis on psychological dimensions of EA and, 14–15; uniqueness of EA compared to other tissue donations and, 13

Min Chueh Chang, 38

Miracle of Life, The (Francis), 268

miscarriages, 10–11, 22, 131, 258, 311, 315

moral contraindications to EA: birth as boundary of new reality and, 132; challenge of determining moral status of EA and, 127; consent to pregnancy and, 137; dignity and, 126; *Donum vitae* and, 140–144, 148; embryos in storage and, 125–127; forms of ET and, 126–127; *Gaudium et spes* and, 132; generative powers of women and, 130; human rights and, 126; image of God and, 144; intrinsic evil of ET as form of pregnancy initiation and, 128–129; IVF and, 126–128, 131, 143–145, 149–150; John Paul II and, 133; laws and mercy of God and, 147–148; magisterium and, 132–136; marital covenant and, 129–130; motherhood and, 129–130, 138, 144; *Mulieris dignitatem* and, 133; nurturing and, pregnancy as, 139–140; order of reason and, 136; organ transplant comparison and, 135; overview of, 125–127; partially procreated children and, 139; *Pastoral Constitution on the Church in the Modern World* and, 132; Pius XII and, 140–141; pro-creation and, 130–131; rescue of embryos and, 125–126, 135, 146–150; status of extracorporeally produced embryos and, 138–139; surrogacy and, 142–143; traditional adop-

tion and, 142; unity of procreative engendering and, 132–141
moral significance of kinship, 224–225
Moschella, Melissa, v, 100, 102, 153n4, 195
motherhood, 92–94, 129–130, 138, 144, 190
Mulieris dignitatem, 119, 133
NaPro (Natural Procreative) Technology, 204
National Catholic Bioethics Center (NCBC), x, 48
National Catholic Bioethics Quarterly (journal), 227
National Embryo Donation Center, 3, 19–20
natural generation, 94–99
natural law: adoption as a spiritual status and social practice and, 219, 235–237; Annunciation and, 247; Aquinas and, 103, 158, 179–185, 190; magisterium and, 27–28; new natural law theory, 59n10, 102–103, 154–155, 182, 187; next steps if EA is illicit and, 154–160; normativity of, 182–185; procreative dimension of marital union and, 182–185
natural teleology, 176–185
naturalistic fallacy, 59
NCBC (National Catholic Bioethics Center), x, 48
New Testament, 33–35, 244
next steps if EA is illicit: abortion and, 154; Aquinas and, 158; artificial wombs and, 156; Catholic bioethics and, 155, 166–168; consequentialism and, 153–154; courage and hope and, 169; dignity and, 165–166; domination of technology and, 159; *Donum vitae* and, 152, 156–157, 165; ectopic embryos and, 163–165; *Evangelium vitae* and, 168–169; evil of cryopreservation and, 156–159; experimentation and, 157; extraordinary and ordinary care distinction and, 161–163; fidelity to truth and, 169; forgiveness for abortion and, 168–169; future of frozen embryos and, 153–155; good of the body and, 158; John Paul II and, 153–154, 166–169; lack of options and, 153–154; leaving embryos in cryopreservation and, 156–157; natural law and, 154–160; new natural law theory and, 154–155; object of cryopreservation violates order of nature and, 157–163; overview of, 151–152; proportionality and, 164; specifying moral objects and, 154–155; thawing and allowing embryos to die and, 163–169; *Veritatis splendor* and, 153–154, 166–168
next steps in EA: CDF and, 318–319; Church's next steps and, 318–320; counseling and, 328–329; development and management of adoption clinics and, 320–332; *Dignitas personae* and, 322; dignity and, 323; *Donum vitae* and, 319–321, 332; *Evangelium vitae* and, 319; guidelines for clinics and, 320–332; impasse on status of EA and, 318–320, 330; John Paul II and, 319; legal context and reform and, 332–333; magisterium and, 318–319; marital status policies and, 324; obtaining embryos policies and, 324–325; open or closed adoption process and, 327–328; other policies and protections and, 329–330; overview of, 317–318, 334; PDG and, 326; research needs

and, 333–334; securing resources and, 330–332; selecting and testing prospective parents and, 326–327; transfer policies and, 325–326
Nightline Christian Adoptions, 41–42
normativity, 179–180, 182–185, 190
O'Donovan, Oliver, 201
Oleson, Christopher, 84–86, 119–120, 176, 186, 190
Option of Adoption Act (1986, Georgia, US), 333
ordinary and extraordinary care distinction, 161–163
organ transplants: definition of, 306; ET and, 102; history of Church's approval of, 306–310; John Paul II and, 309–310; Paul VI as not mentioning, 309; Pius XII and, 306–309; previous condemnation of, 306–309
orphans, prenatal, 220–221
Overall, Christine, 64
Pacholczyk, Tadeusz, xii, 48, 71, 92, 125, 156, 161, 280–282
parenthood. *See also* becoming a parent; children's rights to love and life; protecting the dignity of the child: Christian parenting, 223–224; God's gift of, 253–254; moral equivalence of natural and adoptive forms of, 85–86; relevance and application of the parenthood principle and, 99–100; right to procreate distinguished from to, 65; rights of, 64–67; virtuous parenthood, 87
Pastoral Constitution on the Church in the Modern World, 132
Paul, 33, 76, 222, 257
Paul VI, Pope, 55n3, 122n14, 269–277
Pellegrino, Edmund, 3
personalism, 185–193
personhood: Annunciation and, 241–243, 253, 256–257; becoming a parent and, 89; EA and, xi; Francis and, 242; of frozen embryos, xi; rescue of embryos and, 312; Supreme Court and, xi
Pinchus, Gregory, 38
Pius XII, Pope: moral contraindications to EA and, 140–141; organ transplants and, 306–309; procreative dimension of marital union and, 174
Pontifical Academy of Life, 46–47
prenatal orphans, 219–221
procreative dimension of marital union: abortion and, 190, 192; analogies with other animals and, 183; Aquinas and, 179–185, 190; Catholic bioethics and, 193; conjugal act as including procreation and gestation and, 187; extended inseparability and, 177–178; generation and gestation distinction and, 178; gestational intimacy and, 185–186, 190–191; inclusion of procreation and gestation and, 187; John Paul II and, 176, 185, 186, 188; *Letter to Families* and, 186; marital self-gift and, 186; moral normativity and, 179–180; motherhood and, normativity of, 190; natural inclination for reproduction and, 181; natural law and, 182–185; natural teleology and, 176–185; norms concerning marital intercourse and, 173–174, 178–179; overview of, 173–177; parental intimacy and, 192; personal dimension of the gift and, 190–191; personalism and, 185–193; physical reductionism and, 188; Pius XII and, 174; punctuality and, 178; rescue of embryos

and, 173–175, 193; responses to arguments from personalism and, 187–193; responses to arguments from teleology and, 182–185; right of spouses to become parents and, 180–182; sexual union, generation, and impregnation and, 177–179; *Summa contra Gentiles* and, 181–184; surrogacy and, 174; unparalleled intimacy between mother and child and, 185–186

procreative infidelity, 228–229, 232–238

property, frozen embryos treated as, 23, 33–34, 209, 330–332

protecting the dignity of the child. *See also* children's rights to love and life: agent of implantation and, 216; application to EA of, 208–214; artificial wombs and, 217–218; attitude of dominion and, 203–205; begetting distinguished from making a child and, 200–206; Catholic sexual ethics and, 197–198; clinical language masking injustices and, 204; concluding thought experiment on, 217–218; contraception and, 198–201; definition of reproductive technologies and, 195; *Dignitas personae* and, 206–207; domination of technology and, 207; *Donum vitae* and, 195–201, 204, 206, 211–214, 217–218; extended inseparability and, 214–215; generative faculty and, 206–207, 215; HET as not involving failure to respect dignity and, 196–197, 210–217; heterologous external gestation (HEG) and, 217–218; inseparability norm and, 197–208; instrumentalization necessarily involved in IVF and, 206; integral personal context of conjugal act and, 207; marital fidelity and, 216–217; matching and, 209; NaProTechnology and, 204; overview of, 195–197; postnatal adoption and, 209–210, 214; procreation as not the object of marital sex and, 201–202; psychological dimensions of adoption and, 212–213; reproductive technologies as akin to contraception and, 199–200; rescue of embryos and, 197, 211; response to counterarguments and, 214–217; right to procreation and, 202–203; screenings and, 209; selection and, 209–210; Snowflakes and, 209–210; standard IVF protocols and, 203–205; thawing process and, 213; truly marital intercourse and, 197–198, 201–202; wet-nursing objection and, 215–216

Purdy, Jean, 38

Ratzinger, Joseph Cardinal, 28

references to scripture. *See* scriptural references

Reilly, Christopher, xii, 71–72, 146, 317

reproductive integrity, 105, 110–114

rescue of embryos: adoption as a spiritual status and social practice and, 228–231; artificial wombs and, 315; association with IVF and, 303–304, 314; becoming a parent and, 100–102; Catholic Church and, 265; charity and, 310; complicity with evil and, 302–303; cryopreservation and, 302; definition of, 299; definition of LOT and, 297; dignity and, 313–314; donation of bodies for gestation and, 315–316; *Donum vitae* and, 298, 301–302; EA terminology contrasted with, 299; feminine act of admission and, 107, 112; gestation and, 300–301; HET and, 298–300; history of Church's approval of LOT and, 306–310; humanizing the terminology and, 298–300; impasse on status of EA and, 316; IVF and, 303–304, 314; moral contraindications to EA and, 125–126, 135, 146–150; morality of kinds of action and, 304–305; overview of, 297–298; personhood and, 312; practical concerns with, 310–312; procreative dimension of marital union and, 173–175, 193; promoting rescue and, 312–316; protecting the dignity of the child and, 197, 211; responding to usual objections and, 300–304; *sensus fidelium* and, 305; shipping of embryos and, 313–314; surrogacy and, 301–302; Theology of the Body and magisterium and, 270–271, 280–281; Theology of the Body arguments and, 118

Rex, Elizabeth Bothamley, v, 100–102, 265

rights to love and life. *See* children's rights to love and life

Robertson, Charles, 81, 135, 176, 179–182, 215

Rulli, Tina, 65, 67

salvation history, 242–243, 253

screenings, 8, 14, 22, 209

scriptural references: Genesis (2:23–25, 121; 4:1, 245; 48:5, 32); Exodus (22:22, 220); 2 Maccabees (7:1, 256; 7:20–31, 256; 7:39–42, 256); Matthew (1:18–25, 247, 252; 5:27–28, 272; 6:9–14, 222; 6:33, 76; 12:7, 268; 12:10–11, 268; 19:8, 272; 22:30, 272; 25:40, 240, 250, 295; 25:45, 220, 240; 28:19, 255); Mark (9:37, 278); Luke (1:31-35, 244; 1:34, 105; 1:38, 105; 1:41–45, 247; 10:16, 25; 10:29, 276, 295; 14:11, 254; 14:26, 221); John (3:3, 222; 3:5, 222; 14:6, 254; 15:1–11, 250; 19:25–29, 256); Acts (7:21, 33); Romans (5:20, 257; 8:14–16, 222; 8:15, 33, 96; 9:4, 33); 1 Corinthians (10:13, 45); Galatians (4:3–7, 222; 4:5, 33); Ephesians (1:5, 33); Philemon (1:23–24, 76; 2:6–8, 254); James (1:27, 67); Revelation (21:4, 169)

self-gift, 118–124, 185, 192, 253, 256

self-identity, 222–223

sexual ethics, 54–55, 59–60, 173–174, 197–198

Shpall, Sam, 73

Sisters of Life, 112

Smith, Janet, xiii, 154–155, 297

Snowflakes program, 19n6, 20, 209–210

social context and experience of EA and ED. *See also* medical aspects of EA: altruism and, 18; ambiguous legal status of embryos and, 17–18; anonymous donation and, 20; experience of adopting couples and, 21–23; experience of donor couples and, 18–20; FDA and, 21–22; financial barriers and, 21; infertility counseling and, 21; informed consent and, 19–20; insurance coverage and, 21; legal status of ED and EA and, 20, 23–24; overview of, 17–18; parental responsibility and, 18–19; pregnancy likelihood and, 23; reasons for EA and ED and, 18–21; screenings and, 22; stem cells and, 18; uncertain future and, 24; underinformed nature of donors and, 19

social practice of adoption *See* adoption as a spiritual status and social practice
spiritual status, adoption as. *See* adoption as a spiritual status and social practice
stem cells, 18, 312
Steptoe, Patrick, 38
Strege, Hannah, 41, 248, 270, 294
Strege, John, 248, 254
Strege, Marlene, 248, 249, 254
Summa contra Gentiles (Aquinas), 181
surrogacy, 142–143, 151, 174, 231–233, 301–303, 323, 333
Swift, Adam, 64–65
teleology, 55–56, 59–60, 176–185
Theology of the Body and magisterium: absurd fate resolution and, 293–294; adoption of abused and neglected children, 278–279; artificial contraception as not respecting, 274–275; artificial wombs condemned and, 279–283; *Catechism of the Catholic Church* and, 266, 273–279, 283; CDF and, 282; cryopreservation condemned and, 267, 279–283; defense of marriage and, 270–279; *Dignitas personae* and, 267–268, 293–294; *Donum vitae* and, 266–268, 275–279, 293–294; *Evangelium vitae* and, 286; *Humanae vitae* and, 270–277; leaving embryos frozen and, 280–281; liceity of ET defends morality of EA and, 293–294; overview of, 268–270, 294–295; preface and, 265–268; procreative meaning of marital act and, 270–279; rescue of embryos and, 270–271, 280–281; summary of Theology of the Body and, 270–279; teachings of the magisterium and, 270–273; voice of the embryo and, 268–269
Theology of the Body arguments: Catholic sexual ethics and, 115–118; conjugal act and, 122–124; definition of procreation and, 115–117; *Dignitas personae* and, 117; gift of the self and, 118–124; *Gratissimam sane* and, 124; hermeneutic of the gift and, 118–124; human body's spousal meaning and, 124; moral status of EA according to, 115–124; *Mulieris dignitatem* and, 119; overview of, 115; personal structure of the woman and, 120; procreation as self-gift and knowledge and, 123; rescue of embryos and, 118; scholastic format of chapter on, 115
Therese of Lisieux, 76
Thomas Aquinas, St. *See* Aquinas, Thomas, St.
Thomson, Judith Jarvis, 190
Tollefsen, Christopher, v, 89–91, 95, 108
Tonti-Filippini, Nicholas, 83–86, 158, 160–161, 173, 176, 185–186, 197n4, 207n23
transfer of embryos. *See* embryo transfer (ET)
transplants of organs. *See* organ transplants
Trinity, 76, 95, 244–249, 272
unbaptized infants, 77–78
US bishops' Committee on Doctrine, 31
US Food and Drug Administration FDA (FDA), 18, 21–22
Veritatis splendor (John Paul II), 153–154, 166–168
virginity, 106, 244–245
voice of the embryo, 268–269

voluntary embryo transfer (VET), 34, 38–39
Watt, Helen, 230–231, 235–238
Weaver, Darlene Fozard, ii, 58, 212n35
West, Christopher, 271
West, Ryan, 67

"What Should We Do with the Frozen Embryos?" (Pacholczyk), 281–282
Williams, Thomas, 98n35, 100–102
Wojtyla, Karol, 270. *See also* John Paul II

About the National Catholic Bioethics Center

The National Catholic Bioethics Center (NCBC) is an independent, nonprofit, academic research institute dedicated to applying Catholic moral theology and ethical tradition to bioethical questions. Our society faces unprecedented scientific developments that touch upon the mysteries of life and pose serious ethical challenges. The NCBC was established in 1972 to reflect on these issues and to promote and safeguard the dignity of the human person in health care and the life sciences. The NCBC is governed by a board of directors composed of Catholic cardinals and bishops and prominent Catholic pro-life laity. At the heart of the NCBC is its team of expert ethicists, who are assisted by a dedicated support staff, fellows, interns, and members and other benefactors. All of the NCBC's work is done in conformity with the official teachings of the Catholic Church, teachings drawn from a moral tradition that acknowledges the unity of faith and reason and builds on the solid foundation of the natural law.

The NCBC provides consultation on Catholic institutional ethics and witness to many US bishops, the US Conference of Catholic Bishops, Catholic health care systems and hospitals, dicasteries of the Holy See, and international nonprofit health care and social service organizations. NCBC ethicists also respond to individuals' telephone and email questions 24-7, fielding over fifteen hundred consults every year from patients, family members, and health care professionals facing difficult medical decisions. Further, the NCBC offers educational training programs in the Catholic moral tradition and its application to clinical and research situations. Finally, the NCBC is a leading publisher of books and articles on Catholic health care ethics and produces a wide range of electronic resources for professionals and the public.

The NCBC envisions a world in which the integral understanding of the human person underlying Catholic teaching on respect for human life and dignity is better understood and more widely embraced in America and worldwide. For more information, visit the NCBC's website at www.ncbcenter.org.

www.ingramcontent.com/pod-product-compliance
Lightning Source LLC
Chambersburg PA
CBHW070847111125
35242CB00009B/19